A.C.T.H.–
a practical review of progress to date

برکت بخا نخبک آتی د کتر ا وهب تقریم میگردد

روضاطبی

٤٧،١،١٤

A.C.T.H.–
a practical review of
progress to date

Edited by R. Schuppli, Basle

Hans Huber Publishers
Bern Stuttgart Vienna

An international symposium
Dubrovnik, 23rd–24th April 1973

Manuscripts coordinated and translated under the supervision of:

Dr. C. ADAMS
Mr. I. C.W. BIGLAND, M.A.
Dr. W. JOCHUM
Dr. H. KARRER
Dr. G. KESSLER
Dr. R. LUDWIG
Mr. H. D. PHILPS, M.A.

ISBN 3-456-00377-3

Contents

List of authors

Dr. J. Aubert, Clinique de Pneumo-Phtisiologie, Faculté mixte de Médecine et de Pharmacie, Université Aix-Marseille, B.P. 29, F-13274 Marseille Cédex 2 (France)

Prof. H.J. Bauer, Direktor der Neurologischen Klinik und Poliklinik, von-Siebold-Strasse 5, D-34 Göttingen (German Federal Republic)

Dr. T.B. Binns, ciba laboratories limited, Wimblehurst Road, Horsham, Sussex (England)

Dr. H. Boissière, 155 rue de la Pompe, F-75016 Paris (France)

Prof. J. Charpin, Clinique de Pneumo-Phtisiologie, Faculté mixte de Médecine et de Pharmacie, Université Aix-Marseille, B.P. 29, F-13274 Marseille Cédex 2 (France)

Dr. R. Deguillaume, ciba-geigy limited, Klybeckstrasse 141, CH-4000 Basle (Switzerland)

Dr. P.A. Desaulles, ciba-geigy limited, Klybeckstrasse 141, CH-4000 Basle (Switzerland)

Dr. J. Gelzer, ciba-geigy limited, Klybeckstrasse 141, CH-4000 Basle (Switzerland)

Prof. G. Geyer, Vorstand der I. Medizinischen Abteilung, Kaiser-Franz-Joseph-Spital, Kundratstrasse 3, A-1100 Vienna (Austria)

Prof. M. Giordano, Direttore dell'Istituto di Reumatologia dell'Università di Napoli, Clinica Medica, Piazza L. Miraglia, I-80135 Naples (Italy)

Priv.-Doz. Dr. J. Girard, Endokrinologische Abteilung, Universitätskinderklinik und Poliklinik, Römergasse 8, CH-4005 Basle (Switzerland)

Prof. G. Giusti, Direttore della Clinica delle Malattie Infettive, 1ª Facoltà di Medicina, Università di Napoli, Via D. Cotugno 1 (Ospedale Gesù e Maria), I-80135 Naples (Italy)

Prof. D. Gross, Chefarzt der Klinik für Rheumatologie und Rehabilitation, Stadtspital Triemli, Birmensdorferstrasse 497, CH-8055 Zurich (Switzerland)

Dr. W.J. Irvine, D.Sc., F.R.C.P., M.R.C. Path., Endocrine Clinic, Department of Therapeutics, Royal Infirmary, Edinburgh EH3 9YW (Scotland)

Prof. H. Jesserer, Vorstand der II. Medizinischen Abteilung, Kaiser-Franz-Joseph-Spital, Kundratstrasse 3, A-1100 Vienna (Austria)

Prof. F. Kogoj, Direktor Instituta za Klinička Medicinska Istraživanja, Dermatološka Klinika, Šalata 4, YU-41000 Zagreb (Yugoslavia)

Dr. P. E. Lucchelli, CIBA-GEIGY S.p.A., Servizio Studi e Ricerche Cliniche, Via Piranesi 44, I-20137 Milan (Italy)

Prof. P. Massias, Hôpital Antoine Béclère, 157 rue de la Porte de Trivaux, F-92140 Clamart (France)

Dr. K. L. Möller, Östra Sjukhuset, Smörslottsgatan 1, S-416 85 Gothenburg (Sweden)

Prof. R. Oberholzer, Head of the Medical Department, CIBA-GEIGY LIMITED, Klybeckstrasse 141, CH-4000 Basle (Switzerland)

Prof. F. Piccinino, Clinica delle Malattie Infettive, 1ª Facoltà di Medicina, Università di Napoli, Via D. Cotugno 1 (Ospedale Gesù e Maria), I-80135 Naples (Italy)

Prof. E. Polli, Direttore della Clinica Medica I, Università di Milano, Via F. Sforza 35, I-20122 Milan (Italy)

Dr. H. V. Price, Department of Child Health, The Welsh National School of Medicine, Heath Park, Cardiff CF4 4XN (Wales)

Dr. W. Rittel, CIBA-GEIGY LIMITED, Klybeckstrasse 141, CH-4000 Basle (Switzerland)

Prof. R. Schuppli, Vorsteher der Dermatologischen Universitätsklinik, Petersgraben 9, CH-4000 Basle (Switzerland)

Prof. C. van der Meer, Academisch Ziekenhuis der Vrije Universiteit, De Boelelaan 1117, NL-1011 Amsterdam (Netherlands)

Prof. K. F. Weinges, Medizinische Universitätsklinik und Poliklinik, D-665 Homburg/Saar (German Federal Republic)

Prof. R.-J. Wüthrich, Neurologische Universitätsklinik, Socinstrasse 55, CH-4051 Basle (Switzerland)

Address of chief coordinator:
Dr. C. Adams, Head of the Medical and Pharmaceutical Information Service, CIBA-GEIGY LIMITED, Klybeckstrasse 141, Basle, Switzerland

Opening address

by R. Schuppli*

To begin with, I should like to bid you all a hearty welcome to this symposium. The readiness with which you accepted the invitation to participate in it can, I suspect, be ascribed to two reasons: firstly, the topic with which we shall be dealing is of sufficient importance to interest specialists in widely varying branches of medicine and, secondly, the prospect of being able to spend a few days in one of the most beautiful spots on the continent of Europe no doubt also served as an inducement.

As a physician, one certainly cannot be accused of exaggeration in describing our present day and age as the "golden epoch" of therapeutics. The truth of this assertion can perhaps best be appreciated by those among us who are old enough to remember what it was like to practise medicine at a time when there were no sulphonamides, no corticosteroids, no antibiotics, and no cytotoxic agents, and who themselves actually experienced the feelings of hopelessness which at that time many serious illnesses still engendered in those confronted with their treatment. But the mounting abundance of highly active drugs also entails certain dangers. When, as has been the case during recent years, new therapeutic methods are being introduced in increasingly rapid succession, it inevitably becomes more and more difficult for the individual doctor to gain—in the light of his own personal impressions and experience—an adequate idea of their effectiveness and possible hazards. Hence his ever-increasing dependence upon information reaching him from other sources and hence, too, the steadily growing importance of ways and means of imparting this information. In this connection, symposia of the kind at which we are now gathered together have proved particularly valuable. In contrast to giant international congresses, they afford an opportunity for a genuine exchange of information and knowledge based on direct personal contacts.

As a therapeutic agent, A.C.T.H. provides a particularly good topic for a symposium. Indications for its use are to be found in many different fields of medicine, and specialists who in the normal course of their work would have no contact with one another are all equally interested in obtaining a precise knowledge of its mechanism of action. The fact that a body of information on A.C.T.H. has thus had to be built up piecemeal may indeed perhaps be one of the reasons for the chequered history of A.C.T.H. therapy. In the initial period following its introduction some 20 years ago, it was resorted to on quite a large scale, but the allergic manifestations provoked by the A.C.T.H. extract-preparations then available—manifestations sometimes so serious as to endanger the patient's

---

* Director of the Dermatologische Universitätsklinik, Basle, Switzerland.

life—subsequently resulted in the drug's use becoming more and more restricted. The reputation it acquired as a strongly allergenic substance probably also explains why synthetic A.C.T.H. was at first likewise regarded with scepticism and employed rather hesitantly. Only during the last two to three years, in fact, does it finally seem to have gained therapeutic acceptance. Even now, however, when it can be considered as certain that A.C.T.H. has a major contribution to make in the realm of drug therapy, its use still poses many open questions which can only be resolved by thrashing them out in discussion: there is the problem of hormonal interactions, for example, or the problem of combining A.C.T.H. with corticosteroid therapy—to mention only two points that have yet to be clarified.

I hope that, by the time we come to the end of this symposium, perhaps at least a few of these questions will have been answered.

Recent chemical studies in the field of A.C.T.H.

by W. Rittel *

Investigations on the structure of porcine, ovine, bovine, and human A.C.T.H. which were undertaken during the period from 1954 to 1961 revealed that in this hormone the amino acid sequence displays peculiar—if not bizarre—species-specific differences.

Each of these four A.C.T.H. molecules consists of a chain of 39 amino acids in which the sequences 1–24 and 34–39 are identical. In the sequence 25–33, on the other hand, the amino acids were believed to be arranged as shown in Figure 1. Though the four different types of A.C.T.H. feature similar amino acids in the sequence 25–33, the order in which these amino acids appear varies appreciably from molecule to molecule. Curiously enough, in the case of the porcine molecule, two different formulae were proposed for the amino acids 25–30; it was arbitrarily assumed, however, that here the formula suggested by Howard et al.[6] was the correct one. Today we know that neither of them was accurate.

Species	Authors	Sequence								
		25	26	27	28	29	30	31	32	33
Hog	Howard et al.[6] (1955) Shepherd et al.[19] (1956)						NH$_2$ |			
		-Asp-	Gly-	Ala-	Glu-	Asp-	Glu-	Leu-	Ala-	Glu-
Hog	White and Landmann[22] (1955)	-Gly-	Ala-	Glu-	Asp-	Asp-	Glu-	Leu-	Ala-	Glu-
										NH$_2$ |
Bovine	Li et al.[11] (1958)	-Asp-	Gly-	Glu-	Ala-	Glu-	Asp-	Ser-	Ala-	Glu-
										NH$_2$ |
Sheep	Li et al.[12] (1955)	-Ala-	Gly-	Glu-	Asp-	Asp-	Glu-	Ala-	Ser-	Glu-
							NH$_2$ |			
Man	Lee et al.[9] (1961)	-Asp-	Ala-	Gly-	Glu-	Asp-	Glu-	Ser-	Ala-	Glu-

Fig. 1. Structures proposed for the amino acid sequence 25–33 in various types of A.C.T.H. (before revision of the formulae).

* Research Department, Pharmaceutical Division, CIBA-GEIGY LIMITED, Basle, Switzerland.

One clue, suggesting that these markedly differing formulae might possibly not be correct, could have been deduced from data on the biological activities of the naturally occurring A.C.T.H. peptides. These activities are, in fact, virtually identical—a finding which it would be difficult to account for if the substances in question really did differ so radically in a portion of their amino acid chain. Although it is true that partial sequences from the chain, ranging from 1–18 to 1–24, suffice to produce full stimulation of the adrenal cortex (RAMACHANDRAN et al.[14]; HOFMANN et al.[5]; KAPPELER and SCHWYZER[8]), structural differences—even if located outside the active portion of the chain—may well exert a perceptible influence on biological activity as measured in the intact animal, because two peptides of markedly different structure are unlikely to behave identically with respect to their metabolism in the tissues or plasma, their binding, or their transport.

The chemistry of these species-specific variations in the structure of the A.C.T.H. molecule is a problem with which we have had to deal in our laboratories in connection with work on the synthesis of A.C.T.H. analogues. It is a well-known fact that naturally occurring A.C.T.H. and fragments thereof exert in man an action which is only of brief duration. As therapeutic agents they are therefore employed chiefly in the form of depot preparations. It was for this reason that several years ago we embarked on the synthesis of chemically modified A.C.T.H. peptides. The object of such work was to produce preparations endowed with an inherently prolonged duration of effect. Already at quite an early stage, it was discovered that the corticotrophic activity of A.C.T.H. fragments could be greatly enhanced by replacing L-serine in position 1 by its optical antipode D-serine (KAPPELER et al.[7]; RITTEL[18]). This modification evidently has the effect of inhibiting the breakdown of the molecule by aminopeptidases (BOISSONNAS et al.[3]). We subsequently obtained A.C.T.H. peptides displaying not only a more potent, but also a considerably more prolonged action, by combining the introduction of D-serine in position 1 with replacement of the strongly basic arginines in positions 17 and 18 by the more weakly basic amino acids lysine or ornithine. An example illustrating this combined type of modification is the highly active, short-chain peptide 1-D-serine-17,18-dilysine-A.C.T.H.-(1-18)-octadecapeptide amide (RINIKER and RITTEL[16]), which in man exhibits a duration of effect comparable with that of ®Synacthen Depot (WALSER and MÜLLER[21]). Similarly, it was found possible to achieve a pronounced prolongation of the action of the entire 1–39 sequence of porcine A.C.T.H. by introducing D-serine in position 1.

For possible use in man, however, it was felt that a corresponding analogue (i. e. with D-serine in position 1) featuring the C-terminal sequence of human A.C.T.H. would offer obvious advantages. We therefore decided that it would be interesting to synthesise the D-serine-1 analogue of human A.C.T.H. But the problem then facing us was that LEE et al.[9] had merely described their version of the formula for human A.C.T.H. as a postulated structural formula and had pointed out that it had not been possible to determine with certainty the positioning and number of the side-chain amide groups. Before commencing our attempts to synthesise the analogue in question, we thus found it necessary to re-examine the formula that had been proposed by Lee et al. At this point it should perhaps be mentioned that a human A.C.T.H. molecule whose structure corresponds to that suggested by Lee et al. had been synthesised by an Hungarian research group (Bajusz et al.[1]), but this synthetic material had never been compared or identified with the naturally occurring hormone.

For our own comparative studies we employed a sample of highly purified human A.C.T.H. which was kindly supplied by Organon N.V., Oss (Netherlands). Since it was first assumed that all we should have to do would be to clarify the nature of the amide groups, Riniker began by carrying out in our laboratories a series of deamidation experiments on human A.C.T.H. of natural origin. In these experiments he used natural porcine A.C.T.H. and synthetic peptides (sequence 22–39) as model substances. His results, which are outlined in Figure 2, revealed at once that both of the naturally occurring A.C.T.H. peptides undergo deamidation at a much faster rate than their postulated structural formulae would have led one to expect*. For example, the model peptide A shown in Figure 2, which features an amide group in position 30 (glutamine) in accordance with what used to be accepted as the structural formulae of porcine and human A.C.T.H., remains practically stable under basic conditions. When another amide group is added in position 25, however (model peptide B), deamidation becomes accelerated. But it still fails to attain the rate observed in the case of the hormones of natural origin. These findings indicated that the formulae proposed for human and porcine A.C.T.H. could not be correct. Riniker therefore then resorted to the use of trypsin in order to break down human A.C.T.H., and from the resultant mixture he separated out the various fragments (sequences 1–8, 9–15, 16–21, 17–21, and 22–39) by countercurrent distribution. Fragment 22–39 was now subjected to the stepwise

Peptide	Half-life (hours) in deamidation experiment
Natural porcine A.C.T.H.	~ 1
Natural human A.C.T.H.	~ 1

$$NH_2$$
A*: H-Val-Tyr-Pro-Asp-Gly-Ala-Glu-Asp-Glu-Leu-...Phe-OH   > 100
        22 23 24 25   26 27 28 29 30 31   39

$$NH_2 \qquad\qquad NH_2$$
B*: H-Val-Tyr-Pro-Asp-Ala-Gly-Glu-Asp-Glu-Ser- ...Phe-OH   ~ 20
        22 23 24 25   26 27 28 29 30 31   39

* The two peptides A and B, which were employed for purposes of comparison, were prepared by Mr. P. Sieber.

Fig. 2. Deamidation rate for various A.C.T.H. peptides in 1N aqueous ammonia (pH 11.3) at 25 °C.

* A similar observation was also reported by an Hungarian research team (Gráf et al.[4]).

Species	Authors	Sequence								
		25	26	27	28	29	30	31	32	33
Hog	*Riniker*[15] (1971) *Riniker* et al.[17] (1972)	*NH₂* | -*Asp*-	Gly-	Ala-	Glu-	Asp-	*Glu*-	Leu-	Ala-	Glu- *NH₂* |
Bovine	*Li*[10] (1972)	*NH₂* | -*Asp*-	Gly-	*Ala*-	*Glu*-	*Asp*-	*Glu*-	Ser-	Ala-	Glu- *NH₂* |
Sheep	*Li*[10] (1972)	-*Asp*-	Gly-	*Ala*-	*Glu*-	Asp-	Glu-	*Ser*-	*Ala*-	Glu-
Man	*Riniker*[15] (1971) *Riniker* et al.[17] (1972)	*NH₂* | -*Asp*-	*Gly*-	*Ala*-	Glu-	Asp-	*Glu*-	Ser-	Ala-	Glu-

Fig. 3. Revised formulae for the structure of the amino acid sequence 25–33 in various types of A.C.T.H. The differences as compared with the old formulae (cf. Figure 1) are indicated in italics.

process of Edman degradation; this was carried out under conditions designed to ensure that no rearrangement would occur in the alkali-sensitive peptide, since errors in elucidating the sequence of amino acids had evidently arisen in the past as a result of such transpositions. This degradation procedure resulted in the establishment of the new amino acid sequence for the 25–33 portion of the human A.C.T.H. chain as outlined in Figure 3 (RINIKER[15]; RINIKER et al.[17]). In the new formula for human A.C.T.H., four of the amino acids occupy new positions as compared with the old formula. A corresponding, though somewhat less radical, correction also had to be made in the formula for porcine A.C.T.H. (for the new formula, see Figure 3).

The fact that human A.C.T.H. of natural origin undergoes deamidation so readily can now be ascribed to the presence of an asparaginyl-glycyl sequence (Asn-Gly) in positions 25 and 26*. This deamidation involves the rearrangement shown in Figure 4, in which a mixture of α and β aspartyl-peptide results from the Asn-Gly sequence (SIEBER et al.[20]).

Four of the above-mentioned fragments obtained by breaking down human A.C.T.H. with the aid of trypsin, i.e. sequences 1–8, 9–15, 16–21, and 17–21, were employed in the CIBA laboratories in Horsham (England) in order to check the correctness of the formula for the 1–21 portion of the human A.C.T.H. chain (BENNETT et al.[2]). These studies confirmed that the structure postulated by LEE et al.[9] for this part of the molecule was correct. The structural formula of human A.C.T.H. has thus now been fully elucidated. We have meanwhile

---

* Here, as well as in Figures 3 and 4, the abbreviations "Asn" or $\overset{\text{``NH}_2\text{''}}{\underset{\text{Asp}}{|}}$ are employed to indicate the asparaginyl group (= β-amide of aspartic acid); "Asp" signifies an aspartic acid (= aspartyl) group, i.e. a free β-carboxyl group.

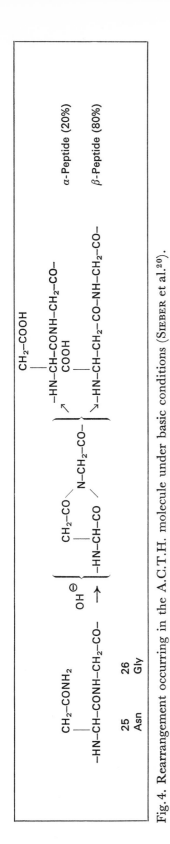

Fig. 4. Rearrangement occurring in the A.C.T.H. molecule under basic conditions (Sieber et al.[20]).

produced the entire molecule by total synthesis and established that it is identical with the naturally occurring hormone (Sieber et al.[20]). An accurately defined standard preparation of human A.C.T.H. is therefore now for the first time available with which to undertake biological and immunological research.

Our experiments on the production of the D-serine analogue will be reported elsewhere.

In the light of our findings, Li[10] has recently revised the formulae for bovine and ovine A.C.T.H. which had been worked out in his laboratory. In the case of these two peptides as well, appreciable corrections in the formulae proved necessary (cf. Figure 3). The new sequences now bear a much closer resemblance to the corresponding sequences in the revised formulae for porcine and human A.C.T.H., the species-specific differences between the four A.C.T.H. molecules being confined, in fact, solely to the three positions 25, 31, and 33. Moreover, since the ovine A.C.T.H. used by Li when revising the structural formula was an artefact generated during the process of isolation (Li et al.[13]), it is possible that untreated and unchanged ovine A.C.T.H. may be even more closely related to human A.C.T.H. The A.C.T.H. precursor giving rise to ovine α-corticotrophin under alkaline conditions probably also features an asparagine group in position 25. It thus seems very likely that untreated ovine A.C.T.H., and bovine A.C.T.H., too, differ from human A.C.T.H. only insofar as they contain one additional amide group.

Finally, it should be pointed out that, although the findings discussed here have no important bearing on the practical aspects of A.C.T.H. therapy, they do at least shed a little more light on what has hitherto been a rather obscure chapter in the history of A.C.T.H.

References

1 Bajusz, S., Medzihradsky, K., Paulay, Z., Láng, Z.: Totalsynthese des menschlichen Corticotropins (α_h-ACTH). Acta chim. Acad. Sci. hung. 52, 335 (1967)

2   BENNETT, H.P.J., LOWRY, P.J., McMARTIN, C.: The sequence determination of regions 6–7, 10–14 and 17–20 of natural human adrenocorticotrophin (ACTH). Biochem. J. (printing)

3   BOISSONNAS, R.A., GUTTMANN, S., PLESS, J.: Synthesis of D-Ser¹-Nle⁴-(Val-NH₂)²⁵-β-corticotropin (1-25), a highly potent analogue of ACTH. Experientia (Basle) *22*, 526 (1966)

4   GRÁF, L., BAJUSZ, S., PATTHY, A., ERZSÉBET, B., CSEH, G.: Revised amide location for porcine and human adrenocorticotropic hormone. Acta biochim. biophys. Acad. Sci. hung. *6*, 415 (1971)

5   HOFMANN, K., YAJIMA, H., YANAIHARA, N., LIU, T.-Y., LANDE, S.: Studies on polypeptides. XIII. The synthesis of a tricosapeptide possessing essentially the full biological activity of natural ACTH. J. Amer. chem. Soc. *83*, 487 (1961)

6   HOWARD, K.S., SHEPHERD, R.G., EIGNER, E.A., DAVIES, D.S., BELL, P.H.: Structure of β-corticotropin: final sequence studies. J. Amer. chem. Soc. *77*, 3419 (1955)

7   KAPPELER, H., RINIKER, B., RITTEL, W., DESAULLES, P., MAIER, R., SCHÄR, B., STAEHELIN, M.: Synthesis and biological activity of peptides related to ACTH. In Beyerman, H.C., Linde, A. van den, Maassen van den Brink, W. (Editors): Peptides, Proc. VIIIth Europ. Peptide Symp., Noordwijk, The Netherlands, 1966, p. 214 (North-Holland, Amsterdam 1967)

8   KAPPELER, H., SCHWYZER, R.: Die Synthese eines Tetracosapeptides mit der Aminosäuresequenz eines hochaktiven Abbauproduktes des β-Corticotropins (ACTH) aus Schweinehypophysen (Vorläufige Mitteilung). Helv. chim. Acta *44*, 1136 (1961)

9   LEE, T.H., LERNER, A.B., BUETTNER-JANUSCH, V.: On the structure of human corticotropin (adrenocorticotropic hormone). J. biol. Chem. *236*, 2970 (1961)

10   LI, C.H.: Adrenocorticotropin. XLV. Revised amino acid sequences for sheep and bovine hormone. Biochem. biophys. Res. Commun. *49*, 835 (1972)

11   LI, C.H., DIXON, J.S., CHUNG, D.: The structure of bovine corticotropin. J. Amer. chem. Soc. *80*, 2587 (1958)

12   LI, C.H., GESCHWIND, I.I., COLE, R.D., RAACKE, I.D., HARRIS, J.I., DIXON, J.S.: Amino-acid sequence of alpha-corticotropin. Nature (Lond.) *176*, 687 (1955)

13   LI, C.H., GESCHWIND, I.I., DIXON, J.S., LEVY, A.L., HARRIS, J.I.: Corticotropins (ACTH). I. Isolation of α-corticotropin from sheep pituitary glands. J. biol. Chem. *213*, 171 (1955)

14   RAMACHANDRAN, J., CHUNG, D., LI, C.H.: Adrenocorticotropins. XXXIV. Aspects of structure-activity relationships of the ACTH molecule. Synthesis of a heptadecapeptide amide, an octadecapeptide amide, and a nonadecapeptide amide possessing high biological activities. J. Amer. chem. Soc. *87*, 2696 (1965)

15   RINIKER, B.: Revised amino acid sequences of porcine and human ACTH. In: Int. Symp., Polypeptide hormones, Liège 1971 (printing)

16   RINIKER, B., RITTEL, W.: Die Synthese des corticotrop hochaktiven [1-D-Serin, 17,18-dilysin]-β-corticotropin-(1-18)-octadecapeptidamids. Helv. chim. Acta *53*, 513 (1970)

17   RINIKER, B., SIEBER, P., RITTEL, W., ZUBER, H.: Revised amino-acid sequences for porcine and human adrenocorticotrophic hormone. Nature new Biol. (Lond.) *235*, 114 (1972)

18   RITTEL, W.: Techniques for the synthesis of ACTH and MSH peptides and analogues. In Back, N., Martini, L., Paoletti, R. (Editors): Pharmacology of hormonal polypeptides and proteins, Proc. Int. Symp., Milan 1967, p. 35 (Plenum Press, New York 1968)

19   SHEPHERD, R.G., WILLSON, S.D., HOWARD, K.S., BELL, P.H., DAVIES, D.S., DAVIS, S.B., EIGNER, E.A., SHAKESPEARE, N.E.: Studies with corticotropin. III. Determination of the structure of β-corticotropin and its active degradation products. J. Amer. chem. Soc. *78*, 5067 (1956)

20 SIEBER, P., RITTEL, W., RINIKER, B.: Die Synthese von menschlichem adreno-corticotropen Hormon (a_h-ACTH) mit revidierter Aminosäuresequenz. Helv. chim. Acta *55*, 1243 (1972)

21 WALSER, A., MÜLLER, T.: The adrenocorticotropic effect in humans of several synthetic peptides related to $\beta^{1\text{-}24}$ corticotrophin. In Margoulies, M. (Editor): Protein and polypeptide hormones, Proc. Int. Symp., Liège 1968, p. 487 (Excerpta med. Found., Amsterdam 1969)

22 WHITE, W. F., LANDMANN, W. A.: Studies on adrenocorticotropin. XI. A preliminary comparison of corticotropin-A with β-corticotropin. J. Amer. chem. Soc. *77*, 1711 (1955)

Discussion

R. SCHUPPLI: Speaking as a medical man, I find it rather difficult to keep up with these developments in the field of structural analysis and to grasp their implications. For this reason I'd just like to ask how reliable the results are that you have described, Dr. RITTEL. This question interests me, for example, in connection with M.S.H., i.e. with melanocyte-stimulating hormone, as well as in connection with possible side effects. It has been our impression that at one time Synacthen used to produce skin pigmentation much more frequently than it does now. Is it conceivable that the structure of this synthetic A.C.T.H. may perhaps be subject to slight variation?

W. RITTEL: I think that when considering the structural formulae of the naturally occurring A.C.T.H. hormones and of Synacthen we have to distinguish between two different problems. In the case of the natural A.C.T.H. hormones to which I referred in my paper, the structural formula is arrived at from analytical experiments—and, as we have already seen, these analytical experiments may under certain circumstances yield erroneous results. The situation in the case of Synacthen, on the other hand, is quite different. We have synthesised the active substance of this preparation in accordance with the formula for the 1–24 sequence of porcine A.C.T.H. as proposed by SHEPHERD et al.*, which has been accepted as correct. Its structure is arrived at by performing a predetermined sequence of reactions which constitute the various consecutive steps in the process of synthesis. In this process, the individual amino acids are joined together to form specified structural elements, which are then linked up into larger units until the synthesis is finally complete. The procedure by which the molecule is built up is thus so precisely defined and meticulously coordinated that no two production batches can possibly differ in their structure.

H. J. BAUER: The question of melanocyte-stimulating activity in relation to problems of structure, which Dr. SCHUPPLI has raised, is one on which I too should like to comment. A few years ago we carried out clinical studies with DW 75, a trial preparation resembling Synacthen, and found that it displayed a tremendous melanocyte-stimulating effect: our patients all looked as if they had just returned from a skiing holiday. But a comparison between the structural formulae of Synacthen and DW 75 shows that they differ only with respect to the terminal amino acids and to one position in the middle of the two molecules (Figure 1). Would it be generally true to say that seemingly minor structural differences of this kind are capable of causing such enormous differences in the clinical effects?

W. RITTEL: Yes. The DW 75 molecule, which is similar to that of Synacthen, has among other things been modified by replacing the L-serine at the amino end by a D-serine. This modification has the effect of stepping up the experimentally demonstrated activity of A.C.T.H. peptides in general by some five to ten times. In other words, though the modification in question is quite a small one chemically, it has very strong biological repercussions. In animal experiments the melanocyte-stimulating action of such derivatives has been found to be 10–30 times greater than that of unchanged A.C.T.H. peptides.

H. J. BAUER: Do any relationships exist between effects such as melanocyte stimulation and the anti-inflammatory activity or other desirable or undesirable concomitant effects of these peptide hormones?

P. A. DESAULLES: Perhaps I can answer that question from the standpoint of a pharmacologist. The extent to which an A.C.T.H. derivative stimulates melanophore

---

*SHEPHERD, R. G., WILLSON, S. D., HOWARD, K. S., BELL, P. H., DAVIES, D. S., DAVIS, S. B., EIGNER, E. A., SHAKESPEARE, N. E.: Studies with corticotropin. III. Determination of the structure of β-corticotropin and its active degradation products. J. Amer. chem. Soc. 78, 5067 (1956)

M.S.H.

H$_2$N-Ala-Glu-(Lys)$_2$-Asp-Glu-Gly-Pro-	Tyr-	Arg-	Met-Glu-His-Phe-Arg-Try-Gly-	Ser-	Pro-	Pro-Lys-Asp-COOH

A.C.T.H.

H$_2$N-Ser-	Tyr-	Ser-	Met-Glu-His-Phe-Arg-Try-Gly-	Lys-	Pro-	Val-Gly-(Lys)$_2$-(Arg)$_2$-Pro-Val-Lys-Val-Tyr-Pro-Gly-Ala-Glu-(Asp)$_2$-Glu-Leu-Ala-Glu-Ala-Phe-Pro-Leu-Glu-Phe-COOH

Synacthen

H$_2$N-Ser-	Tyr-	Ser-	Met-Glu-His-Phe-Arg-Try-Gly-	Lys-	Pro-	Val-Gly-(Lys)$_2$-(Arg)$_2$-Pro-Val-Lys-Val-Tyr-Pro-COOH

DW 75

H$_2$N-D-*Ser*-	Tyr-	Ser-	*Nle*-Glu-His-Phe-Arg-Try-Gly-	Lys-	Pro-	Val-Gly-(Lys)$_2$-(Arg)$_2$-Pro-Val-Lys-Val-Tyr-Pro-L-*Valinamide*

Fig. 1. Structural formulae of M.S.H., A.C.T.H., Synacthen, and DW 75.

expansion can be precisely determined in pharmacological experiments. Often, however, it is not possible to establish any parallelism between the corticotrophic effect of such a derivative and its influence on melanophore expansion. Various peptides each exhibiting the same corticotrophic activity may differ strongly as regards their melanotropic effect. Moreover, on the basis of pharmacological findings it is extremely difficult, and frequently impossible, to make any valid predictions as to how the melanotropic effect will compare with the corticotrophic effect in man. In this field there is thus still wide scope for further experimental research.

Diagnostic procedures applicable to the hypothalamo-pituitary-adrenocortical axis

by C. van der Meer *

Existing between all the endocrine tissues in the body that collectively constitute the endocrine system are many different interrelationships, which in turn involve a large number of reciprocal effects. It is therefore virtually impossible to examine any one endocrine organ or endocrine axis in isolation, however desirable such an approach might be for the purpose of studying its physiology and pathology. Consequently, it must be borne in mind from the outset that no examination of an endocrine organ or axis can ever be complete or will necessarily always enable one to establish a diagnosis.

There are three organs which participate in the hypothalamo-pituitary-adrenocortical axis. The first of them—the hypothalamus—forms part of the diencephalon and is hence very closely connected with the pituitary; contained in the hypothalamus is an area whose centres stimulate the pituitary, thereby inducing it to secrete the hormones which it produces. The hypothalamus also features a centre—in the ventromedial nucleus—which secretes *corticotrophin-releasing hormone* (C.R.H.). This neurohormone, which is produced by ganglion cells, passes via the ganglionic fibres to the portal region of the pituitary, where it then enters the blood and is directly conveyed to its site of action in the anterior pituitary (Figure 1). The transport mechanism for C.R.H. is thus a highly efficient one.

In contrast to this neurohormone, which has the effect of stimulating hormone secretion from the anterior pituitary, the posterior pituitary hormone, i.e. antidiuretic hormone, though likewise produced by the hypothalamus, is stored in the posterior lobe of the pituitary (Figure 2). As and when it is needed, this antidiuretic hormone is released from the posterior pituitary so that it can exert its effect elsewhere in the body at sites far removed from the pituitary.

By stimulating the pituitary, C.R.H. causes it to produce and release A.C.T.H. *(adrenocorticotrophic hormone)*; this A.C.T.H. induces the adrenal cortex to secrete cortisol and cortisone, which, together with aldosterone, are the main adrenocortical hormones.

The hypothalamo-pituitary-adrenocortical axis can also be regarded as constituting a single unit because its component parts are functionally interlinked with one another by a negative feedback mechanism—a mechanism which can be likened to the thermostat controlling a central heating system. This thermostat is first manually adjusted to the required room temperature. Afterwards, as soon as the temperature in the room drops below the desired level, the thermostat emits a signal to the pump and to the burner, in response to which the water is

*Academisch Ziekenhuis der Vrije Universiteit, Amsterdam, Netherlands.

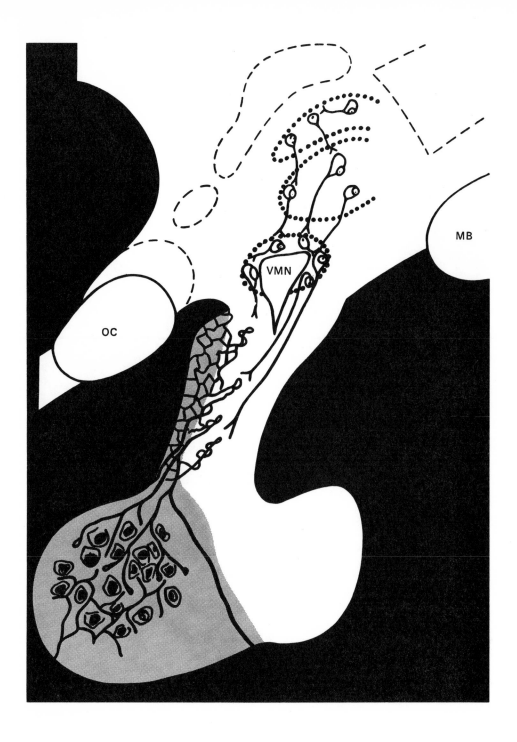

Fig. 1. Diagram of the hypothalamo-anteropituitary axis, indicating the neurovascular pathway linking the hypothalamus with the anterior pituitary via the hypophyseal stalk (OC = optic chiasma; VMN = ventromedial nucleus; MB = mamillary body).

21

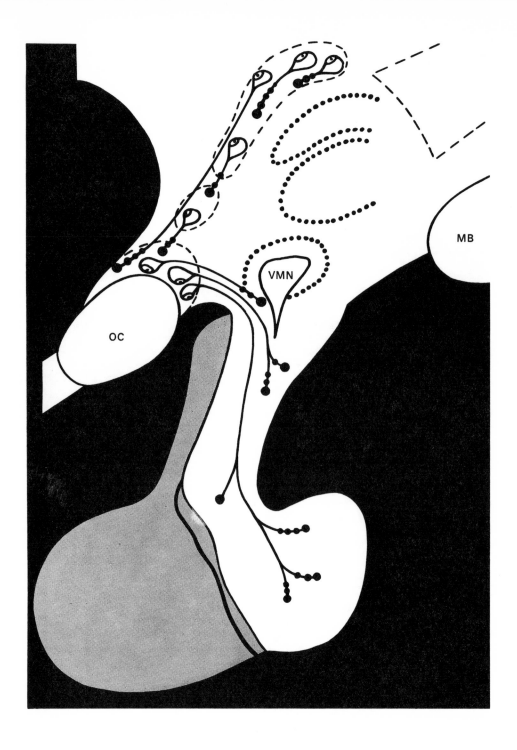

Fig. 2. Diagram of the hypothalamo-posteropituitary axis, indicating the neural pathway linking the hypothalamus with the posterior pituitary.

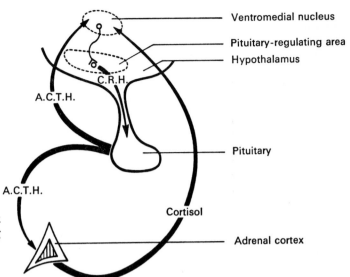

Fig. 3. Diagram of the negative feedback mechanism operating within the hypo-thalamo-pituitary-adrenocortical axis.

then heated up and circulated throughout the central heating system. The radiators proceed to warm the air in the room to the requisite temperature, whereupon the signal ceases. The radiators now cool down again and the air temperature gradually drops until another signal from the thermostat sets the whole process in operation once more.

The functioning of the hypothalamo-pituitary-adrenocortical axis is regulated in much the same manner (Figure 3). A decrease in the concentration of cortisol in the blood has the effect of stimulating the hypothalamus to release larger quantities of C.R.H., so that more A.C.T.H. is secreted and, in turn, correspondingly more cortisol is produced. The resultant increase in the plasma cortisol concentration then inhibits the release of C.R.H. from the hypothalamus, so that the output of A.C.T.H. diminishes. This feedback mechanism is referred to as a negative one, because the rise in the plasma cortisol level triggers off a chain of reactions which counteracts the rise. A further feedback mechanism involving A.C.T.H. and C.R.H. operates between the pituitary and the hypothalamus, although its full significance has not yet been elucidated (Figure 3). It probably serves to correct minor fluctuations occurring within the axis.

To assess the functional status of such an endocrine axis, the diagnostic methods employed must entail:

a) Investigation of the functioning of the individual organs concerned.

b) Investigation of the control mechanism.

It is the hypothalamus that is responsible for regulating hypothalamo-pituitary-adrenocortical function as a whole. For this reason, the control mechanism operating from the hypothalamus is—by analogy with the thermostat which regulates a central heating system—sometimes also referred to as the "adreno-stat". The axis itself is subject to a sleeping-waking rhythm, i.e. the cortisol concentration in the blood attains its maximum immediately after waking and then slowly diminishes (Figure 4). The most pronounced increase in the plasma

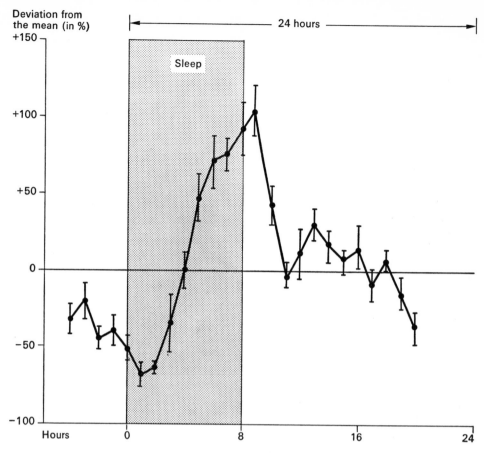

Fig. 4. Normal diurnal rhythm of the plasma cortisol levels. (Figures 4, 5, and 6 are reproduced by courtesy of The Journal of Clinical Endocrinology and Metabolism)

cortisol levels occurs during the period prior to awakening. In persons with a normal sleeping-waking rhythm, the highest cortisol values are recorded in the morning between 8 and 9 a.m. It is during the phase extending from late afternoon to about midnight that the plasma cortisol concentration sinks to its lowest levels. Suggestions to the effect that this rhythm might possibly be dependent on whether the individual is lying or standing, or whether he is kept in darkness or light, have proved to be unfounded. This has been very clearly demonstrated by ORTH et al.*. When test subjects were compelled to adhere to an abnormal diurnal rhythm, e.g. to spend six hours asleep and six hours awake, the 24-hour rhythm of their cortisol production showed two peaks (Figure 5). Other sleeping-waking rhythms also resulted in similar circadian patterns of cortisol secretion (Figure 6). However, since the circadian pattern of the plasma cortisol levels does not undergo an alteration until some ten days after the

* ORTH, D. N., ISLAND, D. P., LIDDLE, G. W.: Experimental alteration of the circadian rhythm in plasma cortisol (17-OHCS) concentration in man. J. clin. Endocr. 27, 549 (1967)

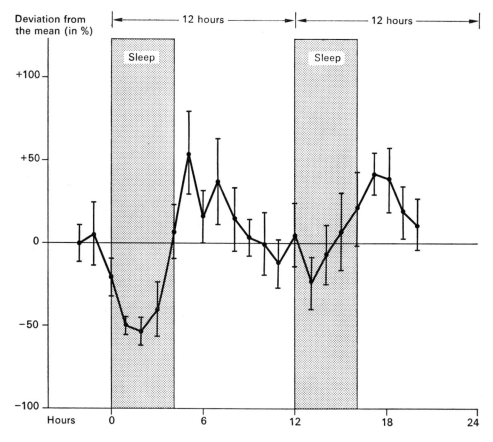

Fig. 5. Pattern of the plasma cortisol levels in the presence of an experimentally accelerated sleeping-waking rhythm.

sleeping-waking rhythm has been changed, it was quite some time before these cause-and-effect relationships were discovered.

The first diagnostic test to be performed on the hypothalamus should be designed to answer the question: does the patient exhibit any sleeping-waking rhythm at all? This rhythm may sometimes be interrupted under the strain of situations involving physical or mental stress. Care must therefore be taken to ensure that the patient is not suffering from stress at the time of the examination. In this connection it should be borne in mind that certain individuals may develop a stress reaction even in response to the puncturing of a vein. In such cases, of course, the plasma cortisol values recorded will not convey an accurate impression of the basic sleeping-waking rhythm of cortisol secretion.

A surgical operation—involving the administration of morphine, anaesthetisation, and the infliction of a trauma—gives rise to a pronounced stress reaction (Figure 7) marked by an increase in the secretion of C.R.H., A.C.T.H., and cortisol. Other hormone systems, too, are involved in this reaction. From the case illustrated in Figure 8, for example, it can be seen that no urine was produced on the day of the operation and that, after the operation, increases

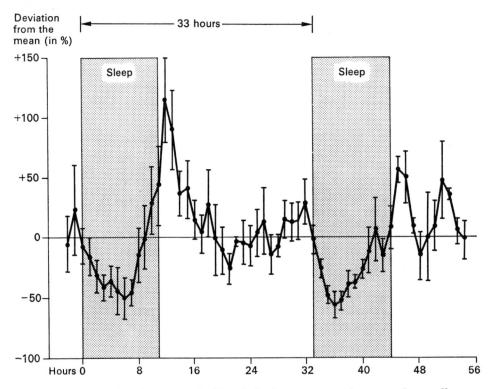

Fig. 6. Pattern of the plasma cortisol levels in the presence of an experimentally prolonged sleeping-waking rhythm.

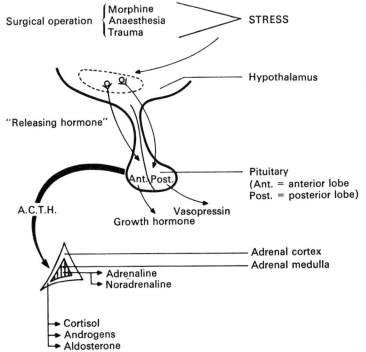

Fig. 7. Diagram illustrating the stress reaction occasioned by surgery.

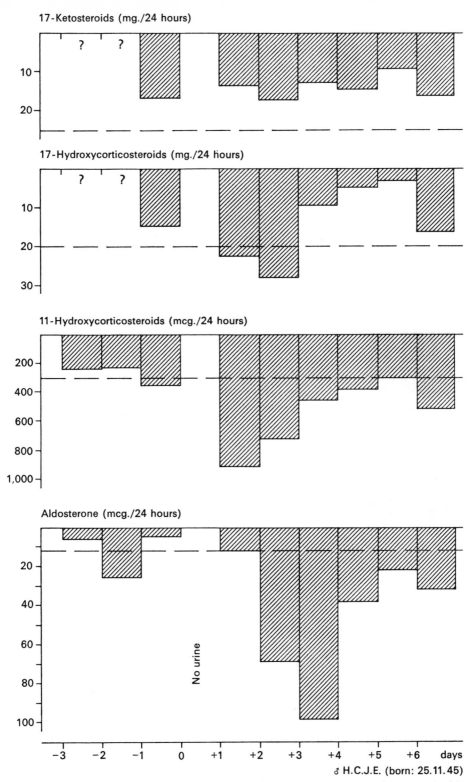

Fig. 8. Urinary excretion of steroids before and during a stress reaction provoked by a surgical operation for removal of an epididymal cyst (Day 0).

27

occurred in the excretion of 17-ketosteroids, 17-hydroxycorticosteroids, and aldosterone in the 24-hour urine.

Also of interest in this connection is an observation which we recently made when we admitted students to our surgical department in order to determine whether a positive nitrogen balance could be induced by means of artificial, i.e. parenteral, feeding. For this purpose they were given infusions, which were set up in such a way that the student was not immobilised during the infusion; total urine collections were made. A few days ago, we discovered very high 17-hydroxycorticosteroid and 17-ketosteroid levels in the urine. We could not account for this sudden rise until we discovered that on the day in question the fiancées of the students had visited them in their rooms—and these visits had evidently imposed a very severe stress on the young men!

One method of deliberately provoking a stress reaction for test purposes involves the induction of hypoglycaemia; here it is important that the blood sugar level should be lowered rapidly. To achieve this, the patient—after his blood sugar level has first been determined—is given insulin intravenously; the blood sugar level is then measured again in order to calculate the decrease. At the same time, a record is made of the plasma cortisol concentration, which should normally rise in response to the rapid decrease in the blood sugar level (Figures 9 and 10). Since this insulin test entails some risk of cerebral damage due to hypoglycaemia, it should be performed only under the supervision of a doctor; and glucose solution, together possibly with glucagon and adrenaline, should be kept in readiness for administration if required.

A stress reaction can also be induced by the injection of a pyrogen. The disadvantage of this method lies in the fact that it causes a very sharp rise in body temperature—usually to levels as high as 41° C.—which makes the patient feel seriously ill. Unfortunately, there is no way in which this febrile response can be prevented. Incidentally, that such pyrogen-induced stress reactions are not attributable solely to the fever, can be indirectly demonstrated with the aid of aetiocholanolone, which is one of the naturally occurring adrenocortical ster-

Time:	Blood samples taken for measurement of:	Infusion:
−30′		NaCl 0.9%
0′	Glucose + cortisol + H.G.H.	Insulin (0.1 U./kg. i.v.)
15′		
30′		
60′		
90′		
120′		
150′		Stop

Cortisol: maximum attained between 30′ and 60′
Normal increase: approx. 10 mcg./100 ml.

H.G.H. (growth hormone): maximum attained between 30′ and 60′
Normal increase: 40 ± 20 ng./ml. plasma

Fig. 9. Insulin-induced hypoglycaemia test.

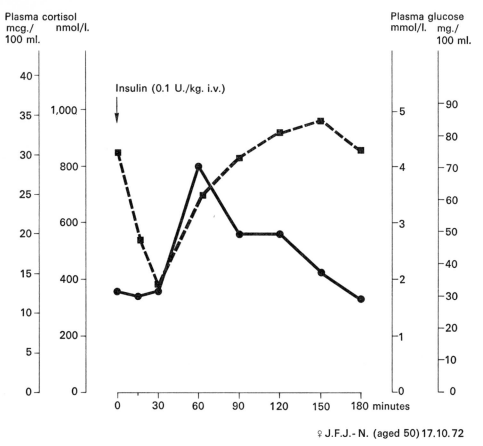

Plasma cortisol mcg./100 ml. nmol/l.

Plasma glucose mmol/l. mg./100 ml.

Insulin (0.1 U./kg. i.v.)

0   30   60   90   120   150   180 minutes

♀ J.F.J.- N. (aged 50) 17.10.72

Fig. 10. Plasma cortisol (●——●) and glucose (■――■) levels recorded during an insulin test (10 mcg./100 ml. cortisol = 276 nmol/l.).

Time:	Blood samples taken for measurement of:	Infusion:
0	Cortisol	250 ml. NaCl 0.9% (0–120′)
120′		
180′		250 ml. NaCl 0.9% + 10 U. lysine-vasopressin (120′–240′)
240′		Stop

Fig. 11. Lysine-vasopressin test.

oids: when this steroid is administered, the body temperature shows a marked rise, but no change occurs in the plasma cortisol concentration.

The simplest solution to the problem of testing pituitary function would be to measure the concentration of A.C.T.H. in the blood before and after an injection of C.R.H. But for this purpose C.R.H. would be required in greater quantities

29

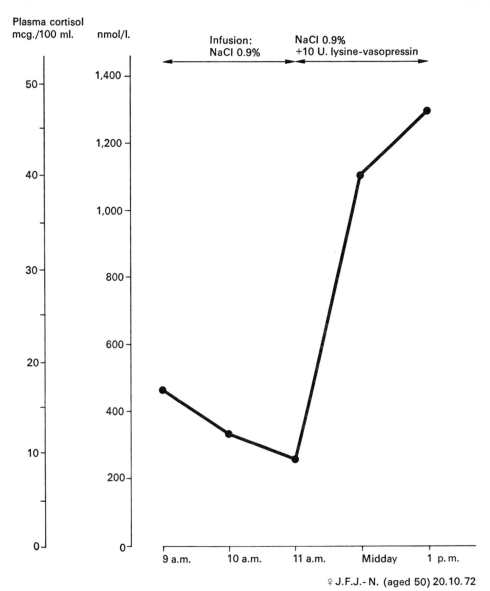

Fig. 12. Plasma cortisol levels recorded during a lysine-vasopressin test.

than are at present available. Moreover, the method of determining A.C.T.H. in the blood by radioimmunoassay has only just emerged from the experimental stage and certainly leaves room for further improvement.

Consequently, it is the lysine-vasopressin test that is currently employed for investigating pituitary function. Vasopressin, a hormone produced by the posterior pituitary, has the effect of raising the plasma cortisol concentration. The test itself is carried out by us as follows:

A physiological saline infusion is started in the morning. Two hours after the start of the infusion the plasma cortisol concentration will normally have reached its base-line level. Within the next two hours 10 I.U. lysine-vasopressin is infused in the saline solution. By the end of these two hours, the plasma cortisol level will—in the presence of normal pituitary function—have risen to at least double the base-line value (Figures 11 and 12).

Since lysine-vasopressin is liable to provoke numerous reactions which are unpleasant for the patient, we have tried—by slowing the infusion rate—to reduce the quantity of lysine-vasopressin administered to such an extent that only mild reactions occur, such as pallor and uncomfortable feelings in the abdomen. These low doses are sufficient to enable one to detect cases in which hypothalamo-pituitary-adrenocortical function is normal. When we calculated the doses by reference to the patient's total body surface, we found that the amount which elicits the aforementioned mild symptoms is roughly the same in every case.

Justified doubts exist as to whether this test really serves as a specific indicator of pituitary function. In the relevant literature emphasis has been placed on the possibility that the action involved may take place via the hypothalamus; but it is very difficult to furnish exact experimental proof of this. Most of the observations reported would seem to suggest that the hypothalamus is in fact the primary site of attack and that the pituitary may be only secondarily involved.

The diagnostic tests employed in the assessment of adrenocortical function, on the other hand, are more specific. A normally functioning adrenal cortex can be made to step up its production of cortisol by means of an A.C.T.H. injection, and the resultant increase in the plasma cortisol concentration can easily be measured.

A.C.T.H. injections, however, have the disadvantage that they may possibly give rise to hypersensitivity reactions, since the A.C.T.H. preparations obtained by extraction from animal pituitaries always remain contaminated to some extent by foreign protein. Synthetic A.C.T.H. preparations, containing only the active substance itself and no accompanying traces of foreign protein, ought therefore—in theory at least—to provoke no hypersensitivity reactions at all; but in practice, they too occasionally produce such reactions, though far more infrequently. There is accordingly everything to be said for employing these synthetic products in preference to A.C.T.H. extract-preparations. Although we have given a large number of synthetic A.C.T.H. (®Synacthen) injections in our hospital, we have so far had only one hypersensitivity reaction.

The so-called Synacthen test of adrenocortical function can be performed in either of two ways:

A. The 30-minute Synacthen test (Table 1 and Figure 13). Here, 0.25 mg. Synacthen is injected intravenously, after a blood sample has first been taken in order to determine the initial plasma cortisol concentration. Thirty minutes later, the plasma cortisol level will have risen sufficiently to permit an assessment of adrenocortical function; if necessary, a further blood sample can be taken after 60 minutes. In 22 out of 26 cases we found the plasma cortisol levels to be higher after 60 minutes than after 30 minutes (Figure 14).

B. The Synacthen infusion test (Figure 15). In this test, a dose of 0.25 mg. Synacthen is infused over a period of six hours. This ensures prolonged stimula-

Table 1. Thirty-minute Synacthen test.

Take blood sample for plasma cortisol determination; then inject 0.25 mg. Synacthen i.v.

After 30 minutes: take another blood sample for plasma cortisol determination.

In the case of a good positive reaction, the plasma cortisol concentration rises after 30 minutes (by at least 10 mcg./100 ml.) to two or more times its initial level.

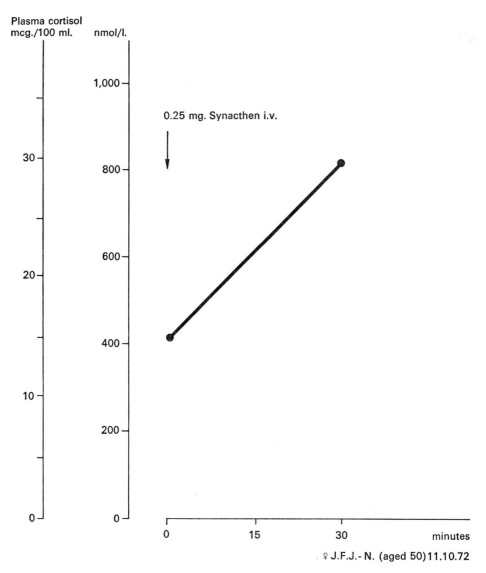

♀ J.F.J.- N. (aged 50) 11.10.72

Fig. 13. Plasma cortisol levels recorded during a 30-minute Synacthen test.

tion of the adrenal cortex, such as may be particularly indicated in cases where secondary adrenocortical hypofunction is suspected, i.e. where the production of cortisol has been arrested owing to a lack of endogenous A.C.T.H. Under

32

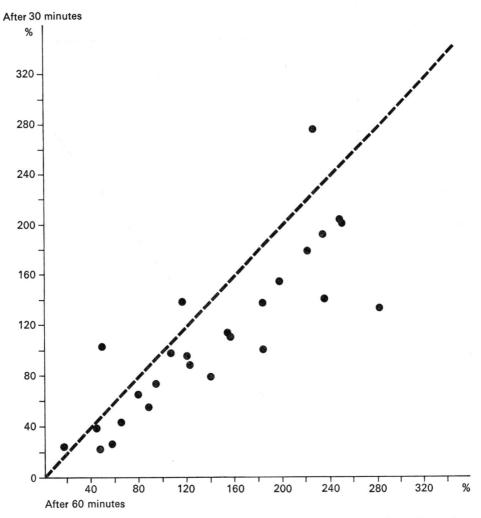

Fig. 14. Rise in the plasma cortisol levels (in %) recorded in the 30-minute Synacthen test after 30 and 60 minutes (N = 26).

these circumstances, the adrenal cortex requires a more prolonged period of stimulation in order to get its cortisol production under way again. In such cases, it is essential that a corticosteroid (e.g. dexamethasone) be given at the same time as the test is carried out, so as to avoid the risk of provoking an addisonian crisis.

Occasionally even the Synacthen infusion test fails to provoke any reaction on the part of the adrenal cortex. This may occur, for example, in a patient who has been undergoing long-term treatment with corticosteroids. If Synacthen Depot is administered in such cases, this usually leads within a few days to restoration of a good response in the 30-minute test or in the infusion test. Sometimes, however, it may be necessary to give daily doses of Synacthen Depot for about one week.

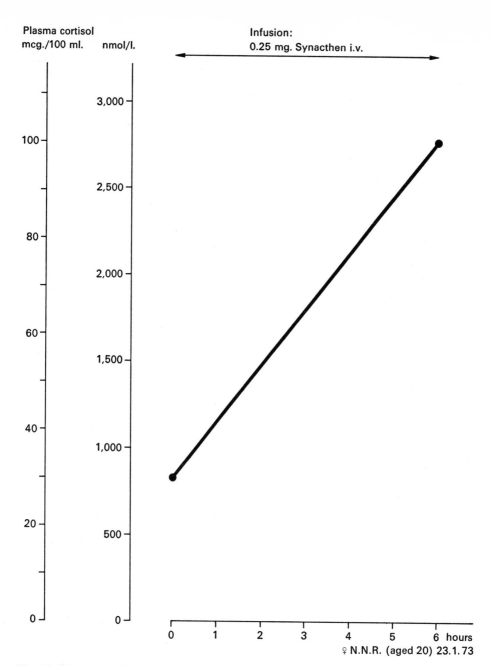

Fig. 15. Plasma cortisol levels recorded during a Synacthen infusion test.

The control mechanism by which the hypothalamo-pituitary-adrenocortical axis is governed can be tested by two possible methods, both of which involve exerting an influence on the production of C.R.H.:

1. The metabolites of steroids originating from the adrenal cortex are determined daily in the 24-hour urine for two days in order to obtain two sets of blank values.

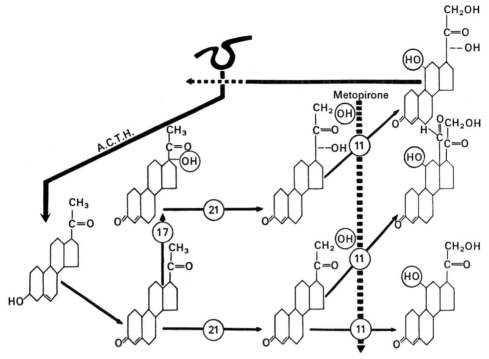

Fig. 16. Diagram indicating how Metopirone suppresses the synthesis of endogenous cortisol by blocking 11β-hydroxylase.

Then, on the third day, the patient is given four or six oral doses of 750 mg. ®Metopirone spread over the day.

Metopirone blocks 11β-hydroxylase in the adrenal cortex (Figure 16), with the result that the production of cortisol practically ceases (to be exact, the output of cortisol from the adrenal cortex is reduced to approximately 3% of normal). This stimulates the hypothalamus, causing it to secrete larger quantities of C.R.H.; under the influence of this C.R.H., the pituitary steps up its production of A.C.T.H., which in turn activates the adrenal cortex. A new hormonal equilibrium is thus established at a higher level of production. Owing to the blockade of 11β-hydroxylase, a very marked increase occurs in the output of steroid precursors, i.e. of substances whose biosynthesis cannot be completed without the intervention of 11β-hydroxylase. These substances display very little, if any, biological activity. They are collectively determined in the urine with the 17-hydroxycorticosteroids. Where the Metopirone test has been performed, the very high urinary 17-hydroxycorticosteroid levels are thus due, not to a rise in cortisol production, but to an increase in the formation of intermediate products. Depending on the laboratory facilities available, it is of course also possible instead to determine the tetrahydro-S fraction; the latter consists of metabolites of 11-desoxycortisol, a precursor which normally becomes transformed into cortisol in the adrenal cortex under the influence of 11β-hydroxylase.

The urine should also be examined again on the second day after administration of the Metopirone, because in some cases it is not until the second day that an

35

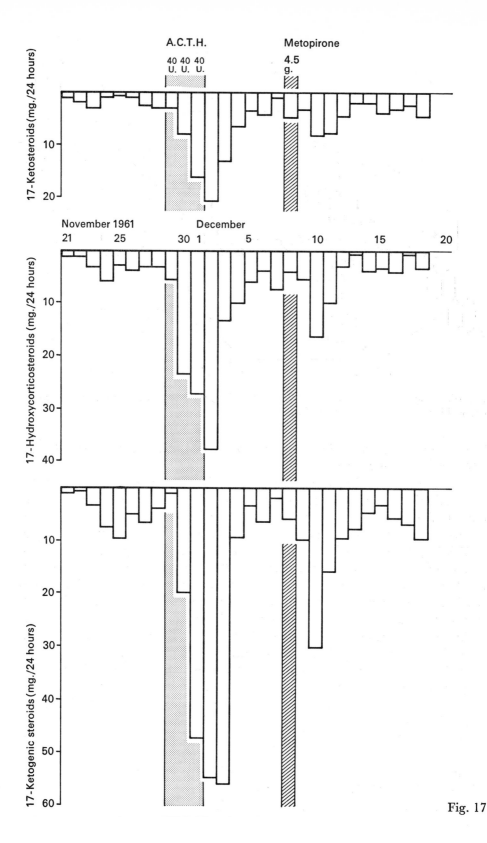

36

Fig. 17

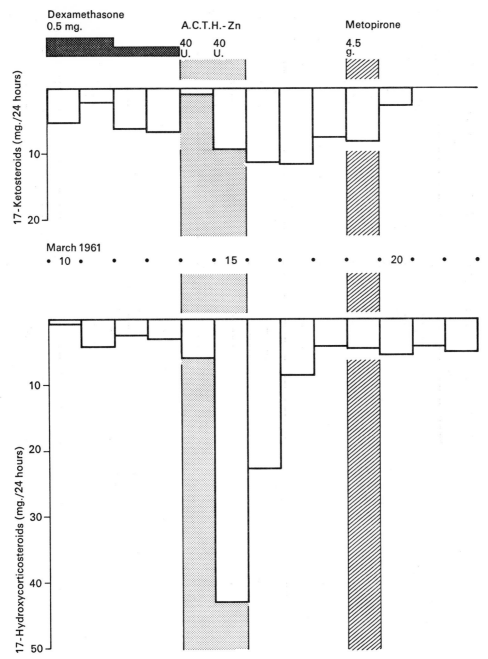

Fig. 18. Excretion of steroids in a 75-year-old male patient (W./heart block) who, after four weeks of treatment with dexamethasone, showed no response in the Metopirone test but a marked reaction to A.C.T.H.

Fig. 17. Excretion of steroids in an 81-year-old female patient (V.V.-V.D.L./hepatitis) who, after four weeks of treatment with betamethasone, still showed a normal response in the Metopirone test and a good reaction to A.C.T.H.

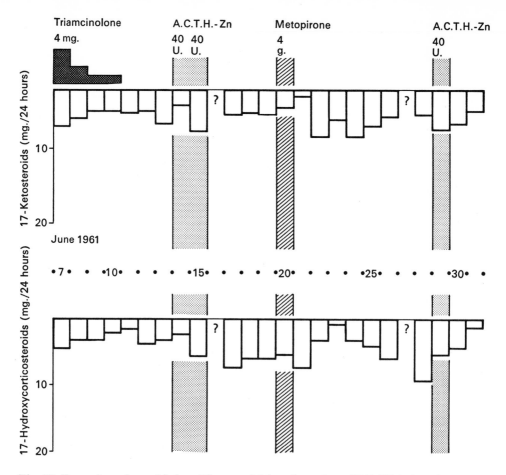

Fig. 19. Excretion of steroids in a 56-year-old female patient (V.D.W./sclerodactylia) who, after seven months of treatment with triamcinolone, showed no response in the Metopirone test and also failed to react to A.C.T.H.

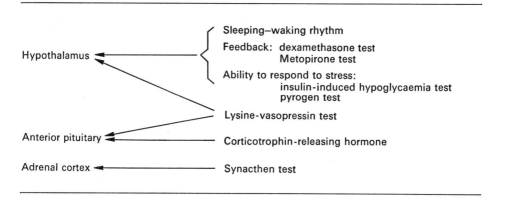

Fig. 20. Battery of tests available for the assessment of hypothalamo-pituitary-adrenocortical function.

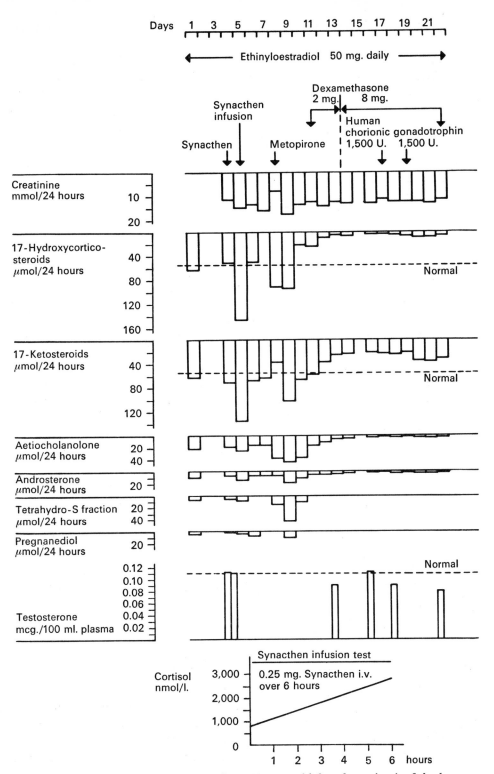

Fig. 21. Example illustrating the use (in a 20-year-old female patient) of the battery of tests outlined in Figure 20.

increase in the 17-hydroxycorticosteroid concentrations can be detected (see also Figure 21).

Illustrated in Figure 17 is a normal response to Metopirone. In this case, the A.C.T.H. test should also elicit a normal reaction. Where, on the other hand, the result of the A.C.T.H. test is normal, but the patient fails to react to Metopirone (Figure 18), this is indicative of secondary adrenocortical hypofunction; in other words, here hypothalamo-pituitary function is impaired.

Figure 19 shows a case in which both the A.C.T.H. test and the Metopirone test yielded a negative result; in this instance, the disorder may well extend to the whole of the hypothalamo-pituitary-adrenocortical axis.

2. The hypothalamo-pituitary-adrenocortical control mechanism can also be tested using dexamethasone. Here, once again, blank values for the cortisol metabolites in the 24-hour urine are first obtained on two successive days; then, on the third day, 2 mg. dexamethasone is given, either orally or intravenously, in fractional doses divided over the day. Dexamethasone, like cortisol, exerts an inhibitory effect on the hypothalamus, with the result that the latter produces less C.R.H., the output of A.C.T.H. and cortisol therefore also being reduced. This reduction is reflected in a decrease in the urinary excretion of steroid metabolites. When these steroid metabolites are determined in the urine, the measurements are not affected by the presence of metabolites resulting directly from the dose of dexamethasone itself; moreover, thanks to the fact that dexamethasone is far more potent than cortisone on a milligramme for milligramme basis, the low dose of 2 mg. in which it requires to be given is such a small quantity that it would in any case have hardly any influence on the measurements.

In cases of hypothalamo-pituitary-adrenocortical hyperactivity, the dexamethasone test can also be carried out with a dose of 8 mg. The battery of tests available is outlined in Figure 20, and a concrete example of their use presented in Figure 21.

Attempts have repeatedly been made to use data obtained from these various tests in order to differentiate between similar clinical pictures, e. g. to distinguish between Cushing's disease as such (basophil adenoma of the pituitary) and Cushing's syndrome (adrenal carcinoma or adenoma). Although it is possible to establish certain guidelines in this connection, they do not always lead to satisfactory results in practice. The best method of differentiating between Cushing's disease and Cushing's syndrome is to determine the blood concentration of A.C.T.H.

The fact that extremely high concentrations of A.C.T.H. are sometimes found in the presence of an ectopic source of production occasionally makes it possible to distinguish a case in which a non-pituitary tumour is acting as a site of ectopic A.C.T.H. production from a case of Cushing's disease. Often, however, such differential diagnosis proves very difficult, with the result that a correct diagnosis can only be established by conducting an intensive search for tumours of this kind.

Discussion

J. GIRARD: Dr. VAN DER MEER's reference to corticotrophin-releasing factor prompts me to ask whether there is any structural affinity between C.R.F. and the 1–24 sequence of the A.C.T.H. molecule.

W. RITTEL: So far as I am aware, nothing is yet known about the chemical structure of the corticotrophin-releasing factor. There was a time when we thought that the 4–10 sequence of A.C.T.H., which also occurs in alpha-M.S.H. and beta-M.S.H., might be identical with corticotrophin-releasing hormone; but unfortunately this has since been disproved.

K.F. WEINGES: Have you ever performed lysine-vasopressin tests in patients receiving corticosteroid therapy, Dr. VAN DER MEER? I ask this for the following reason: a single dose of thyroid hormone, given either in the laevorotatory or in the dextro-rotatory form, totally inhibits T.R.F.-induced secretion of thyroid-stimulating hormone after 48 hours; this suggests that the feedback mechanism operates not only via the hypothalamus but also via the pituitary. I should be interested to know whether similar tests were also performed in the case of A.C.T.H.

C. VAN DER MEER: No, we carried out all our studies without employing any additional drugs or hormones.

T.B. BINNS: The plasma cortisol concentration reflects the level of circulating A.C.T.H. so closely that for many purposes I think it provides an adequate indirect assay of A.C.T.H. But occasions also arise when it is useful to be able to determine the A.C.T.H. level itself, particularly if one has a method of assay sensitive enough to enable one to measure physiological levels. The following slide (Figure 1) shows the levels of endogenous A.C.T.H. in a volunteer after intravenous administration of 100 mg. hydrocortisone. There are two things to which I'd like to draw attention: firstly, the half-life of the endogenous plasma A.C.T.H.—in the early phase, at any rate—was 10.4 minutes; secondly, the final point on the curve is equivalent to 35 femtogrammes per mille (and a femtogramme, I would remind you, is only 10^{-15} gramme). In other words, this method for the bioassay of A.C.T.H., which was recently published by CHAYEN et al.* from the Kennedy Institute of West London Hospital, is fantastically sensitive, far more so than the immunoassay, and so opens up new possibilities for experimenting at physiological levels, even on plasma samples of 0.1 ml.

Now may I show you another slide, also kindly lent to me by Dr. CHAYEN, in which a volunteer was given 800 nanogrammes of Synacthen (Figure 2). The unbroken line represents the plasma A.C.T.H. level, and the interrupted line the plasma cortisol concentration. Unfortunately, this subject was not completely dexamethasone-suppressed; hence the triangle on the left vertical axis just below the figure 5. Here too, however, you can see that there is a rapid rise to just over 100 picogrammes per mille, followed by a sharp decline—the half-life being once again about 10 minutes, though the curve afterwards tends to level off. From the curve showing the plasma cortisol concentration, which was measured simultaneously, you can see that the cortisol level had already started to rise rapidly after five minutes and that it subsequently declined as would be expected.

Just before I left England to attend this meeting, Dr. CHAYEN repeated the same type of experiment using the 1–18 polypeptide (41,795-Ba) to which Dr. RITTEL has already referred. From the preliminary results that Dr. CHAYEN obtained, it seems pretty clear that the half-life of this 1–18 peptide is about 60 minutes. This no doubt accounts for its longer duration of action.

---

*CHAYEN, J., LOVERIDGE, N., DALY, J.R.: A sensitive bioassay for adrenocortico-trophic hormone in human plasma. Clin. Endocr. *1*, 219 (1972)

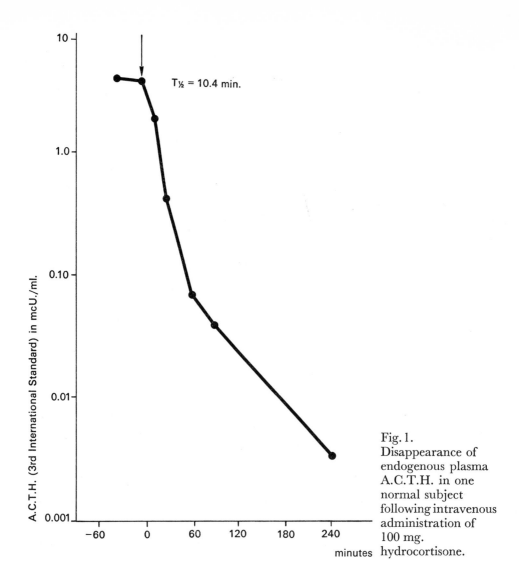

Fig. 1.
Disappearance of endogenous plasma A.C.T.H. in one normal subject following intravenous administration of 100 mg. hydrocortisone.

T½ = 10.4 min.

A.C.T.H. (3rd International Standard) in mcU./ml.

minutes

R. DEGUILLAUME: The various tests of hypothalamo-pituitary-adrenocortical function to which reference has been made certainly constitute valuable aids to the differential diagnosis of disorders affecting the H.P.A. axis, but they do not always prove of decisive value; hence, despite such tests, it is sometimes still difficult to establish a correct diagnosis. Many of these tests have been standardised on the basis of statistical data obtained in healthy volunteers, and on this basis it is relatively easy to draw up what can be considered as normal ranges. When one is dealing with patients, however, the situation becomes quite different. Allow me to cite a few examples to illustrate what I mean.

Except in cases of complete adrenal insufficiency as found in Addison's disease, the 30-minute Synacthen test yields results which are frequently hard to interpret. In Cushing's disease, for instance, a marked rise in the plasma cortisol levels is very often observed, not after 30 minutes, but only after a lapse of as much as two hours. In cases of adrenocortical failure due to treatment with corticosteroids, it is sometimes no easy matter to demonstrate the presence of adrenal insufficiency on the basis of this test: the curves plotted in these patients following stimulation of the adrenal

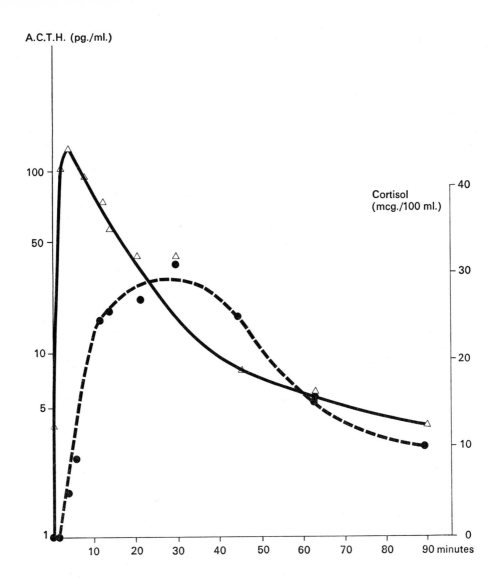

A.C.T.H. (pg./ml.)

Cortisol (mcg./100 ml.)

Fig. 2. Plasma A.C.T.H. (———) and plasma cortisol (———) concentrations in one normal subject following intravenous administration of 800 ng. Synacthen.

cortex tend to encroach on the normal range to such an extent that, when attempting to make a diagnosis in an individual case, one quite often remains in doubt as to how to interpret the response to the test.

As for the test based on inhibition of the pituitary, though it is customarily maintained that no such inhibition can be induced in patients with Cushing's disease, a test performed with a large dose of dexamethasone does in fact generally inhibit the pituitary in these cases, and sometimes even a test in which only a small dose of dexamethasone is employed.

Finally, it is by no means uncommon for the ®Metopirone test to yield results which, within the clinical context of the case under investigation, can only be described as paradoxical. This test is liable to give not only a negative result in a patient with normal pituitary function, but also a false positive result in a patient suffering from

43

manifest pituitary insufficiency—as, for example, in a case reported to us in which complete destruction of the pituitary was subsequently found at autopsy.

J. GIRARD: With regard to the 30-minute Synacthen test, I should like to point out that in paediatrics what we need is a test which not only can be performed quickly, but which also involves the removal of a minimum of blood. In a series of children whom we tested with Synacthen, we found that maximal plasma cortisol levels were not attained until 60 or 120 minutes after the injection. We were thus subsequently able to manage with two blood samples, one taken at time zero and the other after 120 minutes.

As for tests of hypothalamo-pituitary-adrenocortical function, it should be noted that the insulin-induced hypoglycaemia test enables one simultaneously to evaluate both A.C.T.H.-adrenocortical function and growth hormone secretion. The Metopirone test (carried out with an oral dosage of 500 mg. per square metre of body surface) provides similar information. Metopirone stimulates the secretion of growth hormone and leads to an increase in excretion of the tetrahydro-S and tetrahydro-desoxycorticosterone fractions in the 24-hour urine *.

G. GEYER: In cases of Addison's disease the patient may possibly react with an adrenal crisis in the course of an A.C.T.H. test—as I can confirm from personal experience. Can you offer any explanation for this, Dr. VAN DER MEER? So far as I know, in patients suffering from adrenocortical insufficiency, the secretion of A.C.T.H. is already stepped up to a maximum; and I have therefore never been able to understand why in such a case additional exogenous A.C.T.H. should provoke an adrenal crisis.

C. VAN DER MEER: It is indeed difficult to suggest an explanation. According to one hypothesis, in a patient with adrenocortical hypofunction—and consequently with a very low cortisol production—the administration of A.C.T.H. or Synacthen has the effect of completely draining the adrenal cortex of steroids; the production capacity of the adrenal cortex is thus utterly exhausted, with the result that an adrenal crisis may ensue. Whether this explanation is correct, however, is still a moot point.

G. GEYER: I could well imagine that the causes might be of a metabolic nature. A.C.T.H. greatly increases the fatty acid concentration and thus reduces the utilisation of glucose. The adrenal crisis occurring in such cases could therefore be a form of metabolic reaction; it would then not be due at all to exhaustion of the very last corticosteroid reserves, because these reserves would already have been exhausted in response to the very high levels of circulating endogenous A.C.T.H.

W. J. IRVINE: I'd just like to make a brief comment on the diagnosis of Addison's disease with particular reference to the radioimmunoassay of A.C.T.H., because commercial kits are now available with which these assays of A.C.T.H. can be performed very reliably. This, of course, greatly facilitates matters when you are dealing with a patient who is seriously ill, because all you have to do is to take off plasma so that you can measure the A.C.T.H. and cortisol levels, and then start hydrocortisone treatment without delay. Subsequently, you can switch over to dexamethasone and carry out a Synacthen Depot test. If you find a high A.C.T.H. and a low cortisol level, this, coupled with the results of your subsequent test, will leave little doubt about the diagnosis.

May I also suggest that it might well be preferable to use Synacthen Depot instead of ordinary Synacthen when performing tests. I say this because we have found—as I am sure others have, too—that the plasma cortisol response to Synacthen Depot during the first hour or so is very similar indeed to the response obtained with ordinary

---

* STAHL, M., KAPP, J. P., ZACHMANN, M., GIRARD, J.: Effect of a single oral dose of metyrapone on secretion of growth hormone and urinary tetrahydro-11-deoxycortisol and tetrahydro-11-deoxycorticosterone excretion in children. Helv. paediat. Acta 27, 147 (1972)

Synacthen. Synacthen Depot has the advantage as a diagnostic agent of providing a much stronger stimulus to the adrenal cortex and therefore making false negative results less likely, particularly if plasma cortisol is measured not only at one hour but also at five and 24 hours. If the plasma cortisol fails to rise after the first injection of Synacthen Depot, the injection of 1 mg. should be repeated on two subsequent days. In this way a clear distinction will be made between primary and secondary adreno-cortical insufficiency.

Finally, another point I should like to make concerns the often difficult problem of diagnosing Cushing's disease and distinguishing the latter from cases in which the patient is merely depressed, obese, or hypertensive. Here, it has been found most help-ful to resort to the insulin hypoglycaemia test and to measure the patient's plasma cortisol response in this test: in cases of true Cushing's disease, the secretion of cortisol is suppressed, whereas in other cases it remains unaffected.

T. B. BINNS: Before we leave this topic, may I just draw attention to a booklet on tests of hypothalamo-pituitary-adrenal function * which was written for us at CIBA Horsham by Professors JAMES and LANDON, two of the leading British authorities in this field. Clinicians as well as laboratory workers have found this monograph extremely useful, and I should be glad to arrange for a copy to be sent to any of those present who would be interested to receive one.

R. SCHUPPLI: In view of what we have just heard, it would not always appear wise to administer corticosteroids at the same time as A.C.T.H. therapy. In many cases, however, we are obliged to do this, because A.C.T.H. cannot do more than stimulate the adrenal cortex to a maximum. If, in a case of pemphigus for instance, we require 100 to 120 mg. prednisone daily in order to prevent bullous eruptions, we shall not be able to manage with A.C.T.H. alone—at least, not at the beginning. In such cases we often resort to a combination of A.C.T.H. and corticoid therapy, although some-times we have the impression that this results in a mutual inhibitory action instead of a potentiation of the therapeutic effect. I should like to ask the specialists in this field, and Dr. BINNS in particular, how they view this problem. Could it be that concomitant treatment with A.C.T.H. and corticosteroids is contra-indicated?

T. B. BINNS: I don't know that I feel competent to answer that question! I think that under certain circumstances it may perhaps be possible to combine the two; and it would certainly be very advantageous if in this way one could preserve the integrity of the hypothalamo-pituitary-adrenocortical axis. Unfortunately, however, when Professor JAMES** studied this point, he found that, when given in combination with corticotrophin, even relatively small doses of steroids still interfered with the hypo-thalamo-pituitary-adrenocortical axis. I therefore suspect that the scope for such combined therapy is rather limited, but I would defer to Dr. IRVINE's expert opinion on this issue.

W. J. IRVINE: I entirely agree with what Dr. BINNS has just said. I shall have more to say later about the hypothalamo-pituitary-adrenocortical axis in connection with A.C.T.H. therapy. Meanwhile, I would merely state that I consider it most unlikely that its function can be preserved intact by combining oral steroids with A.C.T.H treatment on a long-term basis.

R. SCHUPPLI: But is it your impression that in this respect there may probably be certain differences between the various steroid preparations—for instance, between dexamethasone and prednisone? And, if so, would these differences be sufficiently important to justify changing from one preparation to another?

---

* JAMES, V. H. T., LANDON, J.: Hypothalamic-pituitary-adrenal function tests (CIBA LABORATORIES LIMITED, Horsham, Sussex 1971)
** JAMES, V. H. T.: The investigation of pituitary-adrenal function: effects of cortico-steroid and corticotrophin therapy. Pharmacol. clin. 2, 182 (1970)

W. J. IRVINE: There may be a difference in terms of mineralocorticoid activity, for example, but, so far as I know, there is no difference between these steroids as regards the extent to which they are liable to cause suppression of the hypothalamo-pituitary-adrenocortical axis.

K. F. WEINGES: I think there may be certain differences in this connection, e.g. between prednisolone and dexamethasone. For one thing, the half-life values differ considerably. Prednisolone also becomes bound to some extent with transcortin, whereas no such binding occurs in the case of dexamethasone. I believe that differences in the kinetics of prednisolone and dexamethasone, as well as hydrocortisone, might account for differences in their clinical effects and in their side effects.

Hormonal repercussions of long-term therapy with synthetic A.C.T.H. preparations

by W. J. Irvine, K. S. Wilson, and A. D. Toft *

In recent years the structure of human A.C.T.H. has been established as consisting of 39 amino acids, the biological activity of which is confined to the first 24. Most, but not all, of the immunological activity is dependent on the amino acid sequence 25–39, and species variability occurs within the sequence 25–33. The biologically active sequence 1–24 (tetracosactrin**) was synthesised in 1961, and one potential advantage of such a preparation should be a reduction in hypersensitivity reactions as compared with their incidence in response to porcine preparations of A.C.T.H., e.g. A.C.T.H. gel. Although hypersensitivity reactions to tetracosactrin have been described, their incidence —in terms of doses administered—is estimated to be as low as 1:30,000 (Binns[1]; de Lange and Doorenbos[21]).

Tetracosactrin has a short duration of action amounting to 4–5 hours, with a peak at two hours. While it is of some value in establishing a diagnosis of primary adrenal insufficiency, this preparation has no place in therapy. The limitations imposed by the very brief duration of action of tetracosactrin have been overcome by developing a preparation, known as depot tetracosactrin (®Synacthen Depot), in which the active substance forms a complex with zinc phosphate, as a result of which its absorption is prolonged. When this preparation is given intramuscularly or subcutaneously in a dose of 0.5–1.0 mg., its duration of action is approximately 48 hours, with high levels persisting between the 8th and 24th hour after injection. This time course is somewhat longer than that of A.C.T.H. gel.

Surprisingly enough, the 1–18 fragment of the molecule—substituted at positions 1, 17, and 18 as shown in Figure 1—has a duration of action much longer

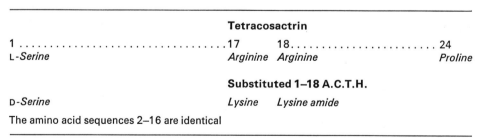

Tetracosactrin

1 17   18. 24
L-*Serine*   *Arginine Arginine*   *Proline*

Substituted 1–18 A.C.T.H.

D-*Serine*   *Lysine   Lysine amide*

The amino acid sequences 2–16 are identical

Fig. 1. Comparison between the amino acid sequences of 1–24 A.C.T.H. (tetracosactrin) and substituted 1–18 A.C.T.H.

*Department of Endocrinology, Royal Infirmary, Edinburgh, Scotland.
**Tetracosactrin = tetracosactide = ®Synacthen.

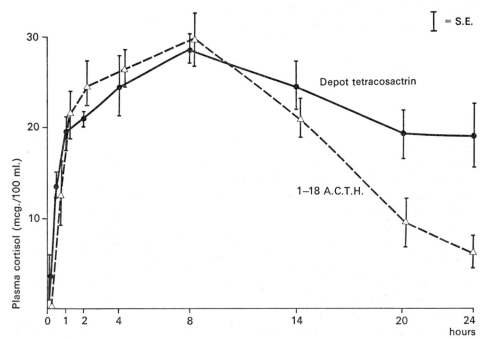

Fig. 2. Plasma cortisol response to an intramuscular injection of 1 mg. depot tetracosac-trin and of 1 mg. substituted 1–18 A.C.T.H., compared in the same five normal male subjects whose plasma cortisol levels had been depressed by pre-treatment with dexamethasone. The plasma cortisol concentrations were estimated by competitive protein binding. Substituted 1–18 A.C.T.H. has a shorter duration of action than depot tetracosactrin. (Data from: IRVINE et al.[12])

than tetracosactrin but shorter than depot tetracosactrin (Figure 2). The dura-tion of action and height of the plasma cortisol peak induced are influenced by the dose and route of administration (Figure 3). In general, if an A.C.T.H. preparation induces high plasma cortisol levels, the total time during which the plasma cortisol remains raised also tends to be prolonged. However, it would appear that, by appropriately selecting the type of synthetic A.C.T.H., its dose, and its route of administration, it may be possible to obtain any desired duration of action from five to 48 hours.

Suppression of the hypothalamo-pituitary-adrenocortical (H.P.A.) axis

One well-recognised complication of prolonged oral steroid therapy is the risk that function of the H.P.A. axis may become suppressed and the probability that such suppression will be prolonged (particularly at the hypothalamo-

Fig. 4. *Above:* Plasma cortisol response over a period of one week, during which two injections of 0.5 mg. depot tetracosactrin are given intramuscularly.
Below: A theoretical alternative and possibly preferable regime in which daily in-jections of a short-acting preparation would enable the early-morning endogenous secretion of A.C.T.H. to occur and hence preserve function of the H.P.A. axis.

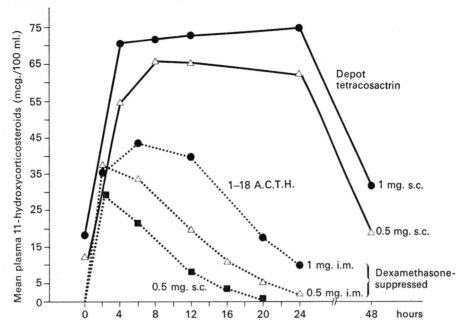

Fig. 3. These curves illustrate that the height and duration of the plasma cortisol response depend upon the type of A.C.T.H. preparation employed, as well as on the dose and route of administration. (Data from: KEENAN et al.[19] and TREADWELL and DENNIS[35])

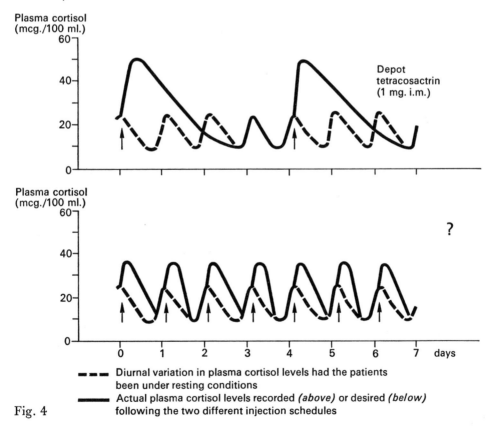

- - - Diurnal variation in plasma cortisol levels had the patients
been under resting conditions

─── Actual plasma cortisol levels recorded *(above)* or desired *(below)*
following the two different injection schedules

Fig. 4

49

pituitary level) if the dosage of oral steroids has been greater than 7.5 mg. prednisone per day (LIVANOU et al.[25]). In certain disease states, in which it is not anticipated that life-long steroid therapy will prove necessary (e.g. certain skin diseases, certain forms of glomerulonephritis, asthma, etc.), the normal practice is to give steroids over periods of clinical relapse and to withdraw or greatly reduce them during periods of natural remission. For the purpose of maintenance therapy in these situations, it would be advantageous to have a preparation that induced elevated plasma cortisol levels of moderate height for a substantial part of each week, but which did not lead to prolonged suppression of the H.P.A. axis.

In this connection it is important to consider how the problem of treatment should be approached: should one use an A.C.T.H. preparation that acts for 48 hours and give it perhaps 2–3 times per week, or should one aim at daily treatment with a shorter-acting A.C.T.H. preparation (Figure 4)?

At present, the data available on the long-term therapeutic use of A.C.T.H. gel or depot tetracosactrin are very limited, and no data exist at all on long-term treatment with the substituted 1–18 polypeptide. MALONE et al.[26] have shown that intermittent oral steroids, given for three consecutive days per week over periods of more than five years, produce the same degree of H.P.A. depression—assessed by the insulin tolerance test—as does daily steroid medication. On the other hand, DALY and GLASS[6] have reported that, in ten patients who had been receiving porcine A.C.T.H. gel for 2–17 years, the plasma cortisol still showed a satisfactory response in the insulin tolerance test, although the levels it attained were lower than in a control group of patients. Our own experience with nine patients who received 0.5 mg. depot tetracosactrin i.m. twice weekly for a period varying between six months and 2½ years indicated that little or no suppression of the H.P.A. axis occurs, particularly if the patient has never previously been treated with oral steroids (Table 1 and Figure 5). Whether this absence of suppression would be maintained if the treatment were continued for longer periods of time, or given in a higher dosage or more frequently, cannot be stated. These preliminary findings are at all events encouraging. It has yet to be explained, however, why intermittent oral

Table 1. Effect of long-term treatment with depot tetracosactrin on the hypothalamo-pituitary-adrenocortical axis.

Number of patients		Duration of therapy	Effects
No previous steroid therapy	3	1½–2½ years	No suppression of H.P.A. axis
Previous steroid therapy	6	6–18 months	Three normal and three marginally subnormal insulin tests
		Dose and frequency	
		0.5 mg. i.m. twice weekly	

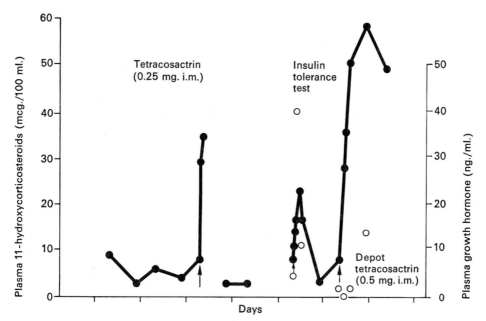

Fig. 5. A study of H.P.A. function in a 30-year-old woman treated with depot tetracosactrin (0.5 mg. i.m. twice weekly for two years) for polymyositis. The diurnal variation of plasma cortisol (●———●) was maintained although the levels were low. The response of the adrenals to 0.25 mg. tetracosactrin i.m. was good. Insulin-induced hypoglycaemia produced a normal rise both in plasma cortisol and in growth hormone (○), indicating normal hypothalamo-pituitary function. The plasma cortisol response to the next therapeutic dose of 0.5 mg. depot tetracosactrin i.m. was good, but no early response in the plasma growth hormone levels was noted. The plasma cortisol levels were estimated by the Mattingly method[27].

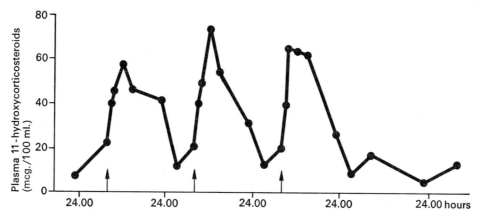

Fig. 6. Plasma cortisol levels estimated by the Mattingly technique in a 24-year-old female subject in response to three daily injections of 0.25 mg. substituted 1–18 A.C.T.H., administered subcutaneously at 08.00 hours. Satisfactory peaks in the plasma cortisol levels were obtained, but the cortisol levels had fallen by 03.00 hours on the following morning, thus permitting endogenous secretion of A.C.T.H. to occur; this endogenous secretion resulted in a rise in the plasma cortisol between 03.00 and 08.00 hours on each of the days following the injection. (From: IRVINE et al.[13])

steroids should produce suppression of the H.P.A. axis, whereas injections of depot tetracosactrin or A.C.T.H. gel apparently do not.

Shown in Figure 6 are the plasma cortisol levels recorded in a young female subject following three daily injections of 0.25 mg. 1–18 A.C.T.H. subcutaneously. Good peaks in the plasma cortisol levels were obtained with a duration of action of some 18 hours, so that the 03.00 hour samples were low and an endogenous rise in plasma cortisol occurred between 03.00 and 08.00 hours, when the next injection was given. There was no cumulative effect with the three successive daily injections, and such a regime should not entail any risk of suppression of the H.P.A. axis.

Effect of treatment with steroids and A.C.T.H. on growth

Another well-known complication of prolonged oral steroid therapy is its inhibitory effect on growth in children (BLODGETT et al.[2]), the cause of which has not yet been fully elucidated. Both HARTOG et al.[11] and FRANTZ and RABKIN[9] have reported that in adults receiving corticosteroids the resting plasma growth hormone level is normal, although the response to hypoglycaemia is diminished. In children who had discontinued long-term steroid therapy at least 12 hours before the performance of an insulin test, MORRIS et al.[28] found essentially normal growth hormone responses. When growth hormone measurements in relation to insulin-induced hypoglycaemia were made in five of our adult patients, treated for periods of six months to 2 ½ years with depot tetracosactrin, all proved to be normal. MORROW et al.[29] have published observations on three juvenile patients with adrenal hyperplasia in whom growth had ceased although they exhibited normal growth hormone responses to insulin hypoglycaemia—a finding which would seem to indicate that the impaired growth is the result of steroid-induced antagonism to growth hormone at tissue level. STRAUCH et al.[34] studied growth hormone releasing mechanisms in adrenal hypercorticism and found that, in patients who did not show a growth hormone response to hypoglycaemia, arginine provoked growth hormone release in six out of nine cases; they suggest that, in the presence of adrenal hypercorticism, a partial growth hormone deficiency is due to inhibition of the secretion of hypothalamic growth hormone releasing factor and that pituitary growth hormone secretion is potentially normal. However, it must be remembered that observations on the release of growth hormone following insulin hypoglycaemia may not reflect its release under physiological conditions.

Plasma growth hormone levels vary considerably in normal subjects according to age, sex, activity, stress, and metabolic factors. The actions of growth hormone, and the control of its secretion, have been reviewed by CATT[4]. After the newborn period, when growth hormone levels are extremely high, the basal level drops to 1–5 ng./ml. in normal subjects, though showing intermittent peaks of secretion which may raise the plasma levels to 25 ng./ml. or more. These spikes of secretion occur most often after activity, during deep sleep (especially in children), and several hours after meals. Such peaks are commoner in women, occurring most frequently in mid-cycle and during oestrogen administration. The greater secretory capacity of the female is accompanied by an increased responsiveness to certain stimuli such as exercise and arginine infusion. Growth hormone secretion during sleep, which has been studied by EASTMAN et al.[7], has been found to show neuro-endocrine rhythmicity, being specifically related to entry into slow-wave sleep (Stages III and IV). Unlike other physiological peaks of its secretion, the sleep-induced increase in growth hormone secretion is not suppressible by hyperglycaemia. Peak plasma growth hormone levels during sleep are not significantly different from levels attained during insulin hypoglycaemia. In a group of ten asthmatic children with steroid-induced growth retardation, two exhibited no increase in plasma growth hormone levels during sleep, three showed subnormal responses, and five had responses within the normal range. Subnormal sleep responses correlated with subnormal responses to arginine and to insulin hypoglycaemia (EASTMAN et al.[7]). In a study of six healthy male subjects, EVANS et al.[8] observed that an intramuscular injection of 1.0 mg. depot 1–24 A.C.T.H. in the morning eliminated the peak of growth hormone release which normally occurs during early slow-wave sleep.

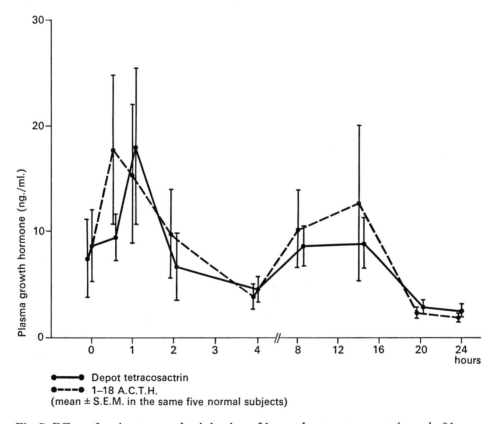

Fig. 7. Effect of an intramuscular injection of 1 mg. depot tetracosactrin and of 1 mg. substituted 1–18 A.C.T.H. on the plasma levels of growth hormone in the same five dexamethasone-suppressed control male subjects as shown in Figure 2.

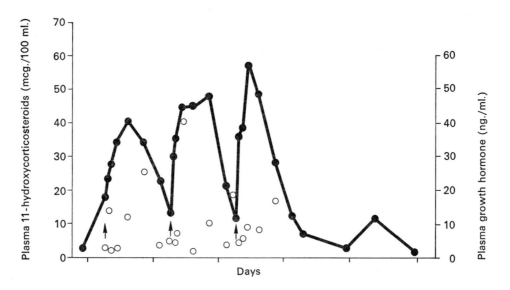

Fig. 8. Plasma cortisol (●——●) and growth hormone (○) responses to three sub-cutaneous injections of 0.5 mg. 1–18 A.C.T.H. in a 24-year-old female subject. A rise in plasma growth hormone was noted within two hours after the first two injections, but starting from a high pre-injection level the plasma growth hormone fell following the third injection.

Although the growth retardation produced by corticosteroids in children is often only temporary, inasmuch as growth recommences when the steroids are withdrawn, in some instances—especially following prolonged steroid therapy—the child's growth may remain permanently stunted (BLODGETT et al.[2]). This effect assumes even greater importance when it is borne in mind that most of the childhood diseases for which steroids are given tend to run a self-limiting course. In a study on the comparative effects exerted by prednisone alone, prednisone plus corticotrophin gel, and corticotrophin gel alone on growth in asthmatic children, FRIEDMAN and STRANG[10] demonstrated that the growth rates in the corticotrophin-treated groups were significantly higher than in the group treated with prednisone alone.

The acute effects of intravenous tetracosactrin on plasma growth hormone levels in normal subjects have been reported by ZAHND et al.[38], who claim to have observed a rise which reached its maximum after periods ranging from 15 to 90 minutes. The findings we obtained with intramuscular injections of 1 mg. depot 1–24 A.C.T.H. and 1 mg. 1–18 A.C.T.H. in five normal male subjects are shown in Figure 7. Although the mean growth hormone levels rose in response to both preparations within one hour, the levels were so variable in different subjects that the changes in the means are not statistically significant. This variability is illustrated in Figure 8, showing the plasma cortisol levels following three daily subcutaneous injections of 0.5 mg. 1–18 A.C.T.H. The open circles represent the values for growth hormone, which are elevated after the first two injections, but lowered from a high pre-injection level after the third injection.

Besides its influence on the integrity of the H.P.A. axis and on growth hormone secretion, other long-term effects of A.C.T.H. therapy have been studied, particularly with regard to their frequency of occurrence as compared with the long-term effects of corticosteroid therapy (Table 2).

Under treatment with corticotrophin, dyspepsia has proved to be less common, and frank peptic ulceration much less frequent. Skin bruising is also far less often observed than with corticosteroids. TREADWELL et al.[36] graded the side effects of steroids and corticotrophins into three categories: mild, moderate, and severe. They report that, both in patients receiving steroids and in those treated with corticotrophin, side effects were just as likely to occur in the young as in the old, but that they arose more often in women than in men at all ages. These authors also found that skin bruising, facial mooning, and dyspepsia were the commonest side effects in the corticosteroid-treated group, and amenorrhoea and acne in the corticotrophin group. Overall, they observed that severe side effects were commoner in patients on corticosteroids, whereas mild or moderately severe side effects were commoner in patients on corticotrophin. Moreover, hypertension, acne, and pigmentation, which are characteristic side effects of A.C.T.H., are overt ones—in contrast to the occult complications of peptic ulceration and osteoporosis seen mainly with oral steroids.

Skin pigmentation has proved to be relatively common with long-term corticotrophin therapy. Two melanocyte-stimulating hormones have been isolated from the pituitary: alpha-M.S.H., containing 13 amino acids, and beta-M.S.H. containing 22 amino acids. Alpha-M.S.H. has a 13 amino acid sequence, and beta-M.S.H. a 7 amino acid sequence, in common with A.C.T.H. (Figure 9). Although alpha-M.S.H. is the more potent of the two in producing melanin pigmentation, beta-M.S.H. appears to be the principal pigmentary hormone in man (LERNER and McGUIRE[23]). A.C.T.H. has intrinsic melanotrophic activity—albeit much less than that of beta-M.S.H.—and it is this which accounts for the diffuse increase in pigmentation that may develop in patients receiving long-term treatment with corticotrophin or depot tetracosactrin above a certain dosage level. Since this effect is dose-dependent, it may be

Table 2. Complications observed in 108 patients treated with oral steroids and 105 treated with A.C.T.H. gel. (From: SAVAGE et al.[33])

	Oral steroids	Corticotrophin
	%	%
Moon face	55	50
Weight increase	27	28
Dyspepsia	54	25
Peptic ulceration	11	2
Bruising	25	4
Hypertension	17	27
Acne	8	29
Pigmentation	4	19

	β-M.S.H.		
1 10	11	17	18. 22
	A.C.T.H.		
1 3	4	10	11. 39

Common peptide sequence

Fig. 9. Comparison between the molecular structure of human A.C.T.H. and beta-M.S.H., illustrating that they have a common 7 amino acid sequence.

advantageous to use small doses of A.C.T.H. repeatedly rather than large doses less frequently.

Hypertension has been found to occur more commonly after long-term cortico-trophin therapy than after treatment with corticosteroids. It is tempting to think that this finding may possibly be related to an increase in aldosterone secretion in response to corticotrophin therapy. It has been shown that patients with impaired pituitary function (LIDDLE et al.[24]) and hypophysectomised animals (LEE et al.[22]) respond less readily than normal subjects to sodium depletion or haemorrhage, which usually induce a marked increase in aldo-sterone secretion. From this it could be inferred that a pituitary hormone—probably A.C.T.H.—is needed for a normal response to these stimuli. However, the relative importance of the role played by A.C.T.H. in the physiological stimulation of aldosterone secretion is uncertain. While pharmacological doses of A.C.T.H. cause an increase in aldosterone production, at physiological dose levels the response in normal subjects is at best small and short-lived (JAMES et al.[16]). In normal subjects the endogenous release of A.C.T.H. that occurs under the stimulus of hypoglycaemia does not affect the plasma con-centration of aldosterone (JAMES et al.[17]). Studies in subjects with pathologically increased A.C.T.H. secretion, e.g. in Cushing's syndrome due to ectopic hyper-secretion of A.C.T.H., have revealed that in these patients plasma aldosterone levels are not increased (LANDON et al.[20]; BROWN et al.[3]). An infusion of as little as 1.4 mU. 1–24 A.C.T.H. per minute (which approaches physiological levels) has been shown to increase the aldosterone secretion rate in normal subjects on a low sodium diet (RAYFIELD et al.[31]). The acute effects of depot tetracosactrin and of substituted 1–18 A.C.T.H. on aldosterone levels in the plasma are outlined in Figure 10. In tissue culture experiments with foetal rat adrenals, KAHRI[18] found that prolonged stimulation with A.C.T.H. caused some glomerulosa cells to become differentiated into fasciculata-reticularis cells. Whether the differentiation is accompanied by a change in function is not known, but this observation possibly offers an explanation for the reduction in aldo-sterone secretion which has been stated to occur after chronic A.C.T.H. ad-ministration (MULROW[30]) and which we have recently demonstrated. The secretion of desoxycorticosterone, on the other hand, appears to be increased following continued therapy with A.C.T.H. (Figure 11)[14].

Corticotrophin has been shown to cause an increase in plasma testosterone in normal women and a decrease in plasma testosterone in normal men (RIVA-

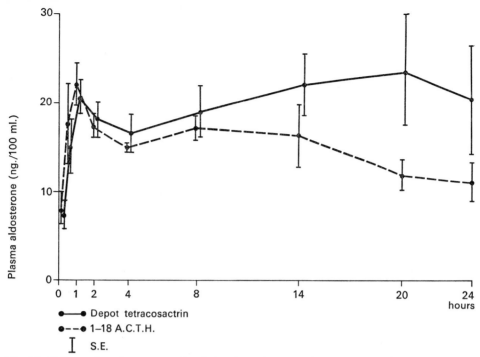

Fig. 10. Effect of an intramuscular injection of 1 mg. depot 1–24 A.C.T.H. and of 1 mg. substituted 1–18 A.C.T.H. on plasma aldosterone levels in the same five normal male subjects as in Figures 2 and 7. Note that an early peak is followed by a more sustained rise and that the overall response is greater with the longer-acting 1–24 A.C.T.H. depot preparation. (Data from: IRVINE et al.[12])

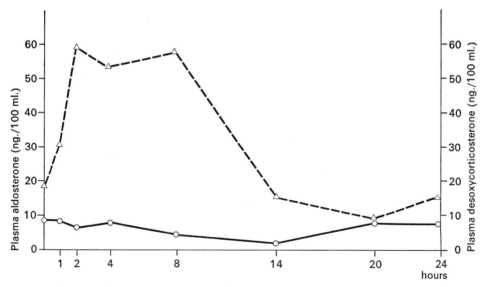

Fig. 11. Plasma aldosterone (○———○) and desoxycorticosterone (△－－－△) levels following intramuscular administration of 1 mg. substituted 1–18 A.C.T.H. in a patient treated with 0.5 mg. depot tetracosactrin i.m. twice weekly for two years. Note the marked rise in the desoxycorticosterone concentration and the absence of a rise in the aldosterone levels. (From: IRVINE et al.[14])

ROLA et al.[32]). In men, however, the urinary 17-ketosteroids are elevated following administration of corticotrophin (CLEVELAND et al.[5]). IRVINE et al.[14,15] have shown that in normal male dexamethasone-suppressed subjects A.C.T.H. causes an increase in plasma androstenedione and a decrease in plasma testosterone, but does not alter plasma luteinising hormone. It would seem that either A.C.T.H. or possibly dexamethasone may inhibit the secretion of testosterone. The weaker adrenal androgens may be metabolised to testosterone in the skin. The increased output of adrenal androgens following stimulation by corticotrophin is reflected in an increased incidence of acne and amenorrhoea, but it may also help in preventing cortisol from exerting a catabolic action. The reported incidence of myopathy, osteoporosis, bruising, skin atrophy, and delayed wound healing is considerably less in corticotrophin-treated patients than in those receiving corticosteroids (WEST[37]; TREADWELL et al.[36]).

Conclusions

In conclusion, depot tetracosactrin—and possibly substituted 1–18 A.C.T.H.—has the advantage over A.C.T.H. gel that it is less likely to cause hypersensitivity reactions and that it can be standardised by weight. There is evidence that depot tetracosactrin may produce less suppression of the hypothalamo-pituitary-adrenocortical axis than oral steroids given continuously or intermittently. Compared with oral steroids, treatment with depot tetracosactrin is less liable to provoke catabolic side effects or to cause dyspepsia. On the other hand, it is more likely to produce hypertension, acne, amenorrhoea, and skin pigmentation.

What we should perhaps aim for is a synthetic A.C.T.H. preparation with an action lasting some 15–18 hours. It is to be hoped that such a preparation would provide an increase in cortisol production of therapeutic value and that at the same time it could be given by daily subcutaneous injection without suppressing endogenous A.C.T.H. secretion early the following morning or inhibiting the release of growth hormone during sleep. A dosage schedule in which such a preparation is administered in small repeated doses could be expected to avoid skin pigmentation, while its influence on the secretion of weak adrenal androgens might counteract the catabolic effect of increased levels of corticosteroids. Doses of 0.25 mg. 1–18 A.C.T.H., given subcutaneously, seem to approximate closely to this type of therapy.

References

1 BINNS, T. B.: Allergy to Synacthen Depot. Lancet *ii*, 1081 (1969); corresp.
2 BLODGETT, F. M., BURGIN, L., IEZZONI, D., GRIBETZ, D., TALBOT, N. B.: Effect of prolonged cortisone therapy on the statural growth, skeletal maturation and metabolic status of children. New Engl. J. Med. *254*, 636 (1956)
3 BROWN, J. J., FRASER, R., LEVER, A. F., ROBERTSON, J. I. S.: Aldosterone: physiological and pathophysiological variations in man. Clin. Endocr. Metab. *1*, 397 (1972)

4   CATT, K. J.: Growth hormone. Lancet i, 933 (1970)

5   CLEVELAND, W. W., AHMAD, N., SANDBERG, D. H., SAVARD, K.: Excretion of testosterone and 17-ketosteroids following administration of HCG and ACTH to normal adult males. Steroids 8, 149 (1966)

6   DALY, J. R., GLASS, D.: Corticosteroid and growth-hormone response to hypoglycaemia in patients on long-term treatment with corticotrophin. Lancet i, 476 (1971)

7   EASTMAN, C. J., MITCHELL, R. P., LAZARUS, L.: Growth hormone secretion during sleep. Proc. endocr. Soc. Aust., Abstr. No. 36 (1971)

8   EVANS, J. I., GLASS, D., DALY, J. R., McLEAN, A. W.: The effect of Zn-tetracosactrin on growth hormone release during sleep. J. clin. Endocr. 36, 36 (1973)

9   FRANTZ, A. G., RABKIN, M. T.: Human growth hormone. Clinical measurement, response to hypoglycemia and suppression by corticosteroids. New Engl. J. Med. 271, 1375 (1964)

10 FRIEDMAN, M., STRANG, L. B.: Effect of long-term corticosteroids and corticotrophin on the growth of children. Lancet ii, 568 (1966)

11 HARTOG, M., GAAFAR, M. A., FRASER, R.: Effect of corticosteroids on serum growth hormone. Lancet ii, 376 (1964)

12 IRVINE, W. J., FRASER, R., TOFT, A. D., WILSON, A., WILSON, K. S., YOUNG, J.: A comparison of the effects of 1–24 ACTH Zn and of substituted 1–18 ACTH on adrenal cortical function in normal subjects. J. Endocr. (printing)

13 IRVINE, W. J., WILSON, K. S., TOFT, A. D.: Adrenocortical stimulation by substituted α1–18 corticotrophin. Lancet i, 1417 (1973)

14 IRVINE, W. J., TOFT, A. D., WILSON, K. S., FRASER, R., WILSON, A., YOUNG, J., HUNTER, W. M., ISMAIL, A. A. A., BAIRD, D. T., BURGER, P. E.: The effect of synthetic corticotrophin analogues on adrenocortical, anterior pituitary and testicular function. (In preparation)

15 IRVINE, W. J., TOFT, A. D., WILSON, K. S., HUNTER, W. M., ISMAIL, A. A. A., BURGER, P. E., BAIRD, D. T.: The effect of synthetic corticotrophin analogues on plasma Δ^4-androstenedione, testosterone and gonadotrophins in normal males. J. Endocr. (printing)

16 JAMES, V. H. T., FRASER, R., LANDON, J.: Plasma steroid assays in the investigation of endocrine function. In Martini, L., Fraschini, F., Motta, M. (Editors): Proc. IInd Int. Congr. horm. Steroids, Milan 1966. Int. Congr. Ser. No. 132, p. 383 (Excerpta med. Found., Amsterdam etc. 1967)

17 JAMES, V. H. T., LANDON, J., FRASER, R.: Some observations on the control of corticosteroid secretion in man. In James, V. H. T., Landon, J. (Editors): The investigation of hypothalamic-pituitary-adrenal function, Proc. Symp., London 1967. Mem. Soc. Endocr. No. 17, p. 141 (Univ. Press, Cambridge 1968)

18 KAHRI, A.: Histochemical and electron microscopic studies on the cells of the rat adrenal cortex in tissue culture. Acta endocr. (Kbh.) 52, Suppl. 108 (1966)

19 KEENAN, J., THOMPSON, J. B., CHAMBERLAIN, M. A., BESSER, G. M.: Prolonged corticotrophic action of a synthetic substituted 1-18ACTH. Brit. med. J. iii, 742 (1971)

20 LANDON, J., JAMES, V. H. T., PEART, W. M.: Cushing's syndrome associated with a "corticotrophin"-producing bronchial neoplasm. Acta endocr. (Kbh.) 56, 321 (1967)

21 LANGE, W. E. DE, DOORENBOS, H.: Corticotrophins and corticosteroids. In Meyler, L., Herxheimer, A. (Editors): Side effects of drugs, Vol. VII, p. 516 (Excerpta med., Amsterdam 1972)

22 LEE, T. C., WAL, B. VAN DER, WIED, D. DE: Influence of the anterior pituitary on the aldosterone secretory response to dietary sodium restriction in the rat. J. Endocr. 42, 465 (1968)

23 LERNER, A. B., McGUIRE, J. S.: Melanocyte-stimulating hormone and adreno-

corticotrophic hormone: their relation to pigmentation. New Engl. J. Med. *270*, 539 (1964)

24 Liddle, G. W., Duncan, L. E., Jr., Bartter, F. C.: Dual mechanism regulating adrenocortical function in man. Amer. J. Med. *21*, 380 (1956)

25 Livanou, T., Ferriman, D., James, V. H. T.: Recovery of hypothalamo-pituitary-adrenal function after corticosteroid therapy. Lancet *ii*, 856 (1967)

26 Malone, D. N. S., Grant, I. W. B., Percy-Robb, I. W.: Hypothalamo-pituitary-adrenal function in asthmatic patients receiving long-term corticosteroid therapy. Lancet *ii*, 733 (1970)

27 Mattingly, D.: A simple fluorimetric method for the estimation of free 11-hydroxycorticoids in human plasma. J. clin. Path. *15*, 374 (1962)

28 Morris, H. G., Jorgensen, J. R., Jenkins, S. A.: Plasma growth hormone concentration in corticosteroid-treated children. J. clin. Invest. *47*, 427 (1968)

29 Morrow, L. B., Mellinger, R. C., Prendergast, J. J., Guansing, A. R.: Growth hormone in hypersecretory diseases of the adrenal gland. J. clin. Endocr. *29*, 1364 (1969)

30 Mulrow, P. J.: The adrenal cortex. Ann. Rev. Physiol. *34*, 409 (1972)

31 Rayfield, E. J., Rose, L. I., Dluhy, R. G., Williams, G. H.: Aldosterone secretory and glucocorticoid excretory responses to alpha 1–24 ACTH (Cortrosyn) in sodium-depleted normal man. J. clin. Endocr. *36*, 30 (1973)

32 Rivarola, M. A., Saez, J. M., Meyer, W. J., Jenkins, M. E., Migeon, C. J.: Metabolic clearance rate and blood production rate of testosterone and androst-4-ene-3,17-dione under basal conditions, ACTH and HCG stimulation. Comparison with urinary production rate of testosterone. J. clin. Endocr. *26*, 1208 (1966)

33 Savage, O., Copeman, W. S. C., Chapman, L., Wells, M. V., Treadwell, B. L. J.: Pituitary and adrenal hormones in rheumatoid arthritis. Lancet *i*, 232 (1962)

34 Strauch, G., Modigliani, E., Luton, J.-P., Bricaire, H.: Partial somatotrophin insufficiency in Cushing's syndrome. Acta endocr. (Kbh.) *60*, 121 (1969)

35 Treadwell, B. L. J., Dennis, P. M.: Comparison of depot tetracosactrin and corticotrophin gel. Brit. med. J. *iv*, 720 (1969)

36 Treadwell, B. L. J., Sever, E. D., Savage, O., Copeman, W. S. C.: Side-effects of long-term treatment with corticosteroids and corticotrophin. Lancet *i*, 1121 (1964)

37 West, H. F.: Ten years of ACTH therapy. Ann. rheum. Dis. *21*, 263 (1962)

38 Zahnd, G. R., Nadeau, A., Mühlendahl, K.-E. van: Effect of corticotrophin on plasma levels of human growth hormone. Lancet *ii*, 1278 (1969)

Discussion

K. F. WEINGES: In Table 2 of your paper, Dr. IRVINE, in which you list complications observed in patients treated with oral steroids or with A.C.T.H. gel, no reference is made to osteoporosis or to disturbances of carbohydrate metabolism. Have you any information on the comparative incidence of these two types of side effect?

W. J. IRVINE: My Table 2, which was taken from a paper by SAVAGE et al., does not include osteoporosis, because these authors were doubtful about the incidence of this complication. But other investigators, including WEST, as well as TREADWELL et al., concluded on the basis of their clinical studies that osteoporosis is distinctly less frequent with A.C.T.H. therapy than with oral steroids. I'm afraid I can't give you much information on carbohydrate metabolism. I presume the point that interests you here is how many patients treated with A.C.T.H. or oral steroids show abnormal responses in glucose tolerance tests. This is a question that I can't answer.

H. J. BAUER: I'd like to add to the question that Dr. WEINGES has just asked. In your Table 2, Dr. IRVINE, you also made no reference to euphoria, which in many cases facilitates treatment, although it makes it more difficult to evaluate the objective response. Once in a while we even see psychotic episodes, and I think that this is another complication which should have been included in the list.
In a series of patients on whom I shall be giving a brief report later, we had one fatality due to a fulminating pulmonary embolism; but we don't know whether this was just a chance occurrence or whether it was perhaps attributable to an increased tendency to thrombosis.
A third problem is that of dizziness setting in immediately after the administration of A.C.T.H. Although this is a side effect which we only encounter occasionally and which as a rule is not a very disturbing one, it may in exceptional cases necessitate the interruption of treatment—as it did in one patient whom I was treating myself. In a recent paper on 1–18 A.C.T.H., RETIENE and SCHULZ * also mention dizziness as a side effect. May I therefore ask if you could comment on this, Dr. IRVINE, on the basis of your experience.
Finally, you stated in your paper that with the 1–18 polypeptide you observed a very much stronger stimulant effect on cortisol production than in response to tetracosactrin. I presume that this difference was to some extent dose-dependent, but I'd be grateful for any comments you might care to offer.

W. J. IRVINE: First of all, I should perhaps emphasise that I haven't tried to cover all the possible complications of treatment with oral steroids and A.C.T.H. I simply picked out certain of the complications and attempted to analyse them biochemically with a view to predicting their occurrence. Moreover, by studying the time course of the biochemical and hormonal changes induced, one may be able to select a dose regime which will minimise the incidence of complications. The side effects of these two forms of treatment are very largely dose-dependent, and one must also bear in mind the fact that, whereas you can achieve steroid blood levels as high as you like by giving oral steroids in appropriately large doses, you cannot increase the plasma cortisol concentration beyond a certain limit by administering A.C.T.H., but you may on the other hand increase the undesirable effects.
I wouldn't know whether the psychological side effects of A.C.T.H. are any better or any worse than those of oral steroids.
With regard to the complication of dizziness which you mentioned, Dr. BAUER, what we have tended to see in subjects receiving 1–18 A.C.T.H. is not so much dizziness,

---

* RETIENE, K., SCHULZ, F.: Human pharmacological studies with a new synthetic corticotrophic peptide consisting of 18 amino acids. XIX. Symp. Dtsch. Ges. Endokr., Berlin 1973, Abstr., Acta endocr. (Kbh.) 72, Suppl. 173: 33 (1973)

but flushing. We have wondered whether this flushing might not possibly be due to an effect of the A.C.T.H. on histamine release and, if so, whether it could perhaps be counteracted by giving an antihistamine. It has been suggested in the literature that substances having a structure such as substituted 1–18 A.C.T.H. might in fact increase the histamine levels—not via a direct allergic mechanism, but simply because they exert an effect on histamine as such. I'm sorry, but I have no information on thrombosis as a possible complication. I can't see any particular reason why A.C.T.H. should induce thrombosis, but if it does, then this could be a problem which ought to be looked into.

In reply to your last point, the 1–18 polypeptide has a much longer effect on the plasma cortisol level than does tetracosactrin when both preparations are given in the same dosage by the same route: for example, 24 hours for 1–18, as compared with five hours for tetracosactrin when each is given in a dose of 0.5 mg.

G. GEYER: You mentioned, Dr. IRVINE, that treatment with A.C.T.H. stimulates the production of adrenal androgens, which in turn might influence the nitrogen balance and thus exert an anabolic effect. Was this merely an hypothesis, or do you actually have some data on the nitrogen balance to indicate that it is a fact?

W.J.IRVINE: It has been reported in the literature[*] that a rise occurs in the ketosteroids in response to A.C.T.H. therapy, but this of course is only indirect evidence. We have recently been measuring androstenedione secretion from the adrenal cortex following treatment with A.C.T.H., and, as I pointed out in my paper, we did in fact find an increase in plasma androstenedione levels in response to the administra- of A.C.T.H.

G. GEYER: Be that as it may, we mustn't forget that most of these adrenal androgens display only very weak anabolic activity!

W.J.IRVINE: Yes, but it's the total quantity of them that matters. You can compensate quite a lot for a weak androgen if you've got enough of it, whereas testosterone—a very potent androgen—will produce an anabolic effect if present only in very low concentrations. Some of these so-called weak androgens are admittedly weak on a weight-for-weight basis; on the other hand, the total quantity of weak androgens may be such that they give rise to quite a strong anabolic effect.

H.JESSERER: The question has been raised as to whether osteoporosis occurs less often in patients treated with A.C.T.H. than in those receiving corticosteroids, and Dr. IRVINE has quoted reports to the effect that its occurrence is a good deal less frequent. In my opinion this is a widespread misconception. You don't observe osteoporosis in a patient until he has been under continuous corticosteroid medication for at least two years. But cases treated uninterruptedly with A.C.T.H. for two years or more are seldom encountered; in such cases as do exist, the risk of osteoporosis is just the same.

W.J.IRVINE: While largely agreeing with what you have just said, Dr. JESSERER, I would point out that it is very difficult to make any dogmatic statements about the incidence of osteoporosis under A.C.T.H. therapy as compared with oral steroid treatment. To make meaningful comparisons you need to treat two matched groups for the same duration of time and with the same equivalent dosage, and here the snag is that it is by no means easy to decide what are equivalent oral steroid dosages for a given regime of A.C.T.H. therapy. What we are hoping to do is to obtain some precise and detailed knowledge as to the biochemical repercussions of treatment with A.C.T.H. If we can demonstrate that A.C.T.H. does indeed exert a significant

---

[*] CLEVELAND, W.W., AHMAD, N., SANDBERG, D.H., SAVARD, K.: Excretion of testosterone and 17-ketosteroids following administration of HCG and ACTH to normal adult males. Steroids *8*, 149 (1966)

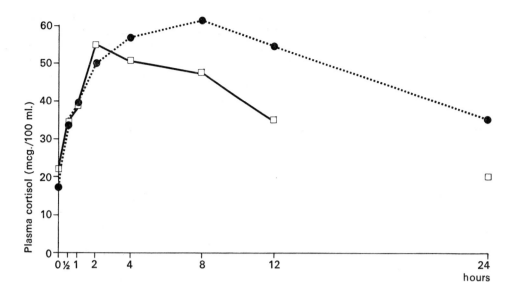

Fig. 1. Plasma cortisol levels following intramuscular injection of 0.25 mg. (●······●) and 0.125 mg. (□———□) Synacthen Depot in nine and ten subjects, respectively.

anabolic effect, this would be an encouraging finding and would provide some objective support for the clinical impression that A.C.T.H. therapy involves less risk of provoking such catabolic side effects as bruising, myopathy, and osteoporosis.

P. MASSIAS: I was particularly struck by the table in Dr. IRVINE's paper comparing the complications encountered with oral steroids and A.C.T.H., because it bears a remarkably close resemblance to a table which I myself have drawn up for an equivalent series of patients. In this connection, I should like to make two observations: firstly, these tables give no indication as to what doses of steroids or of A.C.T.H. were employed; secondly, we never know exactly what quantities of steroids we are getting out of the cortices of our patients when we give them an injection of either 0.5 or 1 mg. of synthetic A.C.T.H.

T. B. BINNS: I'd just like to show one slide which serves to illustrate that quite satisfactory plasma cortisol levels can also be obtained with small doses of A.C.T.H. (Figure 1). I was particularly interested in the data contained in this slide, because this was the first time that we had used such small doses. The square symbols represent doses of 0.125 mg. Synacthen Depot, and the circles 0.25 mg. The two groups were composed of ten and nine subjects, respectively; and the means have quite modest standard errors. You can see that after the 0.125 mg. dose of Synacthen Depot the cortisol level is coming down well at 12 hours. As it would very probably have dipped between the 12th and 24th hour, I didn't feel justified in bridging the gap between these two points by joining them up. These data, by the way, were kindly provided by Dr. HALL and Dr. GRANT at the University Department of Steroid Biochemistry in Glasgow.
Incidentally, it may amuse you to hear that, in another study of this kind performed in two other groups, one girl showed astronomically high plasma cortisol levels. It subsequently transpired that she was on "the Pill"!

J. GIRARD: In connection with the observations which Dr. IRVINE made in his paper when comparing the effects of intermittent steroid therapy and of A.C.T.H. medication on the hypothalamo-pituitary-adrenocortical axis, I should like to ask if he has any comments to offer on treatment with steroids given on alternate days. To my knowledge, such treatment has practically no adverse influence on the hypo-thalamo-pituitary-adrenocortical axis, nor does it affect growth in children with nephrotic syndrome. Admittedly, such patients are not treated over very long periods, but this alternate-day medication is nevertheless given for, say, one month and in some cases even for several months.

Another point I'd like to make is that, when employing long-acting A.C.T.H. prep-arations, it might well be that you do not simply want to raise the plasma cortisol levels but that you are also interested in achieving a biological effect—as in cases of hypoglycaemia, for instance. Consequently, I feel we should bear in mind that plasma cortisol is, after all, merely one parameter and not the only one.

W.J. IRVINE: The literature seems to be somewhat conflicting on the subject of what actually happens during intermittent treatment with oral steroids. For example, when MALONE et al.* gave asthmatics prolonged treatment with oral steroids on three consecutive days a week, they found that it caused marked suppression of hypothalamo-pituitary-adrenocortical function. In another study, however, in which JACOBSON** administered oral steroids on alternate days for a shorter period of time, he claims to have observed no suppression of the hypothalamo-pituitary-adreno-cortical axis, even though he employed much higher doses in some cases (up to 120 mg. prednisone on alternate days, as compared with the 15.5 mg. prednisolone daily on three consecutive days a week used by MALONE et al.). It is at all events certainly true, Dr. GIRARD, that alternate-day treatment with oral steroids, given over periods of several months, has been reported to cause little suppression of the hypothalamo-pituitary-adrenocortical axis. On the other hand, an oral steroid re-gime involving treatment on three consecutive days a week, which perhaps one wouldn't expect to impair the hypothalamo-pituitary-adrenocortical axis, undoubt-edly does if it is continued for a period of several years.

Regarding the use of long-acting A.C.T.H. preparations, I agree with Dr. GIRARD that the plasma cortisol level is, of course, only an indicator. In this connection I should like to repeat that we have treated nine patients for up to two and a half years with Synacthen Depot, and that with the modest dosage of 0.5 mg. twice weekly we have obtained very good therapeutic results and encountered no problems. Though we employed a higher dosage at the start in order to bring the condition under control, we were then able to lower it to the maintenance level. As I have already said, we observed good clinical responses in polymyositis, rheumatoid ar-thritis, and so on, and have so far seen no complications such as hyperglycaemia, glycosuria, or osteoporosis.

R. SCHUPPLI: I'd like to offer a comment on the question of osteoporosis in the light of my own experience. Our patients include some who have been receiving A.C.T.H. for years as treatment for pemphigus or for lepra reactions, and in none of them have we so far ever seen any bone fractures, whereas previously such fractures had occurred in some 90% of the pemphigus patients who had been undergoing corticoid therapy of equivalent therapeutic effectiveness. I think this experience indicates that, as regards the danger of osteoporosis, there really is a difference between long-term corticosteroid therapy and long-term treatment with comparable doses of A.C.T.H. Vertebral fractures in pemphigus patients undergoing treatment with corticosteroids used at one time to be a genuine problem.

---

*MALONE, D.N.S., GRANT, I.W.B., PERCY-ROBB, I.W.: Hypothalamo-pituitary-adrenal function in asthmatic patients receiving long-term corticosteroid therapy. Lancet *ii*, 733 (1970)

**JACOBSON, M.E.: The rationale of alternate-day corticosteroid therapy. Postgrad. Med. *49*, 181 (1971)

Studies on the possible suppressant effect of treatment with A.C.T.H. (depot tetracosactide) on corticotrophic function of the anterior pituitary

by G. GEYER *

From the results of studies in animals and man it can be taken as proven that treatment with corticoids may inhibit corticotrophic function of the anterior pituitary to such an extent that adrenocortical atrophy ensues and that the production and secretion of steroid hormones becomes very greatly reduced. This drug-induced dysfunction of the adrenal cortex is also known to persist for some time after corticoid therapy has been withdrawn.

When treatment is given with A.C.T.H. instead, the question likewise arises as to what effect the medication is liable to have on pituitary-adrenocortical function after the A.C.T.H. has been discontinued. It is at all events certain that the adrenal cortices themselves—far from becoming atrophied as they do following prolonged administration of corticoids—retain their function to the full and, indeed, become so hypertrophic that they are capable of producing an abundant supply of steroids in response to the stimulus of A.C.T.H. On the other hand, it would seem questionable whether, upon completion of a course of A.C.T.H. therapy, the amount of endogenous corticotrophin produced is sufficient to provide for adequate stimulation of these hypertrophic adrenal cortices—particularly since there are reasons for supposing that A.C.T.H. therapy, too, has the effect of suppressing corticotrophic function of the anterior pituitary and of keeping it suppressed afterwards over just as long a period as in response to treatment with corticoids. Such inhibition must presumably be ascribed to the influence of the abnormally high plasma cortisol concentration which is maintained during A.C.T.H. therapy and which can be expected to depress pituitary corticotrophic function to exactly the same degree as treatment with cortisone derivatives. There is also evidence from animal experiments indicating that the administration of A.C.T.H. has other selective inhibitory effects on pituitary-adrenocortical function. KITAY et al.[6], for example, have reported findings which suggest that exogenous A.C.T.H. exerts an extra-adrenal action as a result of which the anterior pituitary is prevented from releasing endogenous A.C.T.H.; and HERRMANN[4] has drawn attention to the fact that, even after only one injection of A.C.T.H., adrenocortical function undergoes a change which exhibits a phasic pattern, i.e. in which the initial stimulation is followed by prolonged inhibition lasting until rebound activation sets in ten days after the injection. HERRMANN explains this phenomenon by reference to certain active substances which he succeeded in extracting from the hypothalamus and pituitary of A.C.T.H.-treated rats and which he has shown to be capable of inhibiting adrenocortical function[5]. It

* I. Medizinische Abteilung, Kaiser-Franz-Joseph-Spital, Vienna, Austria.

has also been observed by STARK et al.[11,12] that in animals pre-treated with A.C.T.H. the reaction of the pituitary-adrenocortical system which normally occurs in response to stress can no longer be elicited; as some of these experimental findings, however, were obtained using an A.C.T.H. extract-preparation, the possibility that other biologically active substances present in the extract may have exerted an influence cannot be entirely excluded.

Since it is impossible for the clinician to assess to what extent such observations are relevant to man and to the problem of treating patients with A.C.T.H., we felt that it would be interesting to undertake a study of our own on the functional status of the corticotrophic system following A.C.T.H. therapy.

Patients, investigational procedure, and methods

The cases studied to date have comprised 12 patients of either sex and from non-selected age groups, who had received A.C.T.H. for at least five months (during which no corticoids were given) as treatment for bronchial asthma. During this period, no rigid dosage schedule was adopted; instead, the doses of A.C.T.H. were adapted to the severity of the symptoms, i.e. the patients received 1 mg. ®Synacthen Depot either every other day or twice a week. After this A.C.T.H. therapy had been withdrawn, the only further treatment administered took the form of sympathomimetic broncholytic agents and antibiotics; it was at this stage that the following programme of tests was carried out in order to determine the extent to which the corticotrophic system was still capable of responding to stimulation:

1. On the 7th, 12th, 20th, and 30th day following the last dose of A.C.T.H., an insulin test was performed and the plasma cortisol measured. For this purpose, the patients were given an intravenous injection of soluble insulin (0.15 U. per kg. body-weight) in the morning on an empty stomach, and samples of venous blood for the plasma cortisol determinations were taken before the injection as well as 30 and 60 minutes afterwards. The plasma cortisol levels were determined fluorimetrically[3]. The blood sugar concentrations were also checked, so as to ensure that the requisite degree of hypoglycaemia (approx. 40 mg.%) had been attained in the test.

2. On the 9th and 10th, 15th and 16th, and 24th and 25th day after the last injection of A.C.T.H., ®Metopirone was administered as a test procedure, the dose being equivalent to 50 mg./kg./day. The 24-hour urine was collected on the day before each test, as well as on each of the two test days, and the urinary excretion of 11-desoxycortisol and its tetrahydro metabolite measured.

Results

1. Insulin test
Only in five out of the total of 48 insulin tests performed were the fasting plasma cortisol levels found to be abnormally low (less than 8 mcg./100 ml.), and only in two of these five instances did the tests yield pathological results inasmuch as the plasma cortisol concentration failed to rise adequately following the

injection of insulin. The overall figures for the fasting plasma cortisol levels averaged 16.5 ±8 mcg./100 ml.—which is within the normal range. In ten out of the 12 patients, the increase in the plasma cortisol concentration measured 30 and/or 60 minutes after the insulin injection was assessed as normal in each of the tests, i.e. it amounted to more than 7 mcg. The mean value for the maximum plasma cortisol concentrations recorded in all these tests which yielded normal results worked out at 28.5 ±12 mcg./100 ml.

In each of two tests, two of the 12 patients showed an inadequate rise in their plasma cortisol concentrations in response to the insulin-induced hypoglycaemia. In one of these patients it was the tests performed on the 7th and 12th day which proved pathological, and in the other patient the tests carried out on the 7th and 20th day. In none of these tests yielding pathological results, however, did the hypoglycaemia itself run an abnormal course.

2. Metopirone test

In healthy subjects, the excretion of 11-desoxycortisol and its tetrahydro metabolite in the urine is normally extremely low (less than 0.5 mg./24 hours). On the first, and particularly on the second day during which Metopirone is given, a sharp rise occurs, the result of the test being assessed as normal if the excretion of these steroids reaches a level of at least 1.5 mg./24 hours.

In nine of the 12 patients studied, the excretion values proved to be abnormally low in the test carried out on the 9th and 10th day following the withdrawal of A.C.T.H.; in the remaining three cases a normal rise was observed. When the test was repeated on the 15th and 16th days, only five of the patients still showed an inadequate response, whereas in the other seven cases the rise in steroid excretion was now normal. The test performed on the 24th and 25th days yielded even better results: only two patients still exhibited an abnormally weak response to Metopirone, whereas the remaining ten showed a normal rise.

Discussion

The results obtained in this study on asthma patients who had been receiving A.C.T.H. therapy for a period of several months reveal that, when the A.C.T.H. is withdrawn, a temporary inability of the plasma cortisol levels to respond adequately to insulin-induced hypoglycaemia is encountered only in a small percentage of cases (two out of 12 patients). From this it would appear that in the great majority of such patients it is still possible, by inducing hypoglycaemia, to provoke a normal reactive secretion of corticotrophin. These observations of ours tally with findings reported by CARTER and JAMES[2] and by REISERT et al.[9]. WALSER et al.[13] also observed a normal endogenous plasma cortisol rhythm following the withdrawal of A.C.T.H. therapy—a fact which likewise suggests that a normal rhythmic secretion of corticotrophin is maintained. As illustrated, however, by the two of our patients who temporarily failed to react normally to hypoglycaemia, it is possible that in exceptional cases the mobilisation of corticotrophin may be transiently impaired following prolonged treatment with A.C.T.H.

At first sight, the findings we obtained in the Metopirone test would seem to be at variance with the results of the insulin tests, insofar as a higher proportion of the patients showed abnormal responses to Metopirone: on the 10th day after the withdrawal of A.C.T.H. therapy, 75% of our patients responded abnormally to Metopirone; almost 42% still exhibited an inadequate reaction on the 16th day; and 16% on the 25th day. These results are in line with the findings reported by BIERICH et al.[1], PLAGER and CUSHMAN[7], and REED et al.[8], but conflict with those of SAVAGE et al.[10].

As regards the seeming inconsistency between the findings we obtained in the insulin test and the results which the Metopirone test yielded in the same patients, we believe that this inconsistency is one of appearance rather than reality. Whereas the insulin test indicated that corticotrophin mobilisation in response to hypoglycaemia was normal in most of the patients, the results of the Metopirone test suggested that in these same cases corticotrophin mobilisation in response to a fall in the plasma cortisol levels is often impaired. It is theoretically possible that these two tests of corticotrophin mobilisation—which, of course, are each based on a different mechanism—may give quite differing results; and in this connection it is interesting to note that differences between the findings they yield are by no means uncommon in patients who have received A.C.T.H. therapy. The functional disturbance which treatment with exogenous A.C.T.H. is liable to provoke in the mechanism responsible for the release of corticotrophin is at all events a rather peculiar one; in cases, by contrast, in which the hypothalamo-pituitary system has sustained anatomical damage as the result of disease, both mechanisms of corticotrophin mobilisation are impaired and, consequently, both tests produce abnormal findings. The disorder occurring after treatment with A.C.T.H., which is a purely functional disorder, evidently affects this control system in a different manner—as revealed by the diverging results obtained not only in the insulin and Metopirone tests, but also often in the vasopressin test[2] as well.

As a practising clinician, one is bound to consider the question as to what prognostic significance these findings may have in patients treated with A.C.T.H. We know from practical experience that, when the A.C.T.H. therapy is discontinued, such patients display no symptoms whatsoever which could be imputed to adrenocortical hypofunction. On the other hand, cases are occasionally encountered in which, after the withdrawal of A.C.T.H., fulminant attacks of fever, status asthmaticus, or haemolysis set in which may provoke very grave states calling for corticosteroid substitution therapy in order to support the circulation. The patients concerned presumably belong to the category of those relatively rare cases which also fail to react normally in the insulin test. Since these abnormal reactions to insulin evidently occur far less frequently after A.C.T.H. therapy than after treatment with corticoids (where they are regularly observed), it seems reasonable to conclude that an abnormal sensitivity to stress is likewise less common following A.C.T.H. therapy. In this connection, however, it must be pointed out that no explanation has yet been offered to account for such a difference in the way in which A.C.T.H. and corticoids affect the pituitary-adrenocortical system.

In our opinion, the insulin test provides a better model of the stress reaction, and affords a more reliable guide to the patient's ability to respond to stress, than does the Metopirone test. The stimulation of corticotrophin secretion to which hypoglycaemia gives rise undoubtedly imitates the physiological response to stress much more closely than the stimulation provoked by Metopirone. This latter form of stimulation is triggered off by an abnormal fall in the plasma cortisol concentration, i.e. by an experimentally induced phenomenon which is without parallel in the physiology and pathophysiology of stress (such a decrease in the plasma cortisol levels is otherwise encountered only in the presence of primary damage to the adrenal cortex or following adrenalectomy). Consequently, we would rather not regard the results of the Metopirone test in patients treated with A.C.T.H. as offering proof that those who show an abnormal response in this test are particularly sensitive to stress.

Summary

In patients with asthma who had undergone several months of treatment with A.C.T.H., tests were carried out with insulin and Metopirone over a period of one month, in order to study the reactivity of anterior pituitary corticotrophic function following withdrawal of the A.C.T.H. Whereas in the insulin test the plasma cortisol concentrations in these cases very seldom showed a below-normal rise in response to the induced hypoglycaemia, in the Metopirone tests performed shortly after the withdrawal of A.C.T.H. therapy the patients frequently exhibited an inadequate reaction. As the interval elapsing between withdrawal of A.C.T.H. and performance of the Metopirone test increased, however, so the number of tests yielding abnormal results progressively decreased. The theoretical and practical implications of these findings are discussed.

References

1 BIERICH, J. R., ECKLER, E., SCHÖNBERG, D.: Die Prüfung der corticotropen Funktion der Hypophyse mit Metopiron. III. Untersuchungen nach langfristiger Behandlung mit ACTH. Endokrinologie 42, 335 (1962)

2 CARTER, M. E., JAMES, V. H. T.: Effect of corticotrophin therapy on pituitary-adrenal function. Ann. rheum. Dis. 29, 73 (1970)

3 DE MOOR, P., STEENO, O., RASKIN, M., HENDRIKX, A.: Fluorimetric determination of free plasma 11-hydroxycorticosteroids in man. Acta endocr. (Kbh.) 33, 297 (1960)

4 HERRMANN, M.: Experimentelle Untersuchungen zur Auswirkung einer einmaligen ACTH-Gabe. Ein Beitrag zur Kenntnis der homöostatischen Regulation. Rev. Anat. Embryol. and Cell. Biol. 39, No. 5 (1967)

5 HERRMANN, M.: Contribution on regulation of corticotrophic partial function. Reference to an active negative regulation. Acta endocr. (Kbh.) Suppl. 173: 30 (1973)

6 KITAY, J. I., HOLUB, D. A., JAILER, J. W.: Inhibition of pituitary ACTH release: an extra-adrenal action of exogenous ACTH. Endocrinology 64, 475 (1959)

7 PLAGER, J. E., CUSHMAN, P., Jr.: Suppression of the pituitary-ACTH response in man by administration of ACTH or cortisol. J. clin. Endocr. 22, 147 (1962)

8 REED, P.I., CLAYMAN, C.B., PALMER, W.L.: Adrenocortical and pituitary responsiveness following long-term, high dosage corticotropin administration. Ann. intern. Med. *61*, 1 (1964)

9 REISERT, P.-M., SCHIPPER, H., VOLLES, E., BAUER, H.: Untersuchungen über die Hypophysenhemmwirkung einer ACTH-Therapie. Klin. Wschr. *48*, 351 (1970)

10 SAVAGE, O., COPEMAN, W.S.C., CHAPMAN, L., WELLS, M.V., TREADWELL, B.L.J.: Pituitary and adrenal hormones in rheumatoid arthritis. Lancet *i*, 232 (1962)

11 STARK, E., ÁCS, Z., MAKARA, G.B., MIHÁLY, K.: The hypophyseal-adrenocortical response to various different stressing procedures in ACTH-treated rats. Canad. J. Physiol. Pharmacol. *46*, 567 (1968)

12 STARK, E., FACHET, J., MIHÁLY, K.: The influence of reserpine on the inhibition of ACTH-secretion induced by exogenous ACTH or a corticoid injection. Arzneimittel-Forsch. *16*, 1574 (1966)

13 WALSER, A., BARTHE, P., SCHÄR, J.: Die Wirkung hoher Dosen von synthetischem ACTH auf die Funktion von Hypothalamus-Hypophyse-Nebennierenrinde. Schweiz. med. Wschr. *98*, 1892 (1968)

Synacthen—why and when?

by F. Kogoj *

Until about ten years ago, repeated attempts had been made to administer corticoids in some form of combination with corticotrophin in cases where it was considered desirable to raise the plasma glucocorticoid levels in order to inhibit mesenchymal reactions. These attempts were prompted chiefly by the idea that additional treatment with corticotrophin would serve to stimulate the adrenals and thus guard against corticoid-induced damage to the adrenal cortex. When it was realised, however, that in patients who have undergone prolonged corticoid therapy a gradual, step-by-step reduction in the dosage is usually sufficient in itself to enable adrenocortical function to recover (Geyer and Reimer[7]) and that the centres in the hypothalamus and anterior pituitary which control the feedback mechanism are affected only to a limited degree, the use of A.C.T.H. as an aid to the restoration of adrenocortical function came to be regarded as obsolete. Moreover, the A.C.T.H. extract-preparations available at the time also displayed two specific drawbacks which complicated their use as therapeutic agents: firstly, they exhibited relatively strong allergenic activity—the incidence of allergic reactions, as reported in the literature, ranging from 3.5 to 38 % (Charpin and Aubert[4])—and, secondly, since they could only be standardised biologically, it was impossible to administer them in exact, unvarying dosages (Schuppli[13,14]; Thieblot and Perrot[16]).

Consequently, in the vast majority of patients requiring glucocorticoid therapy, the usual practice nowadays is to provide the body with a direct supply of exogenous glucocorticoids, for which purpose there exists a wide choice of preparations varying in potency from cortisone to dexamethasone. But the very fact that such highly active cortisone derivatives as dexamethasone are now available should prompt us to bear in mind the warning of Coste[5] that, the greater the therapeutic efficacy of a glucocorticoid preparation, the greater the risk of undesirable effects, including the danger of irreversible damage to the hypothalamo-pituitary-adrenocortical axis.

Meanwhile, however, work on the synthesis of A.C.T.H. polypeptides had been in progress for a number of years. Already in 1963 Schwyzer and Sieber[15] succeeded in synthesising the complete molecule of porcine A.C.T.H. consisting of 39 amino acids, and in 1967 an Hungarian research team (Kisfaludy et al.[10]) reported the successful synthesis of human A.C.T.H.

But the first major result of practical importance yielded by this research was the synthesis (Kappeler and Schwyzer[9]) of a polypeptide containing the first 24 amino acids of the A.C.T.H. molecule, which was subsequently placed

---

* Institut za Klinička Medicinska Istraživanja, Zagreb, Yugoslavia.

at the disposal of the medical profession under the name ®Synacthen. For therapeutic purposes this synthetic polypeptide is now chiefly employed in the form of the long-acting depot preparation (Synacthen Depot). Synacthen possesses all the pharmacological properties of the naturally occurring A.C.T.H. chain composed of 39 amino acids, but its antigenicity is considerably less than that of the A.C.T.H. extract-preparations. Only in isolated cases is Synacthen liable to give rise to allergic reactions (SCHUPPLI[13,14]).

When employed as a mobiliser of cortisol, Synacthen may in principle provoke the same side effects as those occurring in response to the direct administration of glucocorticoids. There are nevertheless certain differences as regards the way in which the two types of treatment are tolerated: some of the side effects which prove a problem with corticoid therapy are either encountered less frequently in patients receiving A.C.T.H. or assume a milder form.

This applies particularly to interference with the control mechanism operating between the hypothalamus and pituitary on the one hand and the adrenal cortex on the other. In patients undergoing relatively short-term treatment with Synacthen Depot, COUTEAUX-DUMONT and LAPIÈRE[6], for example, observed no adverse effects whatsoever on the hypothalamo-pituitary-adrenocortical axis; and WALSER et al.[18] were able to demonstrate that, following treatment for one month with high doses of Synacthen Depot, the hormonal interplay rapidly reverted to normal when the medication was withdrawn.

The use of Synacthen does in fact involve less danger of provoking irreversible disorders of hypothalamo-pituitary-adrenocortical function than in the case of corticoid therapy. One possible explanation for this reduced risk may be that Synacthen—like A.C.T.H. obtained by extraction—is capable of mobilising the entire gamut of adrenocortical steroids, including also the mineralocorticoids, progestogens, oestrogens, and androgens, and perhaps other as yet unidentified biologically active substances as well. The fact that A.C.T.H. has, among other things, the effect of mobilising the adrenocortical androgens has likewise been suggested as the reason why osteoporosis occurs less frequently under treatment with A.C.T.H. than during corticoid therapy.

The comprehensive stimulation of adrenocortical hormone production achieved by employing the pituitary hormone whose specific function it is to stimulate the adrenal cortex no doubt constitutes for the organism as a whole a more physiological process than imposing upon it the strain of treatment with exogenous synthetic glucocorticoids. This would appear to be reflected in the finding that, in contrast to glucocorticoids, neither A.C.T.H. nor Synacthen Depot causes retardation of growth in children. Also deserving of mention in this connection are reports in which it is claimed that A.C.T.H. sometimes elicits good results in cases where glucocorticoid medication has failed to produce the desired response.

Quite a large proportion of these reports relate to the treatment of neurological and dermatological diseases. Here, the suggestion has been raised that corticotrophin as such might also perhaps exert a direct therapeutic effect both on the skin (i.e. on the epidermis) and on neural elements—a possibility which, in view of the fact that the epidermis and the nervous system have a common ectodermal origin, would seem quite conceivable.

It has, moreover, been demonstrated that corticotrophin sometimes produces one side effect in particular which serves as evidence of its direct affinity for the skin: in patients treated with A.C.T.H. or Synacthen, hyperpigmentation occasionally develops in the form of generalised melanoderma, which, to some extent at least, proves reversible. We, too, have seen a case of this kind among our patients. At this point, it should be recalled that the molecule of A.C.T.H. bears a chemical resemblance to that of melanocyte-stimulating hormone (M.S.H.) (CALAS and BONNET[3]) and that the melanocyte-stimulating activity of A.C.T.H. is accounted for by the portion of the amino acid chain which is identical in both A.C.T.H. and M.S.H.

The direct effect exerted by A.C.T.H. on the skin, however, also has certain advantages, as witnessed by the fact that, even when administered to patients over prolonged periods, Synacthen—in contrast to long-term treatment with glucocorticoids—causes no atrophic skin changes. It is possible that the modifications which A.C.T.H. therapy induces in endogenous steroid metabolism may play a role in this connection, particularly since the skin itself also participates in the metabolism of steroids (HSIA and HAO[8]). In skin tests it has been found that administration of Synacthen Depot completely suppresses the local allergic reaction to contact allergens (SARTORIS et al.[12]). In view of this finding, and of other similar observations, such as those reported by BOHNSTEDT and LANZ[2], we consider that in certain dermatological conditions it might be worth while to give local treatment with Synacthen a trial in appropriate cases.

In the light of these various considerations, one general conclusion can also be drawn, namely: there are cogent reasons for supposing that, as an alternative to corticoid therapy, Synacthen can in principle be deemed of equal value. This, of course, does not apply to local treatment with topical corticoids; moreover, the qualification "in principle" is a necessary one, because here too there are exceptions that prove the rule.

In this context, mention should be made of two sets of circumstances which, though of theoretical rather than practical importance, would militate against the use of A.C.T.H. or Synacthen: firstly, if the object of treatment is purely and simply to achieve an enhanced glucocorticoid effect, i.e. if the mobilisation of adrenocortical hormones other than the glucocorticoids has to be avoided at all costs; and, secondly, if for some reason or other parenteral administration of Synacthen proves impracticable.

KORTING[11] states that, since A.C.T.H. is a protein substance, it should not be employed in periarteritis nodosa, a condition which some authors (e.g. VORLAENDER[17]) believe to be due to an auto-aggressive process complicated by the intervention of a virus. What is more, it is only in the acute stages of this disease that KORTING uses glucocorticoids; he likewise utters a warning concerning the dubious effect of corticoid therapy in nodular or allergic vasculitis—a warning which we too have found justified in the light of our own experience. We therefore also exercise caution with regard to the use of Synacthen in these indications.

Needless to say, Synacthen should not be administered to patients suffering from adrenocortical insufficiency (adrenal atrophy, Addison's disease).

Except in conditions such as severe status asthmaticus or very severe pemphigus, where the patient's life is so endangered that glucocorticoids need to be given immediately, or in cases where the body requires very large quantities of corticoids at once, the 30-minute Synacthen test should always be carried out first, in order to gain an impression of the functional status of the patient's adrenal cortex. For this purpose, two blood samples have to be taken, the first immediately prior to an intramuscular injection of 0.25 mg. Synacthen, and the second 30 minutes later; in an emergency, a glucocorticoid can then be given—if necessary intravenously—directly after this second sample has been taken, i.e. without waiting for the result of the plasma cortisol determination; if the patient is afterwards found to have shown a normal response in the 30-minute test, the treatment can then be continued as soon as possible with Synacthen or Synacthen Depot.

We are convinced that—thanks to the synthesis of Synacthen, a polypeptide featuring that portion of the A.C.T.H. molecule which is endowed with the full hormonal activity of corticotrophin, but lacking the portion which makes no contribution to its hormonal effect—a new era has been inaugurated in the field of anti-inflammatory hormone therapy. This judiciously modified form of corticotrophin has opened up a new therapeutic approach, which makes it possible to conform to the currently increasing trend aimed at ensuring as far as is feasible that treatment is adapted to the body's own physiological processes instead of acting independently of or even in opposition to them.

References

1   Bíró, L., Iván, E., Sándor, P., Perényi, T.: Klinisch-pharmakologische Untersuchung des synthetischen ACTH. Ther. hung. *20*, 17 (1972)

2   Bohnstedt, R.M., Lanz, W.: Tierexperimentelle Untersuchungen über einen ACTH-Effekt des Terpentinöls. Naunyn-Schmiedeberg's Arch. exp. Path. Pharmak. *224*, 262 (1955)

3   Calas, E., Bonnet, J.: A.C.T.H.-thérapie en dermatologie. In: A.C.T.H.-thérapie moderne, Coll. thér. CIBA, Marseilles 1969, p. 201 (Kapp & Lahure, Vanves 1970)

4   Charpin, J., Aubert, J.: A.C.T.H.-thérapie et allergie respiratoire, loc. cit.[3], p.105

5   Coste, F.: Historique de l'A.C.T.H.-thérapie, loc.cit.[3], p.7

6   Couteaux-Dumont, C., Lapière, C.M.: ACTH synthétique retard en thérapeutique dermatologique. Arch. belges Derm. *27*, 385 (1971)

7   Geyer, G., Reimer, E.E.: Über kortikotrope Wirksamkeit und Allergenität des synthetischen ACTH-Tetracosactids Synacthen-Depot. Wien. klin. Wschr. *82*, 324 (1970)

8   Hsia, S.L., Hao, Y.-L.: Transformation of cortisone to cortisol. Steroids *10*, 489 (1967)

9   Kappeler, H., Schwyzer, R.: Die Synthese eines Tetracosapeptides mit der Aminosäuresequenz eines hochaktiven Abbauproduktes des β-Corticotropins (ACTH) aus Schweinehypophysen (Vorläufige Mitteilung). Helv. chim. Acta *44*, 1136 (1961)

10 Kisfaludy, L., Bajusz, S., Medzihradsky, K.: Adrenocorticotrop hatásu poly-peptidek és az emberi corticotropin teljes szintézise (Polypeptides with adreno-corticotrophic action and total synthesis of human corticotrophin). Magy. Tud. Akad., Kém. Közl. *28*, 219 (1967)

11 Korting, G. W.: Therapie der Hautkrankheiten, 2nd Ed. (Schattauer, Stutt-gart/New York 1970)

12 Sartoris, S., Pippione, M., Zina, G.: Studio sull'azione inibitrice di un ACTH sintetico sulla reattività cutanea allergica ritardata da contatto. G. ital. Derm. e Minerva derm. *44/110*, 154 (1969)

13 Schuppli, R.: Über die Verwendung von synthetischem ACTH (Synacthen) in der Therapie dermatologischer Affektionen. Dermatologica (Basle) *139*, 243 (1969)

14 Schuppli, R.: Fortschritte in der dermatologischen Therapie. Arch. klin. exp. Derm. *237*, 214 (1970)

15 Schwyzer, R., Sieber, P.: Total synthesis of adrenocorticotrophic hormone. Nature (Lond.) *199*, 172 (1963)

16 Thieblot, L., Perrot, C.: Méthodes de dosage biologiques et cliniques de l'A.C.T.H., loc. cit.[3], p. 67

17 Vorlaender, K.-O.: Immunopathogenese und Therapie der entzündlichen Gefässprozesse aus der Gruppe der Kollagenosen. Derm. Mschr. *158*, 697 (1972)

18 Walser, A., Barthe, P., Schär, J.: Die Wirkung hoher Dosen von syntheti-schem ACTH auf die Funktion von Hypothalamus-Hypophyse-Nebennieren-rinde. Schweiz. med. Wschr. *98*, 1892 (1968)

Discussion

R. Schuppli: Is there anyone here who has had some experience of the contra-indications to which Dr. Kogoj referred in his paper, namely, periarteritis nodosa and allergic vasculitis? I don't somehow think that these are actually genuine contra-indications.

H. J. Bauer: Although I can't claim to have had extensive experience of these conditions, we do quite often use Synacthen in patients suffering from periarteritis nodosa, and we haven't really encountered any adverse effects. If we were to follow up this line of reasoning to its logical conclusion, then we shouldn't employ A.C.T.H. in myasthenia or multiple sclerosis, or for that matter in any other diseases in which we suspect an auto-aggressive mechanism to be involved. As to the possibility that A.C.T.H. may have a direct influence on the nervous system, I can only say that we have no evidence whatsoever to suggest that A.C.T.H. exerts any effects above and beyond those that are in some way or another hormonally mediated.

F. Kogoj: I didn't exactly say in my paper that I considered A.C.T.H. and cortico-steroids to be contra-indicated in periarteritis nodosa and allergic vasculitis. Gluco-corticoids are in fact employed in cases of so-called vasculitis and good responses have been reported. We, too, occasionally use them in these conditions, but with all due caution.
Incidentally, I'd like to take this opportunity to ask to what extent Synacthen should or should not be regarded as a protein substance.

W. Rittel: In answer to your question, Dr. Kogoj, I would point out first of all that from the chemical standpoint a distinction is drawn between a protein and a peptide insofar as, though they both have the same basic chemical structure, they differ greatly with regard to their molecular weight. The term "protein" is applied to substances having a molecular weight of 10,000 or above.
When A.C.T.H. is isolated from a natural source, the extract does of course also contain quite an amount of foreign protein, and the risk that impurities or foreign proteins may fail to be eliminated during the process of isolation is relatively great. We are absolutely certain, however, that no high-molecular protein-like material is present in Synacthen. On the other hand, what Synacthen does also contain are small quantities—amounting to perhaps 1 to 2%—of by-products resulting from the process of synthesis itself, including the methionine-sulphoxide derivative in particular.

W. J. Irvine: I'd certainly subscribe to what's been said about treating auto-immune disorders with A.C.T.H. If we didn't use the drug in these diseases, I fear there wouldn't be many indications left for A.C.T.H. therapy! I don't see any reason why one shouldn't combine oral steroids with A.C.T.H. at the start of treatment. One of the snags with A.C.T.H. medication is the fact that initially you may not get a particularly good response; but then, after the first few injections, the plasma cortisol builds up to a more satisfactory level. For this reason it might well be mis-leading to do a Synacthen test at the beginning of treatment, since the result is unlikely to provide you with an indication as to what response the adrenal cortices are going to give during the following week or the week after that. Although the evidence is a little tenuous, what seems in fact to happen is that during a course of treatment with A.C.T.H. the cortisol response steadily builds up over a period of, say, two or three weeks until it reaches a plateau where it remains stationary. One must therefore beware of carrying out a Synacthen test early on and concluding from the result that the treatment is eliciting rather a poor response in terms of plasma cortisol. Incidentally, I don't believe there is much evidence to suggest that a short course of oral steroids, even if given in a high dosage over a period of several weeks, is likely to have any disastrous effects on the hypothalamo-pituitary-adrenocortical axis. Moreover, since the important thing for the patient is that his condition should be quickly brought under control and a rapid improvement achieved, I feel that treatment with oral steroids is justified at the start; later on you can tail off the steroid medication and maintain the improvement with Synacthen Depot.

A further point I'd like to mention is that the scope of A.C.T.H. is limited by the fact that you cannot stimulate corticosteroid production beyond a certain level. Consequently, you tend to find that it is the more chronic conditions of intermediate severity which prove easiest to control with Synacthen Depot. If the patient has a very severe and/or acute condition, I'm sure you'll find that you need to add oral steroids in order to supplement the therapeutic effect of A.C.T.H.

Finally, I have a question for Dr. RITTEL concerning the substituted 1–18 A.C.T.H. derivative. In this preparation, three of the amino acids have been altered; does he think it likely or unlikely that these alterations in themselves may cause certain complications in terms of antigenicity or of reactions to what is in fact no longer a natural sequence of amino acids?

W. RITTEL: Though I'm not an immunologist, I think that a structural modification of the naturally occurring peptide may in principle involve the risk of an increase in antigenicity. Studies on the antigenicity of A.C.T.H. fragments have, I believe, shown that these peptides act as very weak antigens. As for the alterations in the 1–18 peptide to which you referred, Dr. IRVINE, this derivative is a molecule in which one basic amino acid, i.e. arginine, has been replaced by another, i.e. lysine, in positions 17 and 18; but lysine is just as much a naturally occurring amino acid as arginine. Whether this modification has any influence on the antigenicity of the peptide, is a question which I'm afraid I can't answer.

H. BOISSIÈRE: I should like to ask Dr. KOGOJ what evidence he can quote in support of the statement he made in his paper to the effect that, in contrast to glucocorticoids, neither A.C.T.H. nor Synacthen Depot causes retardation of growth in children. In this connection I have two remarks to make. Firstly, I imagine that very few children have yet been treated with depot A.C.T.H. in doses high enough, and administered over a sufficiently prolonged period, to entail the risk of retarding their growth. Secondly, as for the possibility that synthetic A.C.T.H. may inhibit growth in children, I think this depends on a number of factors, i.e. on whether high doses are employed, whether the injections are given at excessively frequent intervals, and for how long the treatment is prolonged. I shall have more to say about this later when I come to present my paper, in which, among other things, I refer to a 27-month-old child who has now been receiving Synacthen Depot for 17 months in a dosage of 0.5 mg. per week and whose growth is proceeding normally.

F. KOGOJ: A.C.T.H. therapy, too, may of course give rise to disorders of the type that are liable to occur during treatment with glucocorticoids, but they are less frequent and of a much milder nature. In the case of Synacthen, I think the reason for this is that—apart from the allergising properties of the complete A.C.T.H. molecule—this 1–24 peptide exhibits all the other effects of A.C.T.H., including its ability to mobilise the whole gamut of adrenocortical hormones. Even if it were possible to isolate from the entire A.C.T.H. chain only those links that are responsible for stimulating glucocorticoid production, I don't believe that this would prove of much help to the clinician.

M. GIORDANO: With regard to corticosteroid treatment for periarteritis nodosa, I should like to remind you that some 15 years ago KEMPER et al.* suggested that rheumatoid arthritis, if treated over a prolonged period with corticosteroids, might sometimes develop into a collagen disease closely resembling periarteritis nodosa.

---

* KEMPER, J. W., BAGGENSTOSS, A. H., SLOCUMB, C. H.: The relationship of therapy with cortisone to the incidence of vascular lesions in rheumatoid arthritis. Ann. intern. Med. 46, 831 (1957)

These authors claimed that corticosteroid therapy actually aggravated rheumatoid arthritis. I don't know whether, in view of these assertions, corticosteroids ought to be regarded as contra-indicated in cases of spontaneously occurring periarteritis nodosa. On the other hand, periarteritis nodosa is customarily assigned to the category of collagen diseases that by and large are supposed to respond favourably to corticosteroid therapy. I personally haven't had much experience in the treatment of these forms of disease, since they tend to be rather rare in Italy.

F. KOGOJ: Most of the conditions to which the term "collagen disease" is applied consist of various forms of vasculitis and auto-immune diseases. Probably all of us would agree that in such cases treatment with corticotrophin or corticosteroids is in fact capable of producing good results, even though the mechanism underlying their therapeutic effect in these diseases has not yet been fully clarified.

R. SCHUPPLI: Regarding the risk of immunising an organism by altering the amino acids, I don't think that this is a very important factor, because the substances in question are not haptens. They are not proteins like the real albumin molecule, which is a hapten; on the contrary, such haptenic properties as they may exhibit are very, very weak. Using experimental procedures you can never get an immune response with such substances.

J. GIRARD: I don't quite agree with that. Although the human and the porcine 1–39 A.C.T.H. molecules differ only with respect to one amino acid, patients immunised with a porcine A.C.T.H. extract-preparation easily form antibodies that are capable of binding the synthetic 1–39 porcine molecule. I should therefore think that there is at least some potential danger in this connection.

R. SCHUPPLI: But the presence of antibodies doesn't mean disease!

J. GIRARD: No, but once you can detect antibodies you must reckon with the possibility of allergic or anaphylactic reactions or blocking of the biological activity of the respective hormone—and to this extent you have a potential underlying basis for disease.

The role of synthetic A.C.T.H. in clinical practice, and problems connected with its use

by K. F. WEINGES*

Polypeptide hormone preparations employed in clinical practice for diagnostic or therapeutic purposes should, if possible, meet three requirements: firstly, they should have a high degree of purity; secondly, they should display the full biological activity of the hormone in question; and, thirdly, they should exhibit minimal antigenicity.

The adrenocorticotrophic hormone preparation synthesised by KAPPELER and SCHWYZER[17] in 1961 can be regarded as effectively fulfilling these three prerequisites. Produced entirely by synthesis, this preparation—β1–24 tetracosapeptide—is composed of 24 amino acids linked in the same order as the first 24 of the 39 amino acids contained in the naturally occurring A.C.T.H. molecule. Its absolute purity guarantees that the first of the three requirements for clinical use can be met. As for the second requirement, the biological activity of this synthetic corticotrophic peptide is comparable with that of highly purified A.C.T.H. obtained by extraction from natural sources[18, 29, 36].

Shown in Figure 1 is the behaviour of the plasma cortisol levels (determined by a method of competitive protein binding adapted from that of MURPHY[27]) in a healthy 25-year-old man of normal body-weight following injection of the solvent only (0 = blank test), as well as after intravenous (I) and intramuscular (II) administration of 0.25 mg. β1–24 tetracosapeptide (®Synacthen) and after an intravenous injection of 10 mg. hydrocortisone (X). Secretion of endogenous A.C.T.H. had been inhibited by administering a dose of 2 mg. dexamethasone at 11 p.m. on the evening before each of the tests; it is this which accounts for the very low fasting plasma cortisol concentration recorded the next morning at 8 a.m. In response both to intravenous and to intramuscular injection of 0.25 mg. Synacthen, a maximal rise in the plasma cortisol level (to 38.3 and 38.4 mcg./100 ml., respectively) occurred within 90–120 minutes. It is interesting to note that the curves plotted for the plasma cortisol values following intravenous and intramuscular injection of Synacthen do not differ from each other to any marked extent; though this may be partly attributable to the fact that Synacthen is well absorbed by the intramuscular route, the main reasons are probably a) that the hormone becomes more rapidly bound and inactivated when given intravenously and b) that the degree to which the synthesis and secretion of cortisol can be stimulated is limited.

The half-life of endogenous cortisol is about 90 minutes and therefore comparable with that of intravenously administered exogenous hydrocortisone.

* Medizinische Klinik und Poliklinik, Universität des Saarlandes, Homburg/Saar (German Federal Republic).

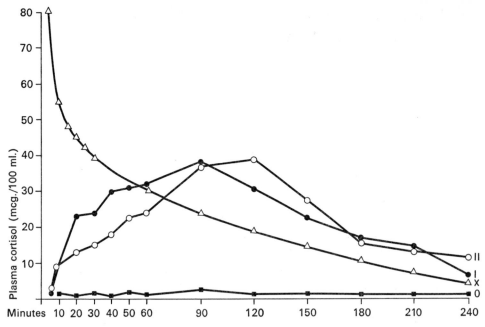

Fig. 1. Plasma cortisol levels (determined by the method of competitive protein binding) in a healthy man of normal body-weight following injection of the solvent only (0), as well as after intravenous (I) and intramuscular (II) injection of 0.25 mg. Synacthen, and after an intravenous injection of 10 mg. hydrocortisone (X). On the evening before each test, 2 mg. dexamethasone was given at 11 p.m.

The biological activity of Synacthen Depot, a long-acting β1–24 tetracosapeptide preparation, will be discussed later in greater detail with reference to the clinical use of this drug.

The antigenicity of A.C.T.H. preparations obtained by extraction and the allergic side effects liable to occur as a result of sensitisation to such preparations are regarded as serious drawbacks to treatment with this hormone. In this connection a distinction has to be drawn between, on the one hand, circulating antibodies which may either lead to frank allergic manifestations or merely have the effect of neutralising the biological activity of the hormone and, on the other hand, what is referred to as cellular immunity, which may be directed against the hormone itself or also against substances accompanying it. This difference is also reflected in the clinical symptomatology in those cases which fail to respond satisfactorily, e.g. whereas in one patient a localised or generalised skin reaction, angioneurotic oedema, or even a state of anaphylactic shock may occur, in another patient the doses of hormone administered may simply exert no biological activity; patients of this latter type are described as being resistant. Allergy and resistance may, of course, also be encountered together in one and the same case.

According to data contained in the literature, the incidence of allergic reactions to A.C.T.H. extract-preparations ranges from 3% to 38%, the differences in

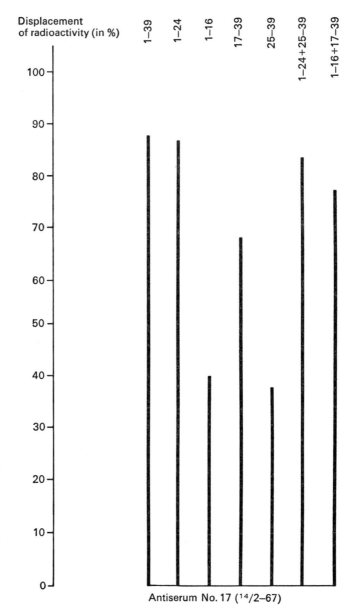

Displacement of radioactivity (in %)

1–39   1–24   1–16   17–39   25–39   1–24+25–39   1–16+17–39

Antiserum No. 17 (^{14}/2–67)

Fig. 2. Competitive inhibition of the binding of porcine I^{131}-A.C.T.H. to porcine A.C.T.H. antibody by various peptide sequences from the A.C.T.H. molecule. All the peptide fragments were incubated in equimolar concentrations. (From FELBER and AUBERT[8])

the percentages quoted being no doubt due to the varying degrees of purity of the extracts employed. Where highly purified preparations are used, allergic reactions occur far less frequently, since it is not so much the foreign A.C.T.H. molecule itself that provokes sensitisation, but rather the foreign proteins with which it is contaminated. It had already been pointed out earlier by several authors[2, 7, 33, 40] that allergy to A.C.T.H. involves a species-specific or organ-specific, but not a hormone-specific, form of sensitisation; and this has since been confirmed in the light of experience with the use of β1–24 tetracosa-peptide[24, 35, 42].

Although the synthetic β1–24 tetracosapeptide causes a much lower incidence of allergic reactions, it nevertheless also appears to display some degree of antigenicity. In patients who had undergone prolonged treatment with Synacthen Depot, GLASS et al.[13], RATCLIFFE et al.[34], and other authors[12] have succeeded in demonstrating the presence of circulating antibodies; but the presence of such antibodies does not enable one to make any direct inferences as to the nature of this antigenicity, particularly since the antibodies may be directed both against the synthetic peptide and against the complete molecule. Furthermore, in rabbits it has proved possible with porcine A.C.T.H. preparations to produce antibodies showing the same avidity for the synthetic N-terminal (1–24) of A.C.T.H. as for the entire molecule with its full complement of 39 amino acids (cf. Figure 2, reproduced from FELBER and AUBERT[8]). Children treated with porcine A.C.T.H. were also found to have developed antibodies displaying a measurable avidity for β1–24 tetracosapeptide[19].

It is not yet possible, however, to reach any final conclusions concerning the immunological properties of A.C.T.H. Further clinical studies will, it is to be hoped, reveal to what extent the relationships between the structure and effects of A.C.T.H. as outlined by SCHWYZER[37] (Figure 3) shed light on the problem of its antigenicity.

With regard to the clinical use of β1–24 tetracosapeptide, a distinction must be drawn between two main fields of indications:

1. Diagnostic tests with Synacthen or Synacthen Depot designed to detect disorders of adrenocortical function.

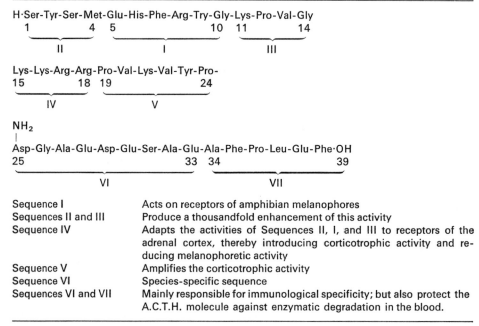

Sequence I	Acts on receptors of amphibian melanophores
Sequences II and III	Produce a thousandfold enhancement of this activity
Sequence IV	Adapts the activities of Sequences II, I, and III to receptors of the adrenal cortex, thereby introducing corticotrophic activity and reducing melanophoretic activity
Sequence V	Amplifies the corticotrophic activity
Sequence VI	Species-specific sequence
Sequences VI and VII	Mainly responsible for immunological specificity; but also protect the A.C.T.H. molecule against enzymatic degradation in the blood.

Fig. 3. Diagrammatic outline of relationships between the structure and effects of A.C.T.H. (Adapted from SCHWYZER[37])

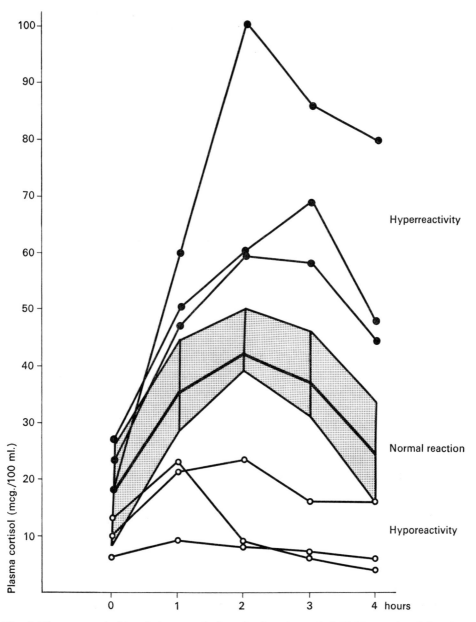

Fig. 4. Plasma cortisol levels in man during the four-hour A.C.T.H. test, i.e. following intramuscular injection of 0.25 mg. Synacthen.

2. Treatment for diseases in which glucocorticoid medication would otherwise appear necessary; for this purpose, it is Synacthen Depot that is almost invariably employed.

The use of Synacthen as a diagnostic aid in the assessment of adrenocortical function poses no problems and has now gained clinical acceptance as a routine examination procedure. The four-hour A.C.T.H. test, in which 0.25 mg.

83

Synacthen is injected intramuscularly, has yielded good results in practice. In this test, the fasting plasma cortisol level is determined at 8 a.m., after which the injection of Synacthen is given and the plasma cortisol then measured hourly over a period of four hours. A rise of 100% corresponds roughly to the norm, as indicated in Figure 4. In cases where the determinations have to be confined to measurement of the 17-hydroxycorticoids (Porter-Silber chromogens) in the 24-hour urine, we have found it preferable to administer an intramuscular injection of 1 mg. Synacthen Depot in the morning; if the patient's adrenal cortices are functioning normally, the 17-hydroxycorticoids in the 24-hour urine will then likewise rise to at least double the blank value (Figure 5).

In patients with adrenocortical dysfunction due to pituitary insufficiency, to prolonged steroid therapy, or to chronic undernourishment of the type associated with anorexia nervosa for example, more prolonged corticotrophic stimulation is needed. In such cases, one should inject 1 mg. Synacthen Depot daily for at least three days and measure the plasma cortisol at 8 a.m., noon, 4 p.m., and 11 p.m. (so as to gain an impression of the circadian rhythm), as well as the 17-hydroxycorticoids in the 24-hour urine. On the second or third day, a pronounced increase usually occurs both in the plasma cortisol levels and in the concentration of Porter-Silber chromogens in the 24-hour urine. Sometimes, however, this increase may not set in until after treatment has been in progress for one week. Needless to say, the 17-ketosteroid concentration in the 24-hour urine (Zimmermann reaction) also rises markedly (cf. Figure 5).

When conducting clinical trials in which the patients are receiving long-term treatment with depot A.C.T.H., one has to consider a variety of aspects. The response to prolonged A.C.T.H. therapy should be compared and contrasted with the response to treatment with one of the standardly employed synthetic glucocorticoids—except, of course, where one is studying some possible effect of A.C.T.H. that is not due to its action on the adrenal cortex.

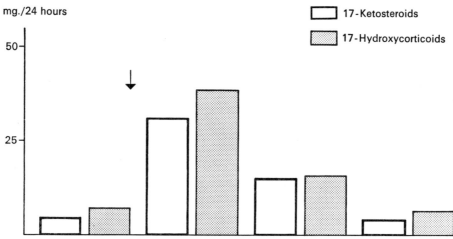

Fig. 5. Excretion of 17-hydroxycorticoids (Porter-Silber chromogens) and 17-keto-steroids (as measured by the Zimmermann reaction) in the 24-hour urine before and after intramuscular injection of 1 mg. Synacthen Depot at 8 a.m. (↓).

The therapeutic indications for treatment with glucocorticoids are based on the anti-inflammatory, anti-allergic, and immunosuppressive effects of these drugs, and on the fact that when prescribed in very high doses in certain haematological diseases they are capable of "stimulating" the bone marrow (provoking an increased release of cells from, or an enhanced production of new cells in, the bone marrow?), diminishing vascular permeability, or exerting a mild cytotoxic action. Cases requiring substitution therapy with hydrocortisone need not be considered in this context.

The undesirable side effects to which glucocorticoid medication is liable to give rise include: inhibition of endogenous A.C.T.H. secretion, which constitutes a particular hazard in situations of stress and leads to adrenocortical atrophy; a marked catabolic action on protein metabolism (resulting in osteoporosis, muscular atrophy, etc.); a diabetogenic effect due to increased gluconeogenesis; and inhibition of glucose utilisation in the periphery. In addition, psychic changes may occur, and inhibition of growth has been observed in children. On the other hand, treatment with glucocorticoids offers advantages inasmuch as these drugs display little or no mineralocorticoid activity and can be administered orally in doses adapted to the patient's individual requirements.

When the possibility of resorting to treatment with A.C.T.H. is weighed in the balance against the clinical and experimental findings that have been obtained with synthetic glucocorticoids, the first question to be asked is whether direct stimulation of the adrenal cortex with A.C.T.H. does not represent a more physiological form of therapy, especially since it steps up the production not only of cortisol but also of adrenocortical androgens and is therefore likely to provoke fewer side effects, at least as far as protein catabolism is concerned.

This is a question to which I cannot yet provide an answer, either on the basis of a careful study of the literature or in the light of personal experience to date. In this context, I am deliberately ignoring experience of a purely clinical nature, though I hasten to add that I certainly do not wish to impugn the validity of this experience. As I see it, however, my own task here is to raise certain fundamental questions which we might profitably discuss.

For example, in what way could the stimulation of endogenous cortisol production and secretion conceivably be made to elicit a better therapeutic effect than the administration of synthetic corticosteroids?

One answer might perhaps be found by reference to possible differences in the kinetics of endogenous and exogenous corticosteroids—in which connection I am not thinking simply of their so-called half-life in the blood. We know that, in contrast to cortisol, synthetic steroids show little or no tendency to become bound to transcortin (corticosteroid-binding globulin)[1]. But no detailed studies on the kinetics either of cortisol or of the synthetic steroids have yet been carried out. Measurement of the half-life values—which is usually performed with the aid of tracer substances—does not provide satisfactory data for this purpose, as can be seen from Figure 6.

The findings obtained to date do indicate, however, that the kinetics both of cortisol and of the synthetic glucocorticoids obey two additively linked exponential functions—a fact which suggests that a two-compartment model is

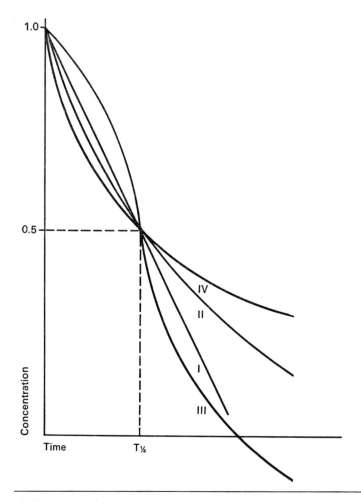

Fig. 6. Diagram illustrating differences in the kinetics of substances which have the same half-life and the same initial concentration.

I Simple type of zero-order reaction (as applicable to ethyl alcohol):

$$\frac{dc}{dt} + k = 0$$

The decrease in the concentration (c) per unit time (t) proceeds steadily and independently of the concentration obtaining at any given moment.
k = reaction-rate constant

II Simple type of first-order reaction (as applicable to buformin):

$$\frac{dc}{dt} + kc = 0$$

The decrease in the concentration per unit time is proportional to the concentration obtaining at the time.

III Complex type of reaction involving several reactions occurring simultaneously (as applicable to glucose):

$$\frac{d^2c}{dt^2} + a\frac{dc}{dt} + bc = 0, \text{ in which } a^2 < 4b$$

a and b = reaction-rate constants

IV Complex type of reaction applicable to cortisol:

$$\frac{d^2c}{dt^2} + a\frac{dc}{dt} + bc = 0, \text{ in which } a^2 > 4b$$

applicable in both instances. But no explanation has yet been found as to why the half-life of cortisol, amounting to some 90–110 minutes, is appreciably shorter than that of prednisolone, methylprednisolone, triamcinolone, betamethasone, and dexamethasone, which works out at 200–300 minutes [25, 30, 32]. The differences in the plasma binding of these substances, and particularly in their tissue affinities and metabolic pathways, are also questions to which no clear-cut answer can be given and which cannot be discussed in detail here. It is therefore impossible to assert that from this angle any one of these steroids in particular exhibits advantages or disadvantages as compared with another, and—for the time being, at least—it is upon clinical experience that we shall thus have to continue basing our assessments of them.

The mild mineralocorticoid effect which cortisol, in contrast to many synthetic glucocorticoids, is known to display, and the stimulant action which it also exerts on corticosterone production (aldosterone production is likewise increased if prolonged treatment with very high doses of A.C.T.H. is given) [11, 23], certainly vary in their repercussions from patient to patient. These, however, are effects that should at all events be taken into consideration during long-term A.C.T.H. therapy, since they are liable to give rise to undesirable manifestations in the form of oedema and hypertension (salt and water retention and possibly also hypopotassaemia) [39]. Diabetogenic effects appear to be less of a problem in patients receiving A.C.T.H., although it should be borne in mind that such effects are largely concentration-dependent or dose-dependent, i.e. in the case of A.C.T.H. therapy they depend upon the endogenous cortisol secretion rate and, in the case of corticoid therapy, upon the daily dosage in which synthetic glucocorticoids are being administered; differences in the way in which the synthetic glucocorticoids are broken down and metabolised could perhaps play an additional role.

It has often been emphasised that one of the advantages of treatment with A.C.T.H. lies in the fact that it also stimulates the production of androgens, whose anabolic activity antagonises the catabolic effects of the glucocorticoids; but this cannot be more than a limited advantage. In the first place, we lack relevant objective clinical findings on the incidence and severity of osteoporosis in patients undergoing long-term A.C.T.H. therapy; and, secondly, we encounter osteoporosis, muscular atrophy, and hirsutism not only in patients with Cushing's disease, in whom production of A.C.T.H. is known to be excessive, but also in patients suffering from adrenocortical carcinoma, a condition associated with considerable increases in the production and secretion of androgens and glucocorticoids. One possible reason for misinterpretations in this connection may be that in very few patients treated with A.C.T.H. has the dosage been carefully individualised by reference to the maximal degree of responsiveness shown by the adrenal cortices and by reference to the extent to which the medication is causing chronic overstimulation of cortisol and androgen secretion.

Since androgenic-anabolic steroids undoubtedly inhibit the catabolic action of glucocorticoids on protein metabolism [22], the fact that corticotrophin stimulates adrenocortical androgen production—even if only to a mild degree—would at least be a minor point in favour of A.C.T.H. therapy. Another possibility which has been discussed is that these androgenic-anabolic steroids may, in addition, antagonise the tendency of glucocorticoids to delay the healing of wounds and to provoke gastric ulcers, and that they may also potentiate the anti-inflammatory and anti-allergic activity of the glucocorticoids. In aplastic anaemia, for example, clinical experience seems to suggest that the use of glucocorticoids together with anabolic steroids offers certain advantages. It is likewise conceivable that androgens may exert a beneficial influence on the psychic changes occurring under treatment with glucocorticoids.

It is still a debatable point, however, as to whether these either antagonistic or potentiating effects, which may accrue from the fact that A.C.T.H. simultaneously stimulates the production both of cortisol and of androgens, are sufficiently important to outweigh the disadvantages of A.C.T.H. therapy in the shape of side effects such as acne, hirsutism, and menstrual disorders in women[3, 20, 39, 41].

Adrenocortical function, as we all know, is controlled by a feedback mechanism. The cortisol secreted by the adrenal cortices under the influence of A.C.T.H. has an inhibitory action on certain regulating centres located in the brain, including probably also the anterior pituitary itself. Incidentally, it should be emphasised that the hypothalamus is not simply one of the elements involved in this A.C.T.H.-cortisol control-circuit, but that it constitutes the centre actually responsible for regulating the secretion of A.C.T.H. Besides the circadian rhythm to which the pituitary-adrenocortical axis is subject, a variety of facilitating and inhibiting impulses emanating from the periphery may also play a role here. It has long been known that synthetic glucocorticoids exert a more potent suppressant effect on hypothalamo-pituitary-adrenocortical function, i.e. that they inhibit endogenous A.C.T.H. secretion more strongly, than does cortisol itself. Long-term treatment with synthetic glucocorticoids may lead to marked atrophy of the adrenal cortices, with the result that various types of stress situation then represent a considerable hazard for the patient. On the other hand, JAMES[16] and IRVINE et al.[15] have demonstrated that, in patients receiving daily doses of A.C.T.H. over a prolonged period, hypothalamo-pituitary-adrenocortical function remains largely unimpaired and that in the insulin test, for example, such patients still respond with a significant rise in their plasma cortisol levels. It would also appear that the circadian rhythm of endogenous A.C.T.H. secretion is not completely abolished under the influence of A.C.T.H. therapy. Though it is conceivable that, by analogy with the negative cortisol-A.C.T.H. feedback, there also exists a positive A.C.T.H.-A.C.T.H. feedback, this has yet to be proved.

In contrast to the inhibitory effect exerted by synthetic glucocorticoids on the secretion of growth hormone (H.G.H.), A.C.T.H. tends if anything to stimulate H.G.H. production[31]; and in patients receiving A.C.T.H. therapy who have been subjected to the so-called hypoglycaemia test or to other forms of stimulation, such as a surgical operation, the increase in the output of H.G.H. has been found to correspond to the norm[5]. In children treated with synthetic glucocorticoids, the inhibitory effect of these drugs on the secretion of A.C.T.H. (and, hence, also on the release of anabolic androgens), as well as on the production of H.G.H., results in growth disturbances which—depending largely on the size of the daily dose administered—may sometimes prove quite severe. In children undergoing prolonged treatment with A.C.T.H. in doses sufficient to ensure an adequate clinical response, e.g. in cases of asthma, nephrotic syndrome, etc., no such inhibition of growth occurs, as has been revealed by the results of comparative studies [5, 10, 26].

Before turning to the role of Synacthen, i.e. of synthetic β1–24 tetracosapeptide, in clinical practice and to the problems which its use may entail, I should first like to make a brief reference to the question of dosage.

In diseases for which long-term treatment with A.C.T.H. is resorted to, the aim of this medication is to step up the production and secretion of cortisol and thereby achieve an anti-inflammatory, anti-allergic, or immunosuppressive effect. For this purpose, biologically active cortisol is required—in other words, cortisol which is not bound to transcortin. It can be reckoned that, in adults who have neither undergone prior treatment with oestrogens nor are suffering

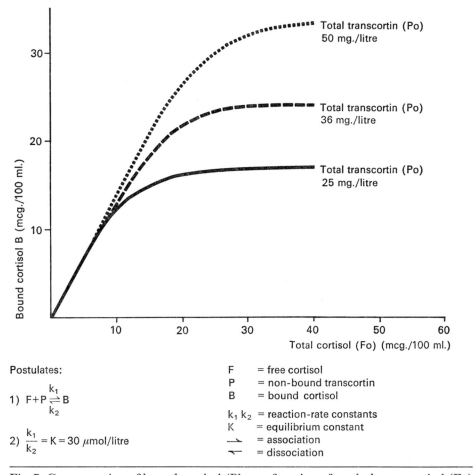

Postulates:

1) $F+P \underset{k_2}{\overset{k_1}{\rightleftharpoons}} B$

2) $\dfrac{k_1}{k_2} = K = 30 \; \mu mol/litre$

F = free cortisol
P = non-bound transcortin
B = bound cortisol

$k_1 \, k_2$ = reaction-rate constants
K = equilibrium constant
→ = association
↽ = dissociation

Fig. 7. Concentration of bound cortisol (B) as a function of total plasma cortisol (Fo) at various total transcortin blood levels (Po).

from liver cirrhosis, the total transcortin concentration averages about 36 mg./litre. The amount of cortisol which this 36 mg./litre is capable of binding works out at approximately 25 mcg./100 ml.; consequently, if the total plasma cortisol concentration is 30 mcg./100 ml., only 5 mcg./100 ml. of this cortisol will be biologically active (Figures 7 and 8).

As indicated in Figure 9, the values change where the total transcortin concentration is either lowered or elevated. From this it can be deduced that, where the adrenal cortex is being subjected to chronic stimulation by means of A.C.T.H. therapy, a plasma cortisol level of between 40 and 60 mcg./100 ml. needs to be attained in order to ensure a requisite concentration of biologically active cortisol.

Unfortunately no representative data are available showing the relationship between, on the one hand, the plasma cortisol levels under treatment with A.C.T.H. and, on the other, the therapeutic effect observed. Although it is known, for example, that maximal plasma cortisol values of 30–60 mcg./100 ml. are recorded two to four hours after a surgical operation[14, 21], more accurate

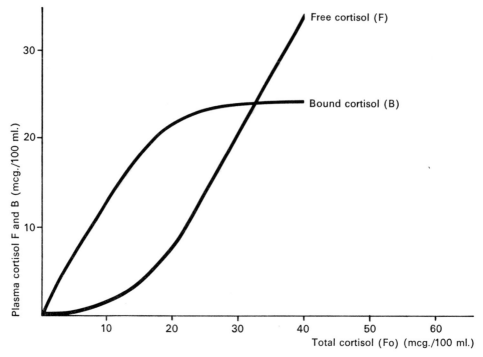

Postulates:

1) $F+P \underset{k_2}{\overset{k_1}{\rightleftharpoons}} B$

2) $\dfrac{k_1}{k_2} = K = 30\ \mu mol/litre$

3) $Po = 36\ mg./litre$

Fig. 8. Concentration of free cortisol (F) and bound cortisol (B) as a function of total plasma cortisol (Fo).

studies will have to be performed in order to provide a sound theoretical basis for the empirical treatment schedules currently employed. Incidentally, no changes in the binding capacity of transcortin, i.e. neither an increase nor a decrease in the concentration of this globulin in the plasma, have been detected during treatment with A.C.T.H.[28].

Figures 10, 11, and 12 show how the plasma cortisol levels behave in response to various doses of Synacthen Depot. These examples indicate, among other things, how important it is that the dosage should also be individually adapted when carrying out long-term A.C.T.H. therapy. A single intramuscular injection of 1 mg. Synacthen Depot causes the plasma cortisol concentration to rise by roughly 100%, the maximal value being attained after about eight hours; thanks to the nocturnal increase in A.C.T.H. secretion which is typical of the nyctohemeral rhythm of adrenocortical activity, an elevated plasma

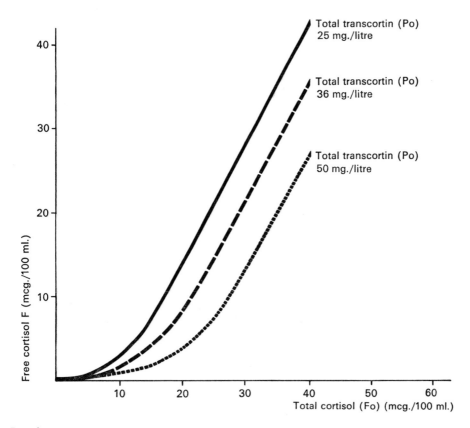

Postulates:

1) $F + P \underset{k_2}{\overset{k_1}{\rightleftharpoons}} B$

2) $\dfrac{k_1}{k_2} = K = 30 \ \mu\text{mol/litre}$

Fig. 9. Concentration of free cortisol (F) as a function of total plasma cortisol (Fo) at various total transcortin blood levels (Po).

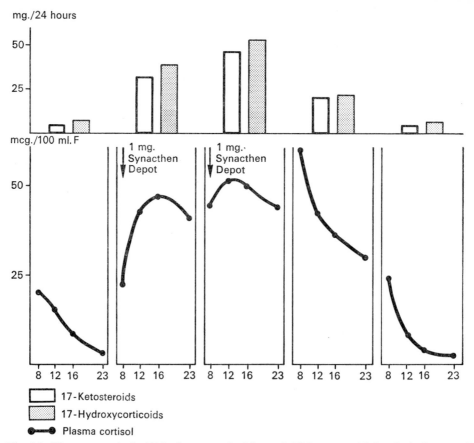

mg./24 hours

mcg./100 ml. F

1 mg. Synacthen Depot

1 mg. Synacthen Depot

8 12 16 23 8 12 16 23 8 12 16 23 8 12 16 23 8 12 16 23

☐ 17-Ketosteroids
▦ 17-Hydroxycorticoids
●━● Plasma cortisol

Fig. 10. Plasma cortisol, 17-hydroxycorticoid, and 17-ketosteroid levels before and after intramuscular injection of 1 mg. Synacthen Depot on each of two successive days.

cortisol concentration may still be recorded after 24 hours. Where 1 mg. Synacthen Depot is administered on each of two successive days (Figure 10), the plasma cortisol concentrations on the second day exceed those measured on the first day and remain for some 40 hours at a higher level than the usual morning values of 15–20 mcg./100 ml.

In our experience, single injections of 2 mg. Synacthen Depot offer no additional advantages, either as regards the degree to which the adrenal cortex is stimulated or with respect to the drug's duration of effect (Figure 11).

Figure 12, relating to a patient who had been receiving Synacthen Depot for three weeks, serves to illustrate that, even where A.C.T.H. therapy has been in progress for only a relatively short time, the responsiveness of the adrenal cortex already shows an increase, as evidenced by the fact that the injection of 0.5 mg. Synacthen Depot given on the 20th day stimulated cortisol secretion to such an extent that the plasma cortisol concentration after eight hours was some four times higher than that recorded in the morning. This phenomenon is attributable to adrenal hypertrophy, which in turn is associated with an enhancement of

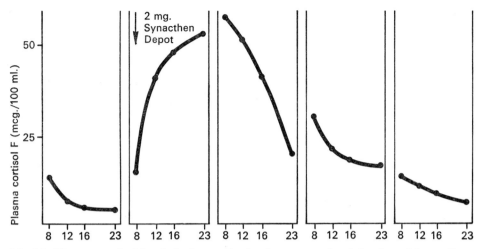

Fig. 11. Plasma cortisol levels before and after intramuscular injection of 2 mg. Synacthen Depot.

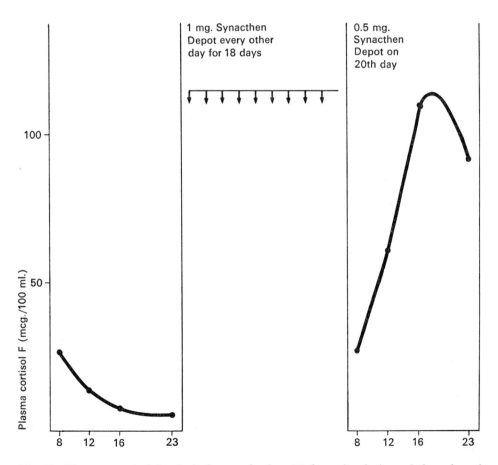

Fig. 12. Plasma cortisol levels before and after 18-day stimulation of the adrenal cortex (1 mg. Synacthen Depot every other day) plus an intramuscular injection of 0.5 mg. Synacthen Depot on the 20th day.

adrenocortical function. SOKOLOFF et al.[38], for example, found that in two patients who had been treated with A.C.T.H. the weight of the adrenals had increased to 27.8 and 28.4 g., respectively; and BRANSOME and REDDY[4] report that in another case examined at autopsy the adrenals weighed as much as 45.5 g. In two infants who died at the ages of eight and nine months after having received intermittent A.C.T.H. therapy alternating with doses of ®Decortin and dexamethasone, respectively, the weight of the adrenals was 19.4 g. and 17.6 g.[6].

Just as adrenocortical atrophy is regarded as a significant hazard of long-term treatment with synthetic glucocorticoids, so must adrenocortical hypertrophy also be borne in mind as a possible risk of prolonged A.C.T.H. therapy. When employing A.C.T.H. it is consequently also essential that the dosage be individually adapted. This individualisation of the dosage can be accurately effected only by checking the plasma cortisol levels; measurement of the Porter-Silber chromogens and 17-ketosteroids in the 24-hour urine also provides additional useful clues. As already mentioned previously, an increase in the total plasma cortisol concentration to 40–60 mcg./100 ml.—or at least to 30 mcg./100 ml.—should in most cases prove sufficient to elicit the desired therapeutic effect, while at the same time also ensuring that the daily rhythm of endogenous A.C.T.H. and cortisol secretion is to some extent maintained.

Since the duration of effect of Synacthen Depot on plasma cortisol levels does not amount to more than about 36 hours, this means that, after having initiated therapy with daily injections, one should administer at least three injections per week as maintenance treatment. As already emphasised, the doses should be individually adapted to the patient's requirements, and in many cases it is certainly possible to reduce them to as little as 0.5 mg. or less. This treatment schedule calling for injections given as frequently as three times a week is, of course, based on purely theoretical considerations and conflicts with numerous clinical reports indicating that, even where the interval between injections is much longer, a satisfactory maintenance effect can often be achieved.

It is still chiefly in the light of clinical experience that the value of long-term A.C.T.H. therapy in a given disease must at present be assessed. In certain indications a great deal of experience has been acquired which merits due attention. Particularly worthy of note are the results obtained in the treatment of asthma, chronic or rheumatoid arthritis, nephrotic syndrome, ulcerative colitis, and Crohn's disease, as well as in the management of skin disorders, e.g. pemphigus, and of neurological conditions such as certain forms of polyneuritis and myasthenia gravis.

Preference should be given to the use of depot A.C.T.H. particularly in cases where treatment with synthetic glucocorticoids either proves unsatisfactory or would have to be given in excessively high daily dosages. It should also be pointed out that fairly prolonged remissions have been observed during and after A.C.T.H. therapy; whatever the explanation for such remissions may be, they certainly cannot be ascribed to a persisting overproduction of endogenous cortisol. Whether, in addition to its stimulant action on the adrenal cortex, A.C.T.H. exerts a peripheral effect as well, is still a moot point.

The use of A.C.T.H. is also assuming increasing importance in patients exhibiting a tendency to gastric ulcers or in cases where gastric ulcers have developed during treatment with glucocorticoids. In this connection it should perhaps be added that patients with Cushing's syndrome do not show a higher susceptibility to gastric ulceration.

In children requiring prolonged treatment, A C.T.H. is likewise preferable to glucocorticoids, because the latter entail the risk of inhibiting growth. Experience to date does not suggest that intermittent alternating administration of A.C.T.H. and steroids offers any significant advantages.

The main problems posed by long-term treatment with A.C.T.H. lie, firstly, in the difficulties encountered in adapting the dosage to the patient's individual requirements and, secondly, in the fact that the drug has to be given by injection and at relatively frequent intervals. Side effects that are liable to restrict the scope of treatment with A.C.T.H. may include, on the one hand, an excessively strong mineralocorticoid action—leading to salt and water retention, a rise in blood pressure, and hypopotassaemia—and, on the other hand, a pronounced androgenic effect resulting in hirsutism, acne, and menstrual disorders in women. The diabetogenic effect of A.C.T.H. therapy, by contrast, appears to be less of a problem than in the case of treatment with glucocorticoids. As for Cushing's syndrome, it should be possible to avoid or minimise mooning of the face, obesity, etc. by appropriately adjusting the dosage.

In cases of A.C.T.H.-induced adrenal hypertrophy, no morphological changes of any importance have yet been detected. Although discrete haemorrhages within the adrenal gland have occasionally been reported, these observations are of no conclusive significance, because such haemorrhages are not necessarily due solely to the fact of the patient's having undergone prolonged treatment with A.C.T.H.

The synthesis of β1–24 tetracosapeptide (Synacthen), which displays the full biological activity of the complete A.C.T.H. molecule, has undoubtedly broadened the scope of therapy for diseases that had previously been treated solely with synthetic glucocorticoids. What would now be most welcome, however, are not more potent A.C.T.H. preparations, but depot formulations possessing a longer duration of effect, which would enable us to manage with intramuscular injections given at less frequent intervals than are at present necessary. In addition, clinico-experimental studies on the correlation between the diurnal plasma cortisol levels and the therapeutic effect of A.C.T.H. medication should be intensified. Moreover, since treatment with A.C.T.H. stimulates the production not only of cortisol but also of anabolic androgens, we likewise require further representative observations on effects attributable to the antagonistic activity of these androgens, particularly with regard to the development of osteoporosis and muscular atrophy. Finally, with the aid of modern methods, we must discover more about the kinetics of cortisol and the synthetic steroids—i.e. about their protein-binding in the plasma, their tissue affinities, the receptors on which they act in the tissues, and their metabolic pathways—so that we shall then have a sound scientific basis to which we can relate our clinical experience.

References

1 ARAKI, Y., YOKOTA, O., KATO, T., KASHIMA, M., MIYAZAKI, T.: Dynamics of synthetic corticosteroids in man. In Pincus, G., Nakao, T., Tait, J.F. (Editors): Steroid dynamics, Proc. Symp. Dynamics of steroid hormones, Tokyo 1965, p.463 (Acad. Press, New York/London 1966)

2 ARNOLDSSON, H.: Allergic reactions to ACTH. Acta allerg. (Kbh.) *12*, Suppl. VI: 122 (1958)

3 BOCK, H.E.: Kortikosteroidtherapie neurologischer Erkrankungen – mit besonderer Berücksichtigung der Nebenwirkungen. Ther. Umsch. *23*, 112 (1966)

4 BRANSOME, E.D., Jr., REDDY, W.J.: Studies of adrenal nucleic acids. RNA, DNA and total protein in human adrenal dysfunction. Metabolism *12*, 27 (1963)

5 CATT, K.J.: Growth hormone. Lancet *i*, 933 (1970)

6 DHOM: Personal communication

7 DUCHAINE, J., SPAPEN, R., JACQUES, M.: L'allergie à l'A.C.T.H. – Etude expérimentale. Rev. franç. Allerg. *2*, 15 (1962)

8 FELBER, J.-P., AUBERT, M.L.: Study on the specificity of antisera used for the radioimmunological determination of ACTH. Measurement of the circadian rhythm of plasma ACTH. In Margoulies, M. (Editor): Protein and polypeptide hormones, Proc. Int. Symp., Liège 1968. Int. Congr. Ser. No. 161, p. 373 (Excerpta med. Found., Amsterdam 1969)

9 FRIEDMAN, M., STRANG, L.B.: Effect of long-term corticosteroids and corticotrophin on the growth of children. Lancet *ii*, 568 (1966)

10 FRIEDMAN, M., STRANG, L.B.: The effects of corticosteroid and ACTH therapy on growth and on the hypothalamic-pituitary adrenal axis of children. Scand. J. resp. Dis. Suppl. 68: 58 (1969)

11 GANONG, W.F., BIGLIERI, E.G., MULROW, P.J.: Mechanisms regulating adrenocortical secretion of aldosterone and glucocorticoids. Rec. Progr. Horm. Res. *22*, 381 (1966)

12 GIRARD, J., HIRT, H.R., BÜHLER, U., ZACHMANN, U., WICK, H., BAUMANN, J.B., STAHL, M.: Long-term treatment with ACTH and allergenic properties of synthetic $\beta^{1\text{-}24}$ corticotrophin. Helv. paediat. Acta *26*, 46 (1971)

13 GLASS, D., NUKI, G., DALY, J.R.: Development of antibodies during long-term therapy with corticotrophin in rheumatoid arthritis. II. Zinc tetracosactrin (Depot Synacthen). Ann. rheum. Dis. *30*, 593 (1971)

14 HAMANAKA, Y., MANABE, H., TANAKA, H., MONDEN, Y., UOZUMI, T., MATSUMOTO, K.: Effects of surgery on plasma levels of cortisol, corticosterone and non-protein-bound cortisol. Acta endocr. *64*, 439 (1970)

15 IRVINE, W.J., CULLEN, D.R., KHAN, S.A., RATCLIFFE, J.G.: Hypothalamic-pituitary-adrenal function in patients treated with long-term depot tetracosactrin. Brit. med. J. *i*, 630 (1971)

16 JAMES, V.H.T.: The investigation of pituitary-adrenal function: effects of corticosteroid and corticotrophin therapy. Pharmacol. clin. *2*, 182 (1970)

17 KAPPELER, H., SCHWYZER, R.: Die Synthese eines Tetracosapeptides mit der Aminosäuresequenz eines hochaktiven Abbauproduktes des β-Corticotropins (ACTH) aus Schweinehypophysen (Vorläufige Mitteilung). Helv. chim. Acta *44*, 1136 (1961)

18 KARL, H.J.: Adrenocorticotrope Wirkung eines vollsynthetischen Tetracosapeptids – $\beta^{1\text{-}24}$Corticotrophin – beim Menschen. Klin. Wschr. *41*, 633 (1963)

19 LANDON, J., FRIEDMAN, M., GREENWOOD, F.C.: Antibodies to corticotrophin and their relation to adrenal function in children receiving corticotrophin therapy. Lancet *i*, 652 (1967)

20 LAULER, D.P., THORN, G.W.: Diseases of the adrenal cortex. In Harrison, T.R., et al. (Editors): Principles of internal medicine, 5th Ed. Vol. I, p. 449 (481) (McGraw-Hill, New York/Toronto/Sydney/London 1966)

21 Le Quesne, L.P.: The response of the adrenal cortex to surgical stress. In Wolstenholme, G.E.W., Porter, R. (Editors): The human adrenal cortex, Ciba Found. Study Group No. 27, p. 65 (Churchill, London 1967)

22 Linèt, O.: Interactions between androgenic-anabolic steroids and glucocorticoids. In Jucker, E. (Editor): Progress in drug research, Vol. 14, p. 139 (Birkhäuser, Basle/Stuttgart 1970)

23 Llaurado, J.G.: Increased excretion of aldosterone immediately after operation. Lancet 268, 1295 (1955)

24 Maeder, E., Schwarz-Speck, M.: Allergieteste mit natürlichem und synthetischem ACTH. Dermatologica (Basle) 129, 59 (1964)

25 Melby, J.C.: Pathophysiology of shock. In Schumer, W., Nyhus, L.M. (Editors): Corticosteroids in the treatment of shock, p. 1 (Univ. Illinois Press, Urbana/Chicago/London 1970)

26 Moulaert, A.J., Gemund, J.J. van: Elimination of severe height growth suppression caused by treatment with betamethasone after switching to ACTH-depot in chronic bronchial asthma. Paediatrica No. 362: 1 (1971)

27 Murphy, B.E.P.: Application of the property of protein-binding to the assay of minute quantities of hormones and other substances. Nature (Lond.) 201, 679 (1964)

28 Murphy, B.E.P., Pattee, C.J.: A study of the binding capacity of corticosteroid-binding globulin in plasma. J. clin. Endocr. 23, 459 (1963)

29 Nelson, J.K., Neill, D.W., Montgomery, D.A.D., MacKay, J.S., Sheridan, B., Weaver, J.A.: Synacthen Depot – adrenal response in normal subjects and corticotrophin-treated patients. Brit. med. J. i, 557 (1968)

30 Nugent, C.A., Eik-Nes, K., Tyler, F.H.: A comparative study of the metabolism of hydrocortisone and prednisolone. J. clin. Endocr. 19, 526 (1959)

31 Pandos, P., Strauch, G., Bricaire, H.: Corticotrophin-induced growth-hormone release. Lancet ii, 527 (1970)

32 Raith, L., Karl, H.J.: Biologische Halbwertszeit, Abbau und Ausscheidung von 16-Methylprednisolon. Klin. Wschr. 44, 298 (1966)

33 Rajka, G.: On the prophylactic possibilities in ACTH allergy. Acta allerg. (Kbh.) 16, 159 (1961)

34 Ratcliffe, J.G., Pritchard, M., El-Shaboury, A.H.: The production of antibodies to porcine corticotrophin and to Synacthen. J. Endocr. 43, 1 (1969)

35 Scheiffarth, F., Götz, H.: Experimentelle Untersuchungen zur Frage sensibilisierender Nebenwirkungen von Tetracosactid. Drug Res. 20, 381 (1970)

36 Schuler, W., Schär, B., Desaulles, P.: Zur Pharmakologie eines ACTH-wirksamen, vollsynthetischen Polypeptids, des β^{1-24}-Corticotropins, CIBA 30'290-Ba, Synacthen. Schweiz. med. Wschr. 93, 1027 (1963)

37 Schwyzer, R.: Relationship of structure to activity of polypeptide hormones, loc. cit.[8], p.201

38 Sokoloff, L., Sharp, J.T., Kaufman, E.H.: The adrenal cortex in rheumatic disease. A.M.A. Arch. intern. Med. 88, 627 (1951)

39 Treadwell, B.L.J., Sever, E.D., Savage, O., Copeman, W.S.C.: Side-effects of long-term treatment with corticosteroids and corticotrophin. Lancet i, 1121 (1964)

40 West, H.F.: Acquired resistance to corticotropins. Ann. rheum. Dis. 15, 124 (1956)

41 West, H.F.: Ten years of ACTH therapy. Ann. rheum. Dis. 21, 263 (1962)

42 Zárate, O., Quinteros, H.: Preliminary report on the therapeutic use of a synthetic corticotrophin. J. Allergy 38, 51 (1966)

Allergenic properties of A.C.T.H.

by J. GIRARD, L. LIPCHITZ, and P.W. NARS*

In the following paper we do not propose to deal with the indications for the diagnostic or therapeutic use of adrenocorticotrophic hormone, since these indications are discussed elsewhere in various contributions to the proceedings of this symposium.

The pharmacological, adrenal or extra-adrenal, effects of A.C.T.H. will be judged as desirable or undesirable, depending on the illness to be treated. On the other hand, immunological responses to the drug, such as localised or generalised allergic or anaphylactic reactions or induction of antibody formation, will without exception be recognised as undesirable side effects. (Deliberate induction of antibodies against a hormone, with the aim of neutralising endogenous overproduction, remains—to our knowledge—wishful thinking rather than a practical possibility.)

If A.C.T.H. is to be given to a patient, *one* of the important considerations in choosing the compound to be used is the degree to which it displays allergenic properties, particularly in cases where repeated administration or long-term therapy are envisaged. Elucidation of the chemical structure of A.C.T.H. obtained from different species revealed that the species-specific segment is restricted to an amino acid sequence of the peptide which is not involved in its biological activity[3, 8, 19, 20, 28]. That foreign proteins and peptides, e.g. A.C.T.H. of animal origin, are potentially antigenic when administered to patients is common knowledge. It is not surprising, therefore, that allergic and anaphylactic reactions after treatment with natural A.C.T.H. of animal origin have frequently been reported[23, 33, 35, 39]. Circulating antibodies have been detected in from 30% to over 60% of patients who have been treated with such substances[7, 15, 24].

Immunological studies have shown that these antibodies are mainly directed against the C-terminal species-specific part of the molecule[8, 24]. (Antibodies directed against impurities present in A.C.T.H. extract-preparations were also reported before highly purified A.C.T.H. became available.) It accordingly seemed reasonable to assume that a peptide containing only the species-nonspecific biologically active N-terminal amino acid sequence, 1–24, would in principle have no antigenic properties. Animal experiments and experience in humans treated with synthetic β1–24 corticotrophin (®Synacthen, tetracosactide CIBA) showed, however, that antibodies against the 1–24 sequence can likewise be induced[1, 9, 11, 13, 14, 25] and that allergic reactions may also occur[4–6, 16, 22, 29, 37].

---

*Abteilung für Endokrinologie der Universitätskinderklinik, Basle, Switzerland.

Personal investigations and data from the literature on the allergenic properties of β1–24 corticotrophin

The induction of antibodies featuring combining sites directed against the 1–24 sequence has been reported after immunisation of rabbits and guinea-pigs with natural A.C.T.H. obtained by extraction[1, 8]. In humans, prolonged treatment with natural porcine A.C.T.H. occasionally induces antibodies with combining sites directed not only against the species-specific 25–33 amino acid sequence but also against the N-terminal 1–24 sequence[8, 24]. (The difference between human and porcine A.C.T.H. is now known to lie only in amino acid position 31[32].) Thus, antibodies directed against the 1–24 sequence can be produced through immunisation with natural A.C.T.H. containing the entire 1–39 molecule.

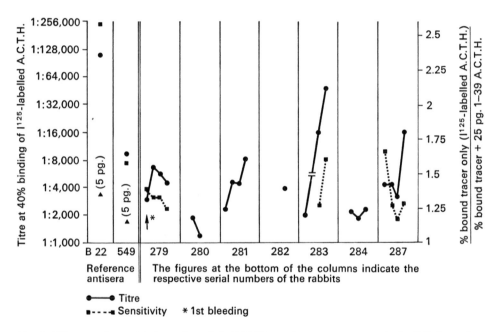

Fig. 1. Titre and sensitivity of anti-A.C.T.H. antisera over a period of 6–8 weeks following the last A.C.T.H. injection. The reference antisera B 22 (kindly donated by Prof. R. Depieds, Laboratoire d'Immunologie, Marseilles, France) and 549 (produced with Synacthen Depot) are shown for purposes of comparison.
Each rabbit was bled at fortnightly intervals after the last injection. The results of the different bleedings are shown separately for each rabbit. Only samples with a titre above 1 : 1,000 and a sensitivity capable of distinguishing 25 pg. of unlabelled A.C.T.H. are shown.
Sensitivity is here defined as the ratio of bound labelled A.C.T.H. only (in %) to bound labelled A.C.T.H. with 25 pg. of unlabelled synthetic 1–39 A.C.T.H. added (in %). The higher the value of this ratio, the greater the sensitivity to 25 pg. A.C.T.H. (For the two reference antisera, the ratio obtained using 5 pg. of unlabelled A.C.T.H. is represented by a triangle.)
All seven antisera (279–284 and 287) were raised in the seven rabbits immunised with natural A.C.T.H. None of 16 rabbits immunised in the same way with Synacthen showed a significant antibody titre.

99

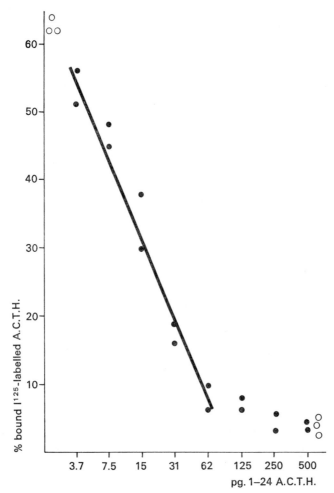

Fig. 2. Standard curve showing the sensitivity to 1–24 A.C.T.H. of an antiserum induced with 1–39 peptide (antiserum B 22 in Figure 1). Final dilution: 1:80,000; incubation time: 48 hours at 4 °C.; incubation volume: 300 mcl.; separating medium: charcoal.

As has been demonstrated by others, and also confirmed in our own laboratory, avid antibodies directed against the 1–24 sequence of A.C.T.H. can also be induced by immunising rabbits and guinea-pigs with synthetic β1–24 cortico-trophin [9, 11, 14]. Antibodies intended for use in radioimmunoassay studies must be of high avidity and should be directed against the biologically active part of the molecule. A recent experiment from our laboratory illustrates the general finding that the 1–39 peptide is a much better antigen than the 1–24 sequence. The course of titre and sensitivity of antisera from seven rabbits immunised with natural corticotrophin are outlined in Figure 1. All the seven animals produced detectable antibodies following three injections. The strong avidity and sensi-tivity of an antiserum induced with 1–39 A.C.T.H. can be seen from Figure 2; in tests in which this antiserum was employed, it was found possible to detect quantities of tetracosactide amounting to less than 4 pg. On the other hand, when the same immunisation schedule was employed to immunise 16 rabbits with Synacthen, no significant antibody titre could be demonstrated in any of the blood samples from these animals. It must be pointed out that these

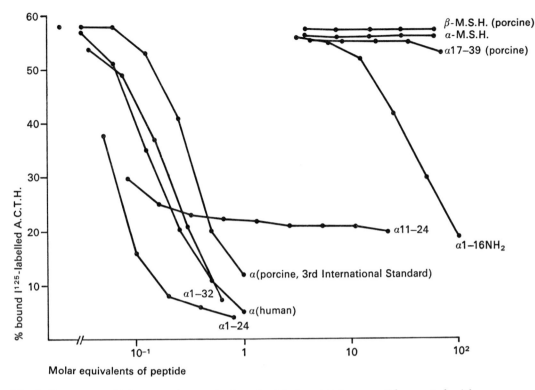

Fig. 3. Extent to which an antiserum induced with depot tetracosactide reacted with various A.C.T.H. fragments and analogues. (The analysis was performed by J. G. RATCLIFFE, Department of Clinical Biochemistry, Royal Infirmary, Glasgow.)

experiments were performed with aqueous solutions of Synacthen and aqueous extracted A.C.T.H.

Using the zinc complex of tetracosactide (Synacthen Depot), however, we and others were able to raise avid antibodies in rabbits and guinea-pigs. The extent to which an antiserum induced by Synacthen Depot in our laboratory reacted with various A.C.T.H. fragments and analogues is shown in Figure 3. The number of animals responding to the Synacthen Depot immunisation, however, was far smaller than the number responding to immunisation with 1–39 A.C.T.H. (cf. Table 1).

Similarly, all reactions—whether clinical or serological—that occur in response to treatment with tetracosactide in humans are without exception observed after prolonged use of the zinc-complex depot preparation. Whether these reactions are due to a specific property of the zinc complex or are an "unavoidable" and non-specific effect of such depot preparations is a question that remains to be answered. Published data, from the literature available to us, concerning patients who—having never previously received treatment with any other A.C.T.H. preparation—developed antibodies or allergic reactions in response to $\beta 1$–24 corticotrophin are summarised in Table 2.

Table 1. Induction of anti-A.C.T.H. antibodies in animals and man.

a) *In animal experiments*	Number of rabbits with antibodies	Number of rabbits immunised
Natural A.C.T.H.	7	7
Synacthen	0	14
Synacthen Depot	2	6

b) *Following therapeutic use*	Number of patients with antibodies	Number of patients studied or showing clinical reactions
Natural A.C.T.H. (*Fleischer* et al.[7])	8	9
Natural A.C.T.H. (*Landon* et al.[24])	13	19
Synacthen Depot (*Glass* et al.[16])	6	18
Synacthen Depot (*Glass* et al.[17])	12	38
Synacthen Depot (*Girard* et al.[14])	3	7
Synacthen Depot (present series)	0	14

Table 2. Reports on allergic responses to depot tetracosactide in patients not previously treated with other A.C.T.H. preparations.

Number of patients investigated	Positive clinical reactions: Localised	Generalised	Circulating antibodies	Reference
		1	n.i.*	*Patriarca*[29]
	1	1	n.i.	*Jensen* and *Sneddon*[22]
		2	n.i.	*Charpin* and *Aubert*[4]**
		1	n.i.	*Uzzan* et al.[37]**
		18	6	*Glass* et al.[16]
7		1(?)	3	*Girard* et al.[14]
14	0	0	0	*Girard* et al. (present series)
38	0	0	12	*Glass* et al.[17]

* Not investigated (by radioimmunoassay)
** Original literature not available; not established with certainty that treatment had consisted exclusively of Synacthen Depot

Our own investigation of 21 paediatric patients on long-term A.C.T.H. therapy was prompted by the suspicion of an adrenal crisis during the unusually fulminant course of an infection in an infant treated for nine weeks with Synacthen Depot[13]. Data on the patients investigated in the present study are given in Table 3. All the children were treated only with Synacthen Depot and had never received any other adrenocorticotrophin preparation. "Side effects" such as extreme cushingoid features, excessive weight gain, and hypertension occurred in all patients to varying degrees, depending on the frequency and dose of the injections. Glycosuria was present in some cases, but no hypernatraemia or hypopotassaemia were observed. Case reports on the patients with A.C.T.H. antibodies have already been published[14]. Further details and follow-up data on children receiving continuing A.C.T.H. therapy will be published in due course.

Table 3. Data on the 21 paediatric patients investigated in the present study.

Patient	Duration of treatment	Dosage of Synacthen Depot	Diagnosis	Anti-A.C.T.H. antibodies
G.S.	3½ weeks	15 times 0.2 mg.	Hypsarrhythmia**	—
B.B.	7 weeks	22 times 0.2 mg.	Hypsarrhythmia	—
S.L.	4 weeks	13 times 0.3 mg.	Hypsarrhythmia	—
B.V.	5 weeks	20 times 0.3 mg.	Hypsarrhythmia	—
B.A.	8 months	77 times 0.3 mg.*	Cerebellar ataxia	—
D.G.	3½ weeks	10 times 0.3 mg. 9 times 0.4 mg.	Hypsarrhythmia	—
S.M.	6 weeks	24 times 0.3 mg.	Hypsarrhythmia	—***
J.K.	5 weeks	8 times 0.2 mg.	Hypsarrhythmia	—***
I.T.	4 weeks	14 times 0.3 mg.	Hypsarrhythmia	—***
E.J.	6 weeks	27 times 0.3 mg.	Hypsarrhythmia	—***
G.N.	4½ weeks	15 times 0.2 mg.	Hypsarrhythmia	—
I.M.	14 weeks	19 times 0.3 mg.	Miliary tuberculosis	—
S.D.	15 weeks	9 times 0.2 mg. 35 times 0.1 mg.	Hypoglycaemia	—
S.S.	8 weeks	11 times 0.2 mg. 7 times 0.3 mg.	Hypsarrhythmia	—
M.J.	9 weeks	26 times 0.3 mg.	Hypsarrhythmia	+
W.S.	3 years	Twice-weekly doses decreasing from 0.5 to 0.005 mg.	Hypopituitarism	+
M.H.	6 months	3 times weekly 1 mg.	Aplastic anaemia	—
M.P.	3 months	21 times 0.2 mg.	Hypsarrhythmia	—
A.M.	3 months	17 times 0.4 mg.	Hypsarrhythmia	—
R.J.	6 months	30 times 0.25 mg.	Hypsarrhythmia	—
B.P.	. . . . No data available.			+

* With a two-month interruption of therapy
** Usual injection schedule used: five injections during the first week, followed by a gradual decrease over five weeks to one injection weekly
*** The first of two blood samples was taken on the day of the first injection of Synacthen Depot.

Materials and methods

Blood samples were taken not earlier than 48 hours after discontinuation of A.C.T.H. therapy. The blood was centrifuged and the plasma frozen until assayed. Synthetic porcine 1–39 A.C.T.H. (supplied by CIBA-GEIGY LIMITED) was used for iodination by the chloramine-T method, and the iodinated A.C.T.H. was purified by cellulose column-chromatography or by adsorption to ®Quso[2, 27, 41]. Each aliquot of labelled A.C.T.H. was repurified with ®Spherosil immediately before use. Damage to the label was checked by chromato-electrophoresis and with dextran-coated charcoal. The immunological reactivity was tested with a standardised excess of rabbit anti-β1–24 corticotrophin[11].

Serial dilutions of the patients' plasmas were performed in 0.06 M. barbitone buffer (pH 8.6) containing human serum albumin (2.5 mg./ml.), mercaptoethanol (0.5%), and Trasylol* (500 U./ml.).

---

* Peptidase inhibitor (®Trasylol Bayer).

Patient and control plasmas were prepared in quadruplicate in a final incubation volume of 250 mcl. containing a maximum amount of 50–100 mcl. of patient plasma. The quantity of labelled A.C.T.H. added in the different assay series was 5 pg., 18.7 pg., and 30 pg., respectively. After incubation at 4 °C. for 48 hours, two of the four series were acidified with 0.5N HCl and left to stand for five minutes. The antibody-bound labelled A.C.T.H. was then separated from the free fraction with dextran-coated charcoal.

For the determination of binding capacity, 50 mcl. of patient plasma was incubated with 18.7 or 30 pg. of labelled A.C.T.H. and increasing amounts of unlabelled antigen, i.e. synthetic β1–24 corticotrophin (Synacthen) and synthetic porcine 1–39 corticotrophin.

Results

Evidence of the presence of antibodies in a plasma sample was accepted as positive on the basis of the following criteria: the percentage of labelled A.C.T.H. bound by the patient's plasma exceeds the non-specific binding capacity of a control plasma by at least 10 %; the binding of labelled A.C.T.H. decreases in serial dilutions of the plasma sample; antigen-antibody binding can be dissociated by acidification; labelled A.C.T.H. can be displaced by an excess of unlabelled antigen.

When we employed these criteria in testing 25 plasma samples from the 21 children treated with Synacthen Depot, we found that three children had developed circulating antibodies capable of binding a significant amount of labelled 1–39 A.C.T.H. (Table 3).

The results of more extensive studies of the plasmas containing A.C.T.H. antibodies are illustrated in Figures 4–6. The binding of labelled 1–39 A.C.T.H. decreases depending on the amount of plasma present (Figure 4). After dissociation of the antigen-antibody binding by acidification, the percentage of labelled A.C.T.H. bound drops to the level of "apparent binding" of the control plasma—a level accounted for by damaged labelled hormone which can be separated off with charcoal-dextran (Figure 5). The binding capacity of the plasma for A.C.T.H. could only be approximately estimated. In our view, the method used does not allow any correction to be made for damage to labelled A.C.T.H. Furthermore, the antibodies could not be shown to have an identical affinity for labelled and unlabelled hormone. The preconditions for calculating

---

Fig. 5. The binding of antigen by antibody can readily be dissociated by acidification, i.e. by lowering the pH to between 2 and 3. As the behaviour of damaged hormone in the charcoal-dextran system of separation is not affected by such a drop in pH, this method is suitable for distinguishing between antibody-bound and damaged hormone in a radioimmunological study. The diluent control and the "apparent binding" of the control plasma are not affected by acidification; the "apparent binding" is accounted for by damaged hormone. The binding of A.C.T.H. to rabbit anti-β1–24 antiserum is dissociated after acidification, and the damage level stays below 3 %. Similarly, the A.C.T.H. bound to the patient's plasma is split after acidification, and the damage level is then comparable to that of the control serum. The binding of A.C.T.H. by the patient's plasma is therefore an antigen-antibody reaction.

Fig. 4. Binding of I^{125}-labelled porcine 1–39 A.C.T.H. by aliquots of the patients' plasmas ranging from 100 to 3.1 mcl. As the amount of plasma present diminishes, so the binding of labelled A.C.T.H. decreases, i.e. from 55%, 58%, and 74% to 16%, 20%, and 22%, respectively. A control plasma gives an "apparent binding" of 12%–15%. In the diluent control, only 1–4% of labelled A.C.T.H. was separated off by adsorption on to charcoal. The difference between the diluent and the control plasma is easily explained by the increased incubation damage due to enzymatic degradation in plasma. Thirty pg. of labelled A.C.T.H. incubated with a 1:4,000 final dilution of rabbit anti-β1–24 antiserum gives a binding of 65%–68%.

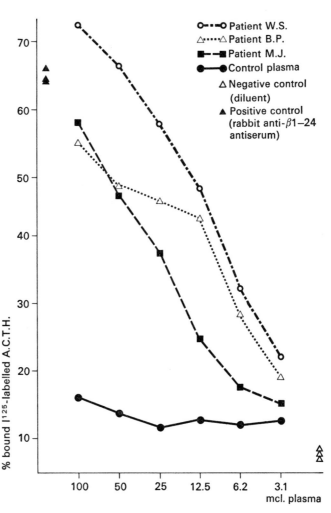

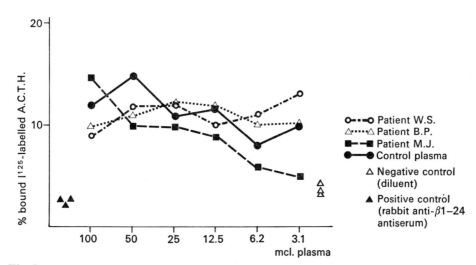

Fig. 5

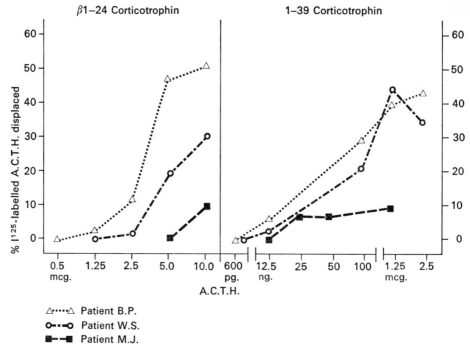

Fig. 6. Displacement of I¹²⁵-labelled porcine 1–39 corticotrophin from binding to patients' plasmas by β1–24 corticotrophin (*left*) and 1–39 corticotrophin (*right*); 50 mcl. of patients' plasmas was used with 18.7 pg. of labelled 1–39 A.C.T.H.
The values referred to in the text were calculated according to the following example: 1.25 mcg. of non-labelled β1–24 corticotrophin does not displace a significant amount of labelled A.C.T.H. from the plasma of patient B.P.; 50 mcl. of this patient's plasma is therefore able to bind at least 1.25 mcg. β1–24 corticotrophin, yielding an estimated minimum binding capacity of 25 mcg. β1–24 corticotrophin per ml. plasma.

an absolute binding capacity were thus not fulfilled. Estimation was therefore based on the minimum amount of unlabelled antigen necessary to displace at least 10% of labelled A.C.T.H. from its binding to 50 mcl. of patient plasma. For the three plasmas investigated, the binding capacities per millilitre of plasma were 25 mcg., 50 mcg., and 100 mcg. β1–24 corticotrophin (Synacthen), respectively (Figure 6). The minimum binding capacity of the entire A.C.T.H. molecule, i.e. of synthetic porcine 1–39 A.C.T.H., was significantly lower, amounting to 250 ng. for two of the plasmas and 1 mcg. for the third (Figure 6).

Discussion

In the following discussion, allergic reactions and the detection of circulating antibodies against Synacthen will mainly be considered in patients who received only synthetic β1–24 corticotrophin and who had not previously been treated with natural A.C.T.H. obtained by extraction. Apart from our own study, we know of only two published reports dealing with the radioimmunological detection of antibodies in patients treated exclusively with Synacthen Depot.

In both series a high incidence of antibody formation was found: six out of 18[16] and 12 out of 38[17] treated patients were reported to have developed antibodies. In the latter series, the criterion used for judging an antibody titre as significant was a binding of labelled 1–24 A.C.T.H. amounting to at least three standard deviations above the mean non-specific binding of a control serum. The actual figures given in this publication, covering data from ten patients, show that the percentage binding of labelled 1–24 A.C.T.H. was below 10% in four of the patients, 14% in one case, and above 20% in the remaining five. When more stringent criteria are applied, however, the incidence of antibodies as reported by GLASS et al.[17] is found to be very similar to that observed in our own series.

The danger of inducing antibodies directed against the species-non-specific biologically active part of the A.C.T.H. molecule lies in the potential risk of binding and inactivating not only exogenous A.C.T.H., but also the patient's endogenous A.C.T.H. Although it would appear logical to assume that antibodies capable of binding the 1–24 fragment will also combine with the entire 1–39 A.C.T.H. molecule, we have obtained contradicting evidence from an animal experiment.

One rabbit (No. 359) immunised with Synacthen Depot developed antibodies capable of binding 50% of 100 pg. labelled 1–39 A.C.T.H. at a final dilution of 1:800. The antiserum obtained from a blood sample taken three months later had to be eight times more concentrated to achieve the same binding. Subsequently the antiserum increased in specificity. It lost its capacity to bind the entire 1–39 A.C.T.H. molecule and was capable only of binding the isolated 1–24 fragment. Similarly, the antibodies detected in the three patients in our series had a much higher binding capacity for the 1–24 fragment than for the entire A.C.T.H. molecule. Hence, it is obvious that an antibody specific for the isolated 1–24 sequence will not necessarily affect the endogenous A.C.T.H. molecule. Neutralisation of the 1–24 fragment by such an antiserum does not imply a binding or neutralisation of the 1–39 molecule.

In the series studied by GLASS et al.[17] the sera were investigated with the labelled 1–24 peptide; no displacement studies using the entire 1–39 molecule were performed. In our series, by contrast, all plasmas were tested with labelled 1–39 A.C.T.H. only; we would therefore not have detected antisera specific for the 1–24 fragment.

Acquired resistance to A.C.T.H. attributed to the presence of antibodies has been reported after the use of extracted A.C.T.H.[38]. LANDON et al.[24], however, found no impairment of adrenocortical function in children receiving corticotrophin therapy, despite the presence of anti-A.C.T.H. antibodies in most of these patients. Acquired resistance due to antibody formation is well known in the case of insulin[18, 40] and has also been reported to occur with growth hormone[30]. But among the large number of patients exhibiting detectable antibodies against human growth hormone, cases in which these antibodies actually block the biological activity of the hormone—leading to an impairment or abolition of its growth-promoting effect—constitute rare exceptions[34]. To our knowledge, there have been no reports of any impairment of the steroidogenic activity of A.C.T.H. following therapy with Synacthen. The steroidogenic action of Synacthen Depot was shown to be intact in one of the three patients from our series who developed antibodies following treatment with this drug. In the one fatal case that occurred, however, adrenocortical insufficiency after discontinuation of A.C.T.H. therapy was suspected[13,14].

A serum A.C.T.H. concentration of 50 pg./ml. is sufficient for maximum stimulation of steroidogenesis[26]. A.C.T.H. values measured radioimmunologically during tests designed to stimulate the release of A.C.T.H. have confirmed that the concentration of endogenous A.C.T.H. lies within the pg./ml. range[2]. The binding capacity of the plasmas from the patients studied by us was far more than sufficient to neutralise endogenous A.C.T.H. in the amounts in which it is normally secreted. FLEISCHER et al.[7] have shown that patients with A.C.T.H. antibodies who receive depot porcine A.C.T.H. to hasten recovery from pituitary-adrenocortical suppression may step up their endogenous A.C.T.H. secretion and thus maintain a normal concentration of "free" A.C.T.H. in spite of the presence of binding antibodies. Although animals immunised with A.C.T.H. are not examined systematically, it is of interest to note that signs of adrenocortical insufficiency in animals with anti-A.C.T.H. antibodies of high avidity and high titre have never been reported.

The presence of circulating antibodies and the occurrence of localised or generalised allergic reactions are two distinct problems. In one series of cases described by GLASS et al.[16], six out of 18 patients showing generalised allergic reactions had circulating antibodies. In another study by the same investigators, none of 12 patients with circulating antibodies had any allergic manifestations[16,17]. RATCLIFFE et al.[31] found circulating antibodies in four out of nine patients with clinical allergies to porcine A.C.T.H. It must also be borne in mind that untoward reactions following administration of A.C.T.H. are not necessarily related to antibodies; systemic and local responses may, for example, be due to an increased vascular permeability produced by synthetic β1–24 A.C.T.H.[21].

As already mentioned, all the patients reported as having exhibited allergic intolerance to Synacthen and/or circulating antibodies had received the long-acting zinc phosphate complex of β1–24 corticotrophin (Synacthen Depot). RATCLIFFE et al.[31] have suggested that the vehicle used for prolonging the action of an A.C.T.H. preparation might affect the conformation or aggregation of the peptide, thereby increasing its antigenicity. It appears that the carboxymethylcellulose preparations are less antigenic than zinc complexes or than the gelatin forms of A.C.T.H.[31].

Patients who have developed allergic reactions to A.C.T.H. therapy, owing to impurities present in the preparation or to hypersensitivity to the extracted A.C.T.H. itself, can in many cases be treated with β1–24 corticotrophin without manifesting any allergic side effects[5,35]. Even under treatment with β1–24 corticotrophin, however, allergic reactions and/or the presence of antibodies are still liable to be observed (Table 4). In patients who have proved allergic to natural A.C.T.H., the possible existence of cross-reacting antibodies should be considered before resuming treatment with synthetic A.C.T.H.

Table 4. Allergic responses to tetracosactide in patients previously treated with natural A.C.T.H.

Number of patients investigated	Positive clinical reactions	Cases exhibiting detectable antibodies	Reference
22		10	*Ratcliffe* et al.[31]*
3	1		*Charpin* et al.[6]
42	4		*Charpin* et al.[5]

*"Many of the subjects had ... received porcine A.C.T.H. previously..."

Under physiological conditions, the A.C.T.H. molecule very probably circulates in the form of the complete 1–39 sequence and not of the 1–24 segment alone. It could thus be anticipated that the 1–24 fragment administered—even though having the same sequence of amino acids as the natural human 1–24 N-terminal—might prove antigenic, since no such substance as an entity unto itself is normally present. Patients who have been treated with only synthetic β1–24 corticotrophin may develop allergic reactions or antibodies which are specific for the isolated 1–24 segment. It is therefore in theory possible that patients specifically allergic to this 1–24 fragment would be able to tolerate the complete human 1–39 molecule. On the basis of these considerations, it would be interesting to study the immunogenic properties of a synthetic human 1–39 A.C.T.H. preparation.

Conclusion

Synthetic β1–24 corticotrophin has been found to be antigenic in both man and animals. However, the incidence of allergic reactions and positive findings of circulating anti-A.C.T.H. antibodies is much lower following treatment with this synthetic polypeptide than after use of the extract-preparations of animal origin that had previously been available. Our experience suggests that both the antigenicity and the steroidogenic action of any A.C.T.H. preparation employed for long-term treatment should be carefully investigated.

References

1 AUBERT, M.L., FELBER, J.-P.: Studies on ACTH-binding antibodies: characterization of immunological specificities. Acta endocr. (Kbh.) *62*, 521 (1969)

2 BERSON, S.A., YALOW, R.S.: Radioimmunoassay of ACTH in plasma. J. clin. Invest. *47*, 2725 (1968)

3 BESSER, G.M., ORTH, D.N., NICHOLSON, W.E., BYYNY, R.L., ABE, K., WOODHAM, J.P.: Dissociation of the disappearance of bioactive and radioimmunoreactive ACTH from plasma in man. J. clin. Endocr. *32*, 595 (1971)

4 CHARPIN, J., AUBERT, J.: Allergie au tétracosapeptide. Marseille-méd. *106*, 881 (1969)

5 CHARPIN, J., AUBERT, J., BOUTIN, C.: The allergenic properties of the newer adrenocorticotrophic hormones. Acta allerg. (Kbh.) *22*, 289 (1967)

6 CHARPIN, J., ZAFIROPOULO, A., AUBERT, J., OHRESSER, P., BOUTIN, C.: Données actuelles concernant l'allergie à l'ACTH. Presse méd. *72*, 3025 (1964)

7 FLEISCHER, N., ABE, K., LIDDLE, G. W., ORTH, D. N., NICHOLSON, W. E.: ACTH antibodies in patients receiving depot porcine ACTH to hasten recovery from pituitary-adrenal suppression. J. clin. Invest. *46*, 196 (1967)

8 FLEISCHER, N., GIVENS, J. R., ABE, K., NICHOLSON, W. E., LIDDLE, G. W.: Studies of ACTH antibodies and their reactions with inactive analogues of ACTH. Endocrinology *78*, 1067 (1966)

9 GELZER, J.: Immunochemical study of β-corticotropin-(1-24)-tetracosa-peptide. Immunochemistry *5*, 23 (1968)

10 GEYER, G., REIMER, E. E.: Über kortikotrope Wirksamkeit und Allergenität des synthetischen ACTH-Tetracosactids Synacthen-Depot. Wien. klin. Wschr. *82*, 324 (1970)

11 GIRARD, J.: Probleme der radioimmunologischen Eiweissbestimmung: Technik and Anwendung. Habil.arbeit, Basle 1971 (not published)

12 GIRARD, J., BAUMANN, J. B., STAHL, M., NARS, P. W., BÜHLER, U., WICK, H.: Experience with insulin-induced hypoglycemia as a provocative test for growth hormone and cortisol secretion in children. Hormones *2*, 338 (1971)

13 GIRARD, J., HIRT, H. R., BÜHLER, U., VEST, M.: Antibodies against the biologically active amino-acid sequence of corticotrophin in an infant treated with synthetic β^{1-24} corticotrophin. Symp. Dtsch. Ges. Endokr. *16*, 293 (1970)

14 GIRARD, J., HIRT, H. R., BÜHLER, U., ZACHMANN, M., WICK, H., BAUMANN, J. B., STAHL, M.: Long-term treatment with ACTH and allergenic properties of synthetic β^{1-24}corticotropin. Helv. paediat. Acta *26*, 46 (1971)

15 GLASS, D., DALY, J. R.: Development of antibodies during long-term therapy with corticotrophin in rheumatoid arthritis. I. Porcine ACTH. Ann. rheum. Dis. *30*, 589 (1971)

16 GLASS, D., MORLEY, J., WILLIAMS, T. J., DALY, J. R.: Allergy to tetracosactrin-depot. Lancet *i*, 547 (1971)

17 GLASS, D., NUKI, G., DALY, J. R.: Development of antibodies during long-term therapy with corticotrophin in rheumatoid arthritis. II. Zinc tetracosactrin (Depot Synacthen). Ann. rheum. Dis. *30*, 593 (1971)

18 HÜRTER, P., KÜHNAU, J., Jr.: Die Aktivität zirkulierender Insulinantikörper bei kindlichen Diabetikern. Helv. paediat. Acta *25*, 154 (1970)

19 IMURA, H., SPARKS, L. L., GRODSKY, G. M., FORSHAM, P. H.: Immunologic studies of adrenocorticotropic hormone (ACTH): dissociation of biologic and immunologic activities. J. clin. Endocr. *25*, 1361 (1965)

20 IMURA, H., SPARKS, L. L., TOSAKA, M., HANE, S., GRODSKY, G. M., FORSHAM, P. H.: Immunologic studies of adrenocorticotropic hormone (ACTH): effect of carboxypeptidase digestion on biologic and immunologic activities. J. clin. Endocr. *27*, 15 (1967)

21 JAQUES, R.: Non-specific effects of synthetic corticotrophin polypeptides. Int. Arch. Allergy *28*, 221 (1965)

22 JENSEN, N. E., SNEDDON, I.: Allergic intolerance to tetracosactrin. Brit. med. J. *ii*, 383 (1969); corresp.

23 KANTOR, S. Z., LARON, Z.: Anaphylactic reaction to ACTH. Ann. paediat. (Basle) *201*, 381 (1963)

24 LANDON, J., FRIEDMAN, M., GREENWOOD, F. C.: Antibodies to corticotrophin and their relation to adrenal function in children receiving corticotrophin therapy. Lancet *i*, 652 (1967)

25 LANDON, J., GIRARD, J., GREENWOOD, F. C.: The specificity of a radioimmunoassay for human plasma ACTH. In Margoulies, M. (Editor): Protein and polypeptide hormones, Proc. Int. Symp., Liège 1968, p. 29. Int. Congr. Ser. No. 161 (Excerpta med. Found., Amsterdam 1969)

26 LANDON, J., JAMES, V. H. T., WHARTON, M. J., FRIEDMAN, M.: Threshold

adrenocortical sensitivity in man and its possible application to corticotrophin bioassay. Lancet *ii*, 697 (1967)

27 LANDON, J., LIVANOU, T., GREENWOOD, F. C.: The preparation and immunological properties of ^{131}I-labelled adrenocorticotrophin. Biochem. J. *105*, 1075 (1967)

28 LI, C. H.: Some aspects of the relationship of peptide structures to activity in pituitary hormones. Vitam. and Horm. *19*, 313 (1961)

29 PATRIARCA, G.: Allergy to tetracosactrin-depot. Lancet *i*, 138 (1971)

30 PRADER, A., WAGNER, H., SZÉKY, J., ILLIG, R., TOUBER, J., MAINGAY, D.: Acquired resistance to human growth hormone caused by specific antibodies. Lancet *ii*, 378 (1964)

31 RATCLIFFE, J. G., PRITCHARD, M., EL-SHABOURY, A. H.: The production of antibodies to porcine corticotrophin and to Synacthen. J. Endocr. *43* 1 (1969)

32 RITTEL, W.: Recent chemical studies in the field of A.C.T.H. In Schuppli, R. (Editor): A.C.T.H.—a practical review of progress to date, Int. Symp., Dubrovnik 1973, p. 11 (Huber, Berne/Stuttgart/Vienna 1973)

33 ROSENBLUM, A. H., ROSENBLUM, P.: Anaphylactic reactions to adrenocorticotropic hormone in children. J. Pediat. *64*, 387 (1964)

34 ROTH, J., GLICK, S. M., YALOW, R. S., BERSON, S. A.: Antibodies to human growth hormone (HGH) in human subjects treated with HGH. J. clin. Invest. *43*, 1056 (1964)

35 SCHWARZ-SPECK, M., MAEDER, E.: Immunologische Untersuchungen mit natürlichem und synthetischem ACTH bei ACTH-Allergikern. Int. Arch. Allergy *24*, Suppl.: 29 (1964)

36 STAHL, M., KAPP, J. P., ZACHMANN, M., GIRARD, J.: Effect of a single oral dose of metyrapone on secretion of growth hormone and urinary tetrahydro-11-deoxycortisol and tetrahydro-11-deoxycorticosterone excretion in children. Helv. paediat. Acta *27*, 147 (1972)

37 UZZAN, D., CHEBAT, J., OLLIERO, H., ISRAEL-ASSELAIN, R.: Traitement des bronchopathies obstructives par le tétracosapeptide retard (corticostimuline synthétique). Presse méd. *77*, 1485 (1969)

38 WEST, H. F.: Ten years of ACTH therapy. Ann. rheum. Dis. *21*, 263 (1962)

39 WOLFROMM, R., HERMAN, D.: L'allergie médicamenteuse à l'ACTH: ses manifestations cliniques, ses moyens de prévention. Sem. Hôp. Paris *43*, 1252 (1967)

40 YALOW, R. S., BERSON, S. A.: Immunoassay of endogenous plasma insulin in man. J. clin. Invest. *39*, 1157 (1960)

41 YALOW, R. S., GLICK, S. M., ROTH, J., BERSON, S. A.: Radioimmunoassay of human plasma ACTH. J. clin. Endocr. *24*, 1219 (1964)

Discussion

J. GELZER: Both Dr. WEINGES and particularly Dr. GIRARD have dealt at length in their papers with the problems of allergenicity and immunogenicity posed by treatment with A.C.T.H. In this connection I should like to state that there is no doubt whatsoever that, if appropriate techniques are used, antibodies can be elicited against all A.C.T.H. preparations known to date and that therefore all these preparations must be regarded as potentially immunogenic and allergenic. The whole question is complicated, however, by the fact that neither from animal experiments nor from clinical studies do we know the relevance of the findings we obtain using immunological methods. It is relatively easy to produce antibodies in an animal experiment; and in such experiments long-acting depot preparations will probably be found to yield higher antibody titres. But in laboratory animals it is virtually impossible to demonstrate any pharmacological effect, such as an alteration in the corticotrophic activity of A.C.T.H., which could be linked with the occurrence of antibodies. This has also been confirmed by Dr. GIRARD.

At this point, I should also like to address a brief remark to Dr. IRVINE who, in the discussion following Dr. KOGOJ's paper, referred to the potential antigenicity of the 1–18 peptide. On the basis of preliminary results obtained by SCHENKEL in our laboratories, I can inform him that in initial experiments performed on mice this peptide was found to behave in the same way as Synacthen, i.e. under the experimental conditions employed no formation of antibodies could be observed. It is therefore probably safe to assume that, with regard to immunogenicity, this 1–18 peptide should not differ markedly from Synacthen and Synacthen Depot.

Now let us come back to the subject of Synacthen Depot. From the immunological standpoint there is no reason why a long-acting preparation should *a priori* display greater allergenicity or immunogenicity than a short-acting one; this is a conclusion backed by wide experience from immunological research with other antigens. Far more important in this connection is the question as to how a given substance behaves in the organism and how it is eliminated. This raises the problem of the pharmacokinetics of A.C.T.H. and of the A.C.T.H. derivatives. One thing is certain: a depot preparation such as Synacthen Depot, which is supplied in the form of a zinc-phosphate complex, will show a distribution pattern differing from that of the water-soluble 1–24 A.C.T.H. derivative, and it might be for this reason that in animal experiments it exhibits greater immunogenicity than the water-soluble preparation.

As far as the clinical implications of this whole problem are concerned, it must be admitted that, despite all the experimental findings that have been obtained, we still do not know—and I don't think Dr. GIRARD has been able to tell us either—whether the immunologically confirmed presence of circulating A.C.T.H. antibodies in a given patient is of any pathognomonic relevance with regard to the possible occurrence of immunological side effects, such as anaphylactic shock or other troublesome and unwanted manifestations in the course of treatment with A.C.T.H. I should be interested to know whether Dr. GIRARD, or perhaps someone else present here, can offer any specific comments on this question. Moreover, it should be added that we also do not know whether those patients who do show signs of allergy or other immunological complications in response to A.C.T.H. therapy have a case history differing in certain specific respects from that of patients in whom antibodies are likewise present but in whom no untoward incidents occur. Thus, it would, for instance, be interesting to learn from Dr. GIRARD, or from others attending this symposium, whether the incidence of side effects has been greater in patients undergoing intermittent treatment with Synacthen than in those receiving tetracosactide continuously, either in the form of Synacthen Depot or in the form of water-soluble Synacthen. From experience of other types of drug allergy (for example, from experience with the antituberculous antibiotic ®Rimactane) we know that the treatment schedule has a tremendously important bearing on the possible occurrence of immunopathological side effects*. I should therefore like to ask Dr. GIRARD and Dr. WEINGES the following two questions: firstly, is anything known about the influence of the treatment schedule on the quality and quantity of the side effects and, secondly, what clinical significance can be ascribed to the presence of immunologically detectable circulating antibodies specifically directed against A.C.T.H. or against portions of the A.C.T.H. chain?

J. GIRARD: Regarding the possible influence of the treatment schedule on the incidence of immunological side effects, my answer would be as follows: in cases of hypsarrhythmia, we start treatment with five injections a week and then gradually reduce the dosage to one weekly injection. Substitution therapy, on the other hand, calls for regular administration of the drug, say, once every two days. The number of patients in whom antibodies have been detected is too small for any conclusions to be drawn as to the influence exerted by the treatment schedule. Moreover, experiments on animals have also failed to indicate what dosage schedules can in general be regarded as certain either to provoke or to prevent antibody formation.

As for the clinical significance of antibodies directed against A.C.T.H., I should like to draw attention to the study by GLASS et al.** in which it is reported that, in six out of 18 patients who had shown a generalised reaction to Synacthen, it also proved possible by radioimmunoassay to demonstrate the presence of antibodies. As mentioned in my—or, rather, our—paper, we have had *one* case in which the clinical picture led us to suspect that an adrenal crisis had supervened; evidence in support of this assumption was also obtained at autopsy: here, despite the fact that the patient had been receiving treatment for nine weeks, only *mild* adrenal hyperplasia was found, and there was no lipid depletion. We were unable, however, to confirm the diagnosis of adrenal failure.

Finally, we succeeded in demonstrating experimentally that antibodies directed against the 1–24 sequence of A.C.T.H. are capable of inhibiting, or even of completely preventing, the binding of Synacthen to the receptors of isolated fat cells.

K. F. WEINGES: From animal experiments and clinical observations it would appear that intermittent doses of polypeptide hormones are more likely to give rise to antibody formation. In laboratory animals a stronger immune reaction can be obtained if the animal is first pre-immunised with subcutaneous or intramuscular injections and then, three weeks later, given an intravenous booster injection. In the case of insulin therapy, too, it has been found that intermittent doses—administered together with oral antidiabetics, for example—tend to evoke antibodies more readily than does continuous treatment with insulin alone, and that in patients receiving such intermittent medication the insulin requirement also increases more rapidly.

The differences with regard to antibody formation that are observed both in animals and in man are probably attributable to the fact that immunological reactivity is, to some extent, genetically predetermined. Consequently, when you try to immunise, say, 100 rabbits, you may only get good antibody formation in perhaps two or three of the animals. The situation is probably much the same in man: in other words, one person—for genetic reasons—will show a stronger immune reaction than another. From the clinical standpoint, however, i.e. so far as treatment with Synacthen is concerned, these differences do not seem to be of any relevance. On the other hand, I doubt whether we have yet acquired sufficient experience in this connection, because the clinical observations available to date do not, to my knowledge, cover

---

*AQUINAS, SR. M., ALLAN, W. G. L., HORSFALL, P. A. L., JENKINS, P. K., WONG HUNG-YAN, GIRLING, D., TALL, R., FOX, W.: Adverse reactions to daily and intermittent rifampicin regimens for pulmonary tuberculosis in Hong Kong. Brit. med. J. i, 765 (1972)

**GLASS, D., MORLEY, J., WILLIAMS, T. J., DALY, J. R.: Allergy to tetracosactrin-depot. Lancet i, 547 (1971)

113

periods of treatment amounting to more than at the most two to three years—whereas from experience with insulin therapy we know that clinically relevant antibody formation, if it occurs at all, does not usually become apparent until a number of years have elapsed. I therefore feel that it is still too early for us to be able to make any valid statements about the precise significance of the antigenic properties of 1–24 A.C.T.H.

You mentioned in your paper, Dr. GIRARD, that no changes had ever been reported in the adrenals of animals which had developed anti-A.C.T.H. antibodies. Have you yourself also examined the pituitaries of such animals and possibly found morphological changes in them?

J. GIRARD: I'm afraid the answer to that question, Dr. WEINGES, is no, because as a rule these animals are not systematically examined after they have been sacrificed. I do know, however, that diabetes insipidus has been provoked in animals by the induction of antibodies directed against antidiuretic hormone. In diabetics, too, antibodies induced by treatment with insulin may block the biological activity of the hormone.

J. AUBERT: It would be interesting to know to what category of immunoglobulin these radioimmunologically detected antibodies belong, because it is not certain that the majority of them are IgE. In 35 patients treated with Synacthen Depot, we have resorted to radioimmunoassay in order to detect antibodies directed against Synacthen. Nine of the patients had become sensitised to Synacthen, but, of these nine, only two were found to have anti-Synacthen antibodies. Of the remaining 26, seven also displayed anti-Synacthen antibodies but were not allergic to Synacthen. Consequently, in a case where anti-Synacthen antibodies are detected by the radioimmunological technique, this does not necessarily mean that the patient will also exhibit hypersensitivity of the reagin-induced type. I think that here there may be a certain analogy with what happens in the case of insulin. Now that it has become possible to obtain highly purified insulin by means of successive recrystallisation, sensitisation of the reagin-induced type is very rarely observed; nevertheless, we know that these highly purified forms of insulin are also capable of inducing antibodies which can be detected radioimmunologically and that these antibodies are occasionally even liable to cause resistance to the therapeutic effect of insulin. I feel this is a point worth emphasising.

T. B. BINNS: May I comment briefly on our experience in the United Kingdom. In just under five years we have received about 50 reports of allergic-type reactions in response to tetracosactrin; this represents, very approximately, something like one incident per 100,000 doses of 0.5 mg. We have the impression—which may be fallacious, and I hope I'm not tempting fate in mentioning it—that the incidence of such reactions has been on the decrease during the past year or two. Curiously enough, there has been quite a striking preponderance of females among the patients in whom these incidents have occurred, but they have not been confined to women nor, for that matter, to patients with an allergic diathesis. It does seem, however, that the persons suffering the most severe reactions are likely to be asthmatic women, and in these cases the reaction usually sets in within about 30 minutes.

As for the laboratory investigations that have been carried out on patients showing reactions of an allergic type to Synacthen Depot, Dr. STANWORTH in Birmingham very kindly examined sera from 18 of these patients and found that the immunoglobulin levels (including IgE) were within normal limits.

Dr. GLASS*, to whose work reference has already been made, also examined the sera from the same patients and showed that serum-binding antibody does not occur more

---

*GLASS, D., NUKI, G., DALY, J.R.: Development of antibodies during long-term therapy with corticotrophin in rheumatoid arthritis. II. Zinc tetracosactrin (Depot Synacthen). Ann. rheum. Dis. *30*, 593 (1971)

frequently in patients who have reacted adversely to Synacthen Depot than in those by whom the preparation has been well tolerated. There appeared in fact to be no correlation at all between the incidence and titre of antibody and the occurrence of allergic-type reactions. Dr. GLASS has also informed me that, in the first two cases of clinical allergy which he had been able to examine, the lymphocyte transformation test proved positive. Meanwhile, however, he has examined three further cases, in two of which the test was negative, while in the third it was equivocal. Thus, for the time being, this whole problem remains unresolved. I can only say that, so far as our experience in Great Britain is concerned, these reactions certainly do seem to fit into a pattern which is recognisable as one of clinical allergy. But quite extensive laboratory investigations have so far failed to yield objective evidence to support the impression that an antigen-antibody interaction is involved.

G. GIUSTI: Since January 1971 we have employed synthetic corticotrophin zinc-phosphate complex to treat a total of 23 patients suffering from chronic active liver disease, the duration of the treatment ranging from four to 29 months. We have observed six adverse reactions to the preparation. As can be seen from Table 1, the symptoms most frequently encountered have been an uneasy feeling, prostration, and fainting. In the first two patients in whom these reactions had occurred, we performed skin sensitivity tests with both Synacthen and Synacthen Depot. Despite the fact that the results of the tests were negative, the next dose of Synacthen Depot again elicited an adverse reaction, and the treatment was therefore discontinued. In the four remaining cases, the synthetic corticotrophin was immediately withdrawn after the first adverse reaction.

I should be interested to know if anyone present can shed some light on the following two questions. Firstly, what is the most suitable test by which to detect possible intolerance to synthetic or natural corticotrophin? Secondly, should Synacthen Depot be withdrawn in the event of adverse reactions of a minor nature, particularly where— as in the case of patients suffering from chronic active hepatitis—alternative therapy is available?

M. GIORDANO: Now that we have come to the end of the first series of papers on the programme, I have a question which I should like to put to those present here, including the rheumatologists in particular. Many authors, and some of the speakers at this symposium too, have reported that, in comparison with corticosteroid therapy, treatment with A.C.T.H. has the advantage of causing little if any interference with hypothalamo-pituitary-adrenocortical function. May I ask precisely what this advantage signifies in clinical terms? It has long been argued that inhibition of adrenocortical function lowers the patient's resistance to infection and to stress—which is

Table 1. Intolerance to tetracosactrin zinc-phosphate complex observed in six (23%) out of 23 cases.

Case No.	Age (years)	Sex	Development of intolerance (months from start of treatment)	Clinical picture soon after the injection*
1	30	M	9th	Uneasy feeling and prostration
2	18	M	12th	Papular rash with itching
3	27	F	6th	Uneasy feeling, dyspnoea, and fainting
4	19	F	5th	Uneasy feeling, vomiting, and headache
5	23	F	12th	Uneasy feeling, vomiting, and fainting
6	21	F	24th	Uneasy feeling and fainting

* All the symptoms listed were of short duration.

115

probably true; the fact remains, however, that this lowering of resistance seldom results in really serious incidents. Corticoid-dependence of the type liable to develop in chronic rheumatics who have received prolonged treatment with corticosteroids is another possible consequence of these corticoid-induced changes in the endocrine system; it is conceivable that suppression of the hypothalamo-pituitary-adrenocortical axis may be basically responsible for the fact that in patients who have been under prolonged treatment with corticosteroids a form of rheumatoid arthritis is sometimes encountered which I myself refer to as "cortisonised" rheumatoid arthritis. After the acutely active phase of the disease has subsided, such patients are not only left with severe lesions of the joints, marked osteoporosis, and atrophy of the skin and muscles, but also suffer from pronounced asthenia, loss of will power, and depression and are unable to tolerate any antirheumatic drugs with the exception of corticosteroids. We don't know to what extent these clinical pictures are indeed provoked by the corticosteroid therapy, nor do we know whether they could be prevented by employing A.C.T.H. and thus avoiding suppression of the hypothalamo-pituitary-adrenocortical axis. If this were in fact the case, then the superiority which A.C.T.H. has so often been claimed to display with regard to its influence on the endocrine system might well also offer a major clinical advantage as compared with corticosteroid therapy.

R. SCHUPPLI: We now have the following three questions to answer: firstly, is there any test by which hypersensitivity to Synacthen can be detected? Secondly, should the occurrence of symptoms such as general weakness be regarded as grounds for discontinuing treatment with Synacthen? And, thirdly, are the weakness and loss of resistance, that are liable to be encountered in cases of rheumatoid arthritis in particular, due to impairment of hypothalamo-pituitary-adrenocortical function?

R. DEGUILLAUME: I don't think that any biological warning test exists which would enable one to guard against side effects of an allergic type in patients receiving Synacthen. Dr. BINNS has clearly shown that no biological evidence has yet been adduced to confirm that these side effects really are of an immunological nature. As for the clinical warning signs, we had reason to believe at one time that grave complications were always preceded by mild allergic manifestations. It would now seem, however, that while this is certainly true in the majority of cases, there may nevertheless be exceptions. One thing is at all events certain: as soon as mild signs of allergy appear—particularly in the form of pruritus or urticaria—treatment with Synacthen Depot should be discontinued at once; the only exceptions to this rule are cases in which flushing occurs a few minutes after the injection—this harmless vasomotor disturbance being probably bound up with an immediate release of histamine.
As for the asthenia sometimes observed in patients treated with Synacthen Depot, this is part and parcel of the problem of adrenocortical exhaustion such as may possibly occur as a result of prolonged treatment. LUTON et al.*, for example, have drawn attention to the possible risk of adrenocortical exhaustion and to the danger of provoking acute adrenal insufficiency when performing an A.C.T.H. test in patients with Addison's disease. But this is a special case. Otherwise I believe that, where one is dealing with a patient whose adrenals are functioning normally, it is extremely doubtful whether adrenocortical exhaustion resulting in clinically manifest asthenia would ever occur. On the contrary, as illustrated by the case outlined in Figure 12 of the paper presented by Dr. WEINGES, what one is far more likely to observe is an increase in the responsiveness of the cortices due to adrenal hypertrophy. So far, in fact, not even in patients receiving prolonged treatment or treatment with high doses have we ever encountered signs of more or less complete adrenocortical exhaustion in response to Synacthen Depot.

---

*LUTON, J.-P., SLAMA, G., TURPIN, G., BRICAIRE, H.: Tentative de stimulation prolongée des insuffisances surrénales par la béta-1–24 corticotrophine retard. Rev. franç. Endocr. clin. *13*, 425 (1972)

J. Aubert: I think I can perhaps give at least a partial answer to some of the questions that have been asked here. First of all, I would point out that, when confronted with an accident in the course of treatment with Synacthen, it is extremely difficult to make a differential diagnosis, i.e. to distinguish between, on the one hand, a phenomenon due to the release of histamine and, on the other, a purely allergic process of the reagin-induced type. Even if the patient develops generalised pruritus or cutaneous oedema, it is not always certain that this is an allergic manifestation. I believe, however, that specific immunoglobulin determinations will soon make it possible to obtain more reliable backing for a differential diagnosis. Secondly, care must be taken to differentiate between the various categories of patient treated with Synacthen: "non-atopic" subjects, for example, run little risk of becoming sensitised to the drug, whereas the risk is much greater in the case of "atopic" subjects, such as asthmatics. Incidentally, treatment for brief periods entails less danger in this respect than very prolonged courses of therapy.

J. Gelzer: I should like to ask Dr. Aubert whether he considers that, with a view to avoiding untoward incidents, "atopic" patients such as the asthmatics he treated should be carefully examined before commencing A.C.T.H. therapy in order to discover whether they are possibly allergic to A.C.T.H. What immunodiagnostic methods, if any, would he suggest for the purpose of such examinations? I think we are all agreed that, though we do not yet know precisely what significance to ascribe to the presence of antibodies, patients who are already found to have circulating antibodies prior to treatment should be assigned to a special category.

J. Aubert: When another synthetic polypeptide—containing 25 amino acids—was placed at our disposal, we found that certain patients who had become sensitised to Synacthen were able to tolerate this synthetic A.C.T.H. preparation without suffering any ill effects.

T. B. Binns: In connection with what Dr. Aubert has just said, I should like to repeat that in our experience these adverse reactions have not been confined to patients with an allergic diathesis or with an atopic disposition, and also that when such reactions had occurred we were unable to find any difference in the immunoglobulins as compared with patients who had not reacted adversely to Synacthen Depot.

J. Girard: Though I am not an immunologist, I think that we can perhaps draw an analogy here with experience obtained in animal experiments: when trying to immunise laboratory animals against peptide hormones it is impossible to predict whether or not a particular animal will respond to a given hormone. In this connection, I should like to refer to one of our patients who developed antibodies when treated with Synacthen; since this was a case of hypopituitarism, the patient was at the same time receiving treatment with growth hormone as well, but he did not produce any antibodies against growth hormone, although I understand the latter to be a far better "antigen". This case also illustrates another point: even if the presence of antibodies has been conclusively demonstrated by the radioimmunoassay technique, this does not necessarily mean that the treatment has to be abandoned. In our patient, in fact, we continued the Synacthen medication, and his adrenals were reacting perfectly well to this drug.

D. Gross: When administering long-term treatment with A.C.T.H. or Synacthen Depot to patients suffering from rheumatoid arthritis one quite often observes a decrease in therapeutic effect as the treatment continues. Is this perhaps due to denaturation of the corticotrophin by antibodies, or is there another explanation for this phenomenon?

J. Gelzer: Could you please explain more clearly what you mean by "a decrease in therapeutic effect", Dr. Gross? Do you mean that you had to give the drug in increasing doses in order to maintain the therapeutic response or to eliminate pain?

D. Gross: What I was referring to is an impression that I have gained from clinical observations. By "a decrease in therapeutic effect" I mean that it becomes increasingly difficult to suppress the signs and symptoms of inflammation and that the patients tend to complain again of increasing pain and swelling; this can to some extent be offset by raising the dosage.

G. Geyer: There is at all events no reason to suppose that a clinically manifest allergy to A.C.T.H. necessarily goes hand in hand with a loss of therapeutic efficacy. I have, for example, measured the secretion of cortisol in response to A.C.T.H. in patients with A.C.T.H.-induced allergies in the form of extensive urticaria or asthmoid reactions; despite these cutaneous and pulmonary manifestations, cortisol secretion remained unchanged.

K. F. Weinges: We have to draw a distinction here between cell-mediated immune reactions and circulating antibodies. A localised allergy is a cell-mediated reaction and has nothing to do with inactivation of the hormone by antibodies. As Dr. Girard has also already mentioned in his paper, no evidence has yet emerged to suggest that any impairment of the biological activity of Synacthen occurs owing to the presence of antibodies; I therefore do not think that a diminution in the drug's clinical effect could be accounted for on this basis.
Even during long-term A.C.T.H. therapy, a normally functioning adrenal cortex does not become exhausted; on the contrary, it hypertrophies and produces more and more cortisol. If cases do occur in which the clinical effectiveness of A.C.T.H. wears off in the course of time, one possible reason might be the fact that the A.C.T.H. is being more quickly bound and inactivated, e.g. as a result of enzyme induction and enzymatic degradation.

J. Girard: Regarding neutralisation of the biological activity of A.C.T.H. by antibodies, I should like to point out that, in comparison with endogenous A.C.T.H. production, the doses of exogenous A.C.T.H. administered for therapeutic purposes are so disproportionally large that the binding capacity of the antibodies would never suffice to neutralise them. Moreover, it has also been demonstrated that in the presence of antibodies endogenous A.C.T.H. is secreted in more abundant quantities, thereby ensuring an adequate supply of free circulating A.C.T.H.
I have a counterquestion to put to Dr. Gross in this connection: do you sometimes also have to raise the dosage in patients treated with corticoids, i.e. is corticoid therapy too, liable to become less effective in the course of time?

D. Gross: Yes, that may certainly happen as well. But, if it does, we interpret this loss of effect differently: in these cases we assume that there must have been an increase in the inflammatory process as such.

H. Jesserer: I should like to add a rider in support of the question Dr. Gross has asked. The example of parathormone provides an analogy to the problem he has raised. Parathormone is unsuitable for the long-term treatment of hypoparathyroidism because it becomes progressively inactivated by immuno-antigenic processes until it finally ceases to have any effect at all. It is thus quite conceivable that, for similar reasons, A.C.T.H. might gradually become less effective in a patient receiving prolonged treatment; the fact that in such a case glucocorticoids may still be capable of exerting an action does not, in my opinion, contradict this hypothesis. Admittedly, of course, the situation as far as parathormone is concerned is different in that this hormone is employed in cases where the parathyroid glands no longer display any activity of their own at all.

T. B. Binns: We all know how difficult it is to get something into the literature, but it may well be even more difficult to get it out again! About ten years ago, Dr. West*in Sheffield published a report on some patients who, after having first derived benefit

---

118 *West, H. F.: Ten years of ACTH therapy. Ann. rheum. Dis. *21*, 263 (1962)

from A.C.T.H. therapy, ceased after a while to respond to the treatment; he concluded that they had become resistant to the effect of A.C.T.H. Nowadays, however, most if not all physicians who have had experience with A.C.T.H.—at least in the United Kingdom—would discount this theory. I at any rate know of no one who believes that corticotrophins may lose their activity in the course of time.

K. F. WEINGES: If a decrease in the effectiveness of A.C.T.H. is encountered in rheumatic patients as frequently as Dr. GROSS has indicated, I think one ought to investigate the problem and measure the plasma cortisol levels in order to find out whether the adrenal cortices have become less responsive, or whether they are still responding satisfactorily but secreting cortisol which is no longer able to act. If the plasma cortisol concentrations are undiminished, one should then consider whether perhaps the transcortin levels have risen—as might, I imagine, be the case in a woman receiving concomitant treatment with oestrogens.

R. SCHUPPLI: I should like now to sum up the main points that have emerged from this discussion on the side effects of A.C.T.H. therapy. First of all, there is no test that enables one to decide in a given case whether or not it is safe to administer Synacthen. In this respect, Synacthen differs radically from the old A.C.T.H. preparations: if a patient was allergic to these, we used to get a positive reaction when we performed a skin test. In three of our patients who had developed severe urticaria and symptoms of shock in response to Synacthen, however, skin tests failed to yield positive results— and the lymphocyte transformation test also proved negative. We simply do not yet know how these allergic complications come about in patients who have been treated with Synacthen.

Now to the second question: what signs and symptoms should prompt one to withdraw Synacthen? Important as a pointer in this connection are the cutaneous manifestations. If a patient complains of itching after an injection of Synacthen, the treatment should be discontinued, because experience has shown that in such cases there is a danger that severe urticaria may develop. These serious reactions don't occur suddenly, but are preceded by certain prodromal symptoms.

As for the question of a loss of effect in the course of treatment with A.C.T.H., this is something that—in dermatological cases, at any rate—we do not see. As I have already indicated, we have treated patients for periods as long as five to six years and have never encountered any diminution in the therapeutic effect. It is conceivable, of course, that a possible decrease in the drug's effectiveness might have nothing to do with immunological factors: for example, some hitherto unknown enzyme could perhaps break down the A.C.T.H.—in which case, the emergence of this enzyme might perhaps be a phenomenon typical only of patients suffering from rheumatoid arthritis. Incidentally, I think we should beware of concentrating our attention too exclusively on the immunological aspects of this whole problem, since various other factors that may also be of relevance might thus escape our notice. Immunology is certainly very important, but it doesn't cover everything.

Synacthen and Synacthen Depot in dermatology

by R. Schuppli*

A perusal of the dermatological literature published during recent years reveals that increasing use is now being made of A.C.T.H. as an alternative to corticosteroids in the treatment of skin diseases. It is also clearly apparent that for this purpose tetracosactide (®Synacthen or ®Synacthen Depot) — the less allergenic synthetic A.C.T.H. derivative—is accorded preference over A.C.T.H. preparations of natural origin. In the following paper an account will be given of the experience which we have acquired with tetracosactide over the past six to seven years in close on 300 patients suffering from various skin disorders. All the conditions in question were chronic affections that had already been treated with other drugs—in some instances for very prolonged periods; in other words, these were cases in which the influence exerted by A.C.T.H. therapy on the disease process could be readily assessed. Patients with skin disorders running a brief clinical course or showing a tendency to spontaneous remission were excluded from consideration.

Skin diseases provide a particularly good yardstick by which to evaluate the effects of a drug. They can be objectively assessed without difficulty, the extent of the lesions can also be measured objectively, and the severity of the inflammation can—at least to a certain degree—likewise be estimated objectively. Moreover, from years of previous experience, both the patient himself and the doctor are often thoroughly familiar with the course which a particular skin disease is wont to run. Finally, in many cases, the disease process can also be objectively studied with the aid of simple skin tests.

Listed in Table 1 are the diagnoses established in the patients we treated with tetracosactide. Here it should be emphasised that, without exception, all these patients were cases in which we had already made prolonged but unsuccessful attempts at treatment by other methods. When we first embarked on this tetracosactide medication in 1966, we employed the drug chiefly in the water-soluble form, which we administered intravenously in doses of 0.25 mg. or 0.5 mg.; since 1967, however, we have been using only Synacthen Depot, injected in intramuscular doses of 1 mg. The treatment is initiated with injections given on alternate days, the interval between the injections later being extended in the light of the clinical response. In the course of the medication, the patients in this series have received total doses ranging from 1 mg. to 186 mg., the average being 11 mg.

In order to arrive at a more or less objective assessment of the response to the treatment, we adopted an arbitrary rating scale with scores of 0 to 3, which

*Dermatologische Universitätsklinik, Basle, Switzerland.

Table 1. Skin diseases treated with Synacthen or Synacthen Depot during the period 1966–1972.

Disease		Number of cases
Eczema		77
— Contact eczema	41	
— Barbers' eczema	12	
— Microbial eczema	12	
— Chronic constitutional eczema	12	
Psoriasis		68
— Psoriasis vulgaris	47	
— Psoriatic arthropathy	11	
— Pustular psoriasis	5	
— Psoriatic erythrodermia	5	
Chronic recurrent urticaria		21
Prurigo simplex chronica		14
Collagen diseases		10
Diffuse pruritus		13
Erythrodermia		7
Pemphigus		15
Dermatitis herpetiformis		8
Reticulosis		8
Alopecia areata totalis		6
Vitiligo		5
Miscellaneous skin diseases		31
Total		283

were assigned as follows: disease completely cleared under treatment with tetracosactide = 3; temporary improvement = 2; no effect = 1; deterioration = 0. A numerical analysis of the therapeutic effectiveness of tetracosactide, based on this rating scale, is presented in Table 2. Given the criteria of efficacy employed in this study, an index figure of less than 2 signifies that the treatment was unsuccessful, whereas a figure of more than 2 indicates that the drug elicited a transient therapeutic response, and one exceeding 2.5 that it produced a sustained curative effect.

From the efficacy-index figures listed in Table 2 for the various skin diseases treated, it can be seen that, though A.C.T.H. is alleged to display some melanocyte-stimulating activity, tetracosactide proved completely ineffective in cases of alopecia areata and vitiligo. It also failed to exert any effect in psoriatic erythrodermia. In psoriasis vulgaris and psoriatic arthropathy, too, we seldom observed any prolonged responses, although in some cases the symptoms of joint involvement may show a transient improvement under the influence of tetracosactide. Cases of pruritus, as well as of chronic recurrent urticaria in which it is impossible to detect the presence of an allergen, likewise rarely show a satisfactory response to tetracosactide. More encouraging results, however, can be obtained in the various forms of eczema. Eczema in hairdressers, caused by contact with nickel, is one example in particular in which the disease can be kept under control by means of tetracosactide injections.

Table 2. Efficacy index for treatment with Synacthen and Synacthen Depot in skin diseases.

Disease	Index
Pemphigus (various forms)	2.6
Dermatitis herpetiformis	2.4
Pustular psoriasis	2.25
Prurigo	2.2
Contact eczema (barbers' eczema)	2.2
Contact eczema (various forms)	2.15
Chronic constitutional eczema	2.1
Microbial eczema	2.05
Neurodermatitis circumscripta (Vidal)	2.0
Psoriatic arthropathy	1.9
Psoriasis vulgaris	1.75
Chronic recurrent urticaria	1.6
Diffuse pruritus	1.6
Psoriatic erythrodermia	1.55
Collagen diseases (incl. especially scleroderma)	1.55
Alopecia areata totalis	1.3
Vitiligo	1.3
Reticulosis	1.3

Occasionally, indeed, one even has the impression that, thanks to treatment with tetracosactide, the patient loses his hypersensitivity to such an extent that he becomes able again to tolerate contact with the allergens which were originally responsible for the eczema. Prurigo, too, though usually refractory to other forms of treatment, generally responds quite well to tetracosactide. One condition that definitely constitutes an indication for tetracosactide is pustular psoriasis. With tetracosactide it is as a rule possible to suppress the acute febrile pustular eruptions, although the underlying psoriatic process itself shows a much less favourable response. It is in diseases characterised by spontaneous vesication that tetracosactide yields the best results, i.e. in dermatitis herpetiformis and especially in the various forms of pemphigus; in this indication, in fact, tetracosactide may well now be regarded as the drug of first choice.*

These findings suggest that, by and large, the therapeutic effects of tetracosactide are closely comparable with those of the corticosteroids. One exception in this connection is alopecia areata, in which even relatively frequent injections of tetracosactide never elicited results as good as those obtained with corticosteroids; this surprising observation calls for further detailed investigation.

The therapeutic activity which tetracosactide exhibits in various forms of skin disease cannot be ascribed to a general anti-inflammatory effect. If this were so, it would be impossible to account for the fact, for instance, that tetracosactide proves less effective in such a markedly inflammatory condition as psoriatic erythrodermia than it does in pustular psoriasis. It seems more likely that its therapeutic properties in dermatological indications are essentially attributable

*For further details, see FISCHER, R.: Über die Anwendung von Synacthen und Synacthen Depot in der Dermatologie. Inaug.-Diss., Basle (in preparation)

to the influence which A.C.T.H.—or the corticosteroids secreted from the adrenal cortex under the stimulus of A.C.T.H.—exerts on immunological processes. This appears to be borne out by the finding that in skin disorders which are known to be largely of immunological origin, such as the pemphigus and eczema groups, the drug's efficacy index works out at a figure of over 2. It might perhaps even be possible to deduce whether or not a skin disease is of immunological origin by reference to how well it responds to treatment with tetracosactide. Especially interesting from this aspect is the example of pustular psoriasis: recent observations have shown that this special form of psoriasis can be provoked by minimal quantities of various substances, including iodine in particular. On the other hand, the failure of chronic recurrent urticaria to respond to tetracosactide suggests that—as already indicated by clinical evidence—this sub-form of urticaria is very probably not due to allergy.

In order to shed light on the question of the extent to which tetracosactide is capable of influencing immunological processes, we have embarked on a study of the effects exerted by this drug on experimentally quantifiable immunological reactions. For this purpose we have selected the following test procedures: a) patch tests; b) tuberculin tests; c) syphilis serum tests; and d) tests to determine the pemphigus antibody titre. Patients in whom these tests are performed receive 1 mg. Synacthen Depot every other day, the tests being repeated at intervals of three to four days (except in the case of the pemphigus antibody titres, which are determined every two to three months). The results so far obtained, which admittedly relate to only a few patients, can be summarised as follows:

a) In patch tests the reaction of the skin becomes weaker under the influence of Synacthen Depot. This is particularly apparent in cases where the test has yielded only a weakly positive result prior to the treatment; in such instances, the tests usually prove negative after Synacthen Depot has been administered.

b) Tuberculin reactions are more difficult to assess. Here again, however, the reaction usually becomes weaker following treatment with Synacthen Depot. In one patient, however, we had the impression that the tuberculin reaction had become more pronounced.

c) In the serum tests, Synacthen Depot fails to modify the reactions in a uniform manner. Whereas, in all the patients we have so far studied, the Wassermann reaction has weakened in response to the treatment, the V.D.R.L.* reaction has tended to become more strongly positive.

d) Treatment with Synacthen Depot has the effect of diminishing the pemphigus antibody titre (measured by the immunofluorescence method); antibodies directed against intercellular substance may disappear completely, whereas antibodies directed against basement membrane tend to react less.

For the moment, the only conclusion emerging from these investigations is that certain immune reactions are indeed affected by tetracosactide, but that it affects them in different ways.

One factor which has a decisive bearing on the usefulness, or otherwise, of a given form of treatment—especially in the management of chronic diseases—is

---

* Venereal Disease Research Laboratory.

Table 3. Side effects observed during treatment with Synacthen or Synacthen Depot.

Side effect	Number of patients	%	Average number of injections given before the side effect appeared
Fluid retention	12	4	12
Hyperglycaemia	9	3	17
Cushingoid signs	6	2	43
Nervousness	6	2	4
Gastric symptoms	5	1.5	18
Mycotic infections	5	1.5	36
Allergy	3	1	15
Miscellaneous	3	1	15

the type and frequency of the side effects that it provokes. In the 283 carefully observed patients with whom the present report is concerned, we have encountered side effects on 49 occasions (in 14% of our cases). The types of side effect, and their incidence, are indicated in Table 3, which calls for the following comments:

Fluid retention may sometimes manifest itself after only a few injections, especially if these are administered daily or every other day. It becomes apparent chiefly in the form of a gain in body-weight, although in some patients it may be most noticeable in certain localised areas of the body, such as the face. Generally, however, fluid retention does not develop until a number of injections have been given; only in two of our cases did it prove so severe as to necessitate the withdrawal of treatment with tetracosactide.

Elevation of the blood sugar levels, which we noted in nine cases, was difficult to interpret, particularly since the patients included seven with frank diabetes who showed no deterioration while in receipt of tetracosactide. In those cases in which a rise in the blood sugar levels did occur, it was usually during protracted therapy. This hyperglycaemia often responded readily to dietary measures; only in four patients did it compel us to discontinue the medication.

A mild form of *Cushing's syndrome* occurred in six patients. The earliest recorded onset of the syndrome was after the eighth injection; as a rule, however, it was only in the further course of prolonged treatment with tetracosactide that this side effect appeared. In no case did it call for withdrawal of the drug.

It is by no means easy to assess the significance of the *"nervous" symptoms* of which six patients complained—symptoms described as a feeling of warmth following injection of the drug, "feverishness", or general nervousness. Since these symptoms were already reported by most of the six patients after the very first injection, they were no doubt largely of a psychogenic nature. Of five patients who complained of *gastric discomfort* during treatment with tetracosactide, only one—in whom the medication was subsequently withdrawn—was found to be suffering from a recurrence of peptic ulceration; in the remaining four cases, the symptoms were probably likewise mainly of nervous origin.

The *mycotic infections* which supervened in the course of treatment in five patients can be ascribed to a decrease in their powers of natural resistance. On the other hand, even in cases receiving protracted treatment, we never observed any bacterial or viral infections. In three patients who developed a genuine form of *allergic urticaria* in response to tetracosactide, the drug had of course to be withdrawn.

On the whole, these side effects were of a mild nature and necessitated discontinuation of the therapy only in ten out of the 49 patients. When a comparison is made between the side effects occurring under Synacthen or Synacthen Depot with those encountered in response to corticosteroid treatment of equivalent duration and therapeutic efficacy, it becomes evident that the side effects of tetracosactide are appreciably less frequent and less severe. In particular, we never encountered any bone fractures—a complication which had been observed almost regularly in patients with pemphigus at the time when we were still employing corticosteroids as treatment for this disease. The incidence of severe stomach disorders, such as gastric ulcers and haemorrhage, is also considerably lower. As for diffuse atrophy of the skin and bruising, these side effects were never met with in any of our patients.

From the results we have obtained, the following conclusions can be drawn: Synacthen Depot has established a firm place for itself in the dermatological field; and, in the treatment of pemphigus in particular, it constitutes the drug of first choice. Generally speaking, in chronic skin conditions treatment with Synacthen Depot is a better alternative to corticosteroid therapy, because the side effects which it provokes are fewer and less serious. In alopecia areata, however, tetracosactide fails to provide a substitute for treatment with corticosteroids. Whether the clinical effectiveness of tetracosactide is attributable purely and simply to the fact that it induces the adrenal cortex to produce and secrete therapeutically active steroids, or whether another mechanism may also be involved, is a question to which an answer is likely to be found chiefly by analysing the effect of this synthetic corticotrophin on various immune reactions and by comparing this effect with that of the corticosteroids.

Discussion

K.F. WEINGES: I should be interested, Dr. SCHUPPLI, to hear more about the dosage schedule you used. Did you have to give an injection every other day in order to maintain an effect, or were you later able to manage with one or two injections per week?

R. SCHUPPLI: In answer to this question, allow me to show you the type of treatment schedule used in a case of pemphigus vulgaris (Figure 1). We had treated this woman with corticosteroids for about one year, the dosage being equivalent to roughly 30 mg. prednisone daily. Indicated at the top of the diagram is the clinical course of the skin lesions. As you can see, there were repeated exacerbations. When a vertebral fracture occurred, we withdrew the corticosteroid therapy from one day to the next and replaced it by Synacthen Depot. We began by giving injections every other day and then prolonged the interval between doses to three, four, and finally five days. Later we were able to increase the intervals even further, i.e. we administered the drug only if and when there was a bullous eruption and then gradually withdrew it. During the past two years or so, this patient has required only three injections, each of which was given when—in response to the stress of exposure to sunlight—a very mild eruption of bullae had occurred. In this case, Synacthen Depot was clearly superior to corticosteroids.

E. POLLI: I should like to ask you a question, Dr. SCHUPPLI, in connection with the slide that you have just shown us illustrating a case of pemphigus. Judging both from this slide and from data in other papers already presented here, it seems to me that no clear-cut correlation exists between the doses of corticosteroids and of A.C.T.H. that are required to produce a therapeutic effect. Could you perhaps offer a comment on this point?

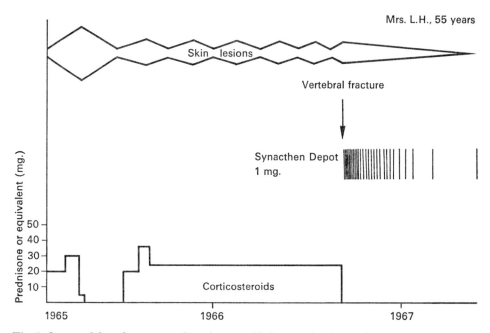

Fig. 1. Successful replacement of corticosteroid therapy by Synacthen Depot following a vertebral fracture in a woman suffering from pemphigus vulgaris.

R. SCHUPPLI: Pemphigus is probably the easiest disease in which to assess equivalence of dosage as between steroids and A.C.T.H. In pemphigus we have found that 1 mg. of synthetic A.C.T.H., given every second day, exerts an effect equivalent to that of 20–25 mg. prednisone daily. We also obtained the same dosage ratios for these two forms of treatment in lepra reactions.

F. KOGOJ: In this connection, I should like to describe from my own experience a case involving a 53-year-old medical colleague who for nine years has been suffering from arthritis confined chiefly to the small joints of the hand and fingers. Antirheumatic agents—with the exception of corticoids—had failed to exert any influence on the clinical course of the condition, which was marked by exacerbations and remissions. Repeated laboratory tests (antistreptolysin titre, Waaler-Rose differential agglutination test, and uric acid determinations) had yielded negative findings. In the spring of 1972 a severe exacerbation occurred, marked by pain and swelling which also spread to the wrist of the right hand; the erythrocyte sedimentation rate was 50/70. The articular lesions were still present in December 1972, when a very small number of papulosquamous eruptions also developed, the clinical and histological appearance of which was suggestive of psoriasis. It was in this condition that I saw the patient for the first time towards the end of February 1973 and diagnosed psoriatic arthropathy. He had five injections of 1 mg. Synacthen Depot at the rate of roughly two a week. A few minutes after the first injection he began sweating profusely, complained of dizziness and nausea, and collapsed; his blood pressure rose to 195/135 mm. Hg. The patient quickly recovered, however, and—unbeknownst to me at the time—resumed the treatment without suffering any further complications and without showing any rise in blood pressure. The results of the medication were highly satisfactory. The pain disappeared after the very first injection, the swelling then subsided too, and the skin lesions became almost invisible. It should also be mentioned that some time before the start of the treatment, as well as a few days after the last injection of Synacthen Depot, the patient had an attack of acute urticaria. Some four weeks following this series of injections, quite a severe exacerbation of the patient's arthritis set in. Despite two injections of Synacthen Depot, the reddening, swelling, and pain have actually increased; the injections are at present being continued. Looking back on this case with the benefit of hindsight, I still believe that the episode occurring after the first injection was not due to an allergic reaction, but that it nevertheless must have been indirectly caused by the Synacthen Depot. I think this may have been the sort of phenomenon that the French refer to as an "autonomic nervous surprise".

R. SCHUPPLI: This is a reaction of the kind that does occasionally occur following any injection; perhaps the likeliest explanation is that the drug was injected into a blood vessel. If you inject a crystalline substance intravascularly, you are liable to get this syndrome of flushing, elevated blood pressure, and collapse.

W. J. IRVINE: I'd like to add a few comments on the daily use of Synacthen Depot. When we started employing Synacthen Depot some time ago, we decided to give it daily for the first two days, in order to get a good response going and to bring the patient's condition rapidly under control. We soon discovered, however, that this daily medication provoked fairly severe fluid retention and electrolyte abnormalities, marked particularly by a fall in the serum potassium levels. The reasons for these phenomena are, of course, now quite clear. As I have already indicated in my paper, Synacthen Depot also stimulates the secretion of aldosterone, this stimulation persisting for a period longer than 24 hours when the drug is given in a dose of 1 mg. Hence, if you use Synacthen Depot on a daily basis, even for only a few days, you get quite a strong build-up of aldosterone—with consequences that become only too obvious. I think it would therefore now be considered inappropriate to administer Synacthen Depot daily, even at the start of treatment; otherwise you almost inevitably run the risk of complications such as I have just mentioned. Where one is anxious to achieve a good initial response, I suggest that the best approach is to combine Synacthen Depot with oral steroids, rather than to increase the frequency of the Synacthen Depot injections.

I also have a theoretical question I wish to raise. From an immunological standpoint one can, of course, draw a distinction between low-dose tolerance and high-dose tolerance. This prompts me to wonder whether one may perhaps be more likely to get an immune reaction against Synacthen Depot by administering the drug intermittently than by giving a continuous course of treatment with either a high or a low dosage.

R. SCHUPPLI: I can't answer your theoretical question, Dr. IRVINE, but I do entirely agree with you in giving A.C.T.H. only every second day at the start of treatment and in combining it, if necessary, with an oral steroid.

R.-J. WÜTHRICH: When commencing medication with Synacthen Depot in cases of multiple sclerosis we have always given the drug daily, but to guard against possible side effects we take appropriate precautions, i.e. we administer potassium substitution treatment, diuretic therapy, etc. Using this approach we have encountered very few problems in the way of side effects such as Dr. IRVINE has just mentioned. Consequently, in the many hundreds of courses of treatment we have given, we have seen no reason to depart from this dosage schedule.

Treatment with synthetic A.C.T.H. in paediatrics

by H. Boissière*

Since its introduction as a therapeutic agent, it is chiefly in adults that ®Synacthen (including the longer-acting formulation known as ®Synacthen Depot) has been employed. In paediatrics, where experience with this drug (β1–24 corticotrophin or tetracosactide) has been less extensive and of more recent date, the number of cases thus far treated has not been sufficient to permit satisfactory guidelines to be laid down for its use in children. On the basis of a series of 224 paediatric cases, taken from the relevant French literature as well as from among our own patients, I believe, however, that it is now possible to draw up a balance-sheet, as it were, which—though still far from complete— nevertheless holds out much promise for the future. The report I am about to present, which will be confined purely and simply to clinical aspects of the use of Synacthen and Synacthen Depot in the management of diseases of child- hood, deals with the indications for such medication, its therapeutic efficacy, and its tolerability.

Cases studied

The 224 cases treated can be divided into the following two groups:

a) 175 cases upon which six reports were already presented in Paris in May 1971 at a colloquium on modern A.C.T.H. therapy over which I had the honour to preside.
b) 49 further cases which have been studied in my own hospital department during the past two years and which serve either to confirm or to shed further light on the indications for tetracosactide therapy and on the findings that had been obtained earlier.

The diseases for which the 224 children were treated can be listed as follows (Table 1):
– Childhood asthma in 39 patients. VIALATTE and PAUPE[10] already reported on 31 of these cases in 1971, the remaining eight being cases treated in my own department. Almost all of these children, whose ages ranged from 18 months to 17 years, were suffering from severe asthma, and six of them from status asthmaticus.
– Acute infective laryngitis, associated with marked dyspnoea, in 11 infants aged six months to three years. Of these cases, six have been taken from the report by JANBON et al.[4] and five were cases of my own.

---

*Hôpital Notre-Dame du Perpétuel Secours, Paris, France.

Table 1. Tabular review of the 224 children treated, indicating the diseases from which they were suffering and distinguishing between cases reported upon in 1971 at the *Colloque thérapeutique CIBA* and the author's own cases.

	1971 Colloque thérapeutique CIBA	1973 Cases treated by the author	Totals
Asthma	31	8	39
Acute infective laryngitis	6	5	11
Dyspnoeic bronchopneumopathy	47	8	55
Infectious diseases	36	9	45
C.N.S. disorders	40	9	49
Haemolytic jaundice of the newborn	10	2	12
Chronic rheumatism	5		5
Miscellaneous		8	8
Totals	175	49	224

– Dyspnoeic bronchopneumopathy of viral origin—with diffuse or focal X-ray findings and disturbances of ventilation—in 55 cases, of which 47 have already been reported upon by the above-mentioned authors from Montpellier[4], the remaining eight being my own patients.

– Severe infections (45 cases) comprising meningo-encephalitis, neurotoxia, purulent meningitis, and severe forms of whooping cough, measles, and chicken-pox. Of these 45 cases, 36 have been taken from the report already referred to[4], and nine were patients treated in my own department.

– Non-infective C.N.S. disorders (49 cases). Of these cases, involving West's syndrome, Lennox's syndrome, or forms of encephalopathy accompanied by convulsions, nine have been reported upon by BRISSAUD et al.[3], seven by SOULAYROL et al.[8], and 24 by BERNARD et al.[2]; nine were cases which I myself observed.

– Haemolytic jaundice of the newborn in 12 cases, of which D'OELSNITZ et al.[6] studied ten and I myself the remaining two.

– Chronic rheumatism in five cases which have been reported by MOZZICO-NACCI and ATTAL[5].

– Finally, eight cases which I myself observed, namely, two of neonatal hypoglycaemia, one of very severe neonatal distress, one of acquired haemolytic anaemia of viral origin, one of infective adenopathy, one of acute sacro-iliac arthritis, and two of generalised eczema.

Some of these 224 children were given treatment with the short-acting formulation of Synacthen, but the vast majority received Synacthen Depot, the size of the single doses ranging from 0.25 to 1 mg. according to age. The duration of the medication and the intervals between doses varied, of course, depending on the severity of the disease and on the effectiveness of the treatment.

The results obtained with tetracosactide must be analysed in the light both of the therapeutic responses observed and of the drug's tolerability.

Therapeutic responses

Global evaluation

Of the 224 patients treated, 179 (80%) showed very good results, as compared with 45 (20%) in whom the response was either negative or mediocre and in whom—owing, among other things, to the irreversible nature of the neurological sequelae—the treatment could nowise be said even to have proved partially successful (Table 2).

The therapeutic effectiveness of tetracosactide, however, has to be assessed by reference to the form of disease treated—a method of assessment which not only reveals profound differences in the drug's action in one type of case as compared with another, but which also provides a better approach to the problem of differentiating between the respective indications for A.C.T.H. and cortico-steroids. Certain conditions respond remarkably well to tetracosactide; these conditions, in which the success rate reaches 90% or more, therefore constitute very good indications for A.C.T.H. therapy. There are other diseases, by contrast, in which such therapy yields success rates equivalent to barely 10% but in which, despite this, tetracosactide still deserves preference inasmuch as it is one of the rare drugs—or possibly the only drug—offering any likelihood of effecting a cure.

Childhood asthma

The cases of asthma treated with tetracosactide consisted of 39 children aged 18 months to 17 years, 31 of whom were suffering from severe asthma, six from status asthmaticus, and two from asthmatiform dyspnoea (Table 3).

The first 11 patients in this series were given short-acting Synacthen, and the remaining 28 Synacthen Depot. Depending on the patient's age, the dosage for

Table 2. Global evaluation of results obtained in children treated with tetracosactide.

Number of cases	Number of good responses	Number of failures
224	179 (80%)	45 (20%)

Table 3. Results obtained with Synacthen or Synacthen Depot in childhood asthma.

Age groups and number of patients per group		Type of asthma		Type of Synacthen employed		Results	
≤6 years	14	Severe asthma	31	Synacthen	11	Good response	36
6 to 12 years	15	Status asthmaticus	6	Synacthen Depot	28	Poor response	3
12 to 17 years	10	Asthmatiform dyspnoea	2				
Total	39		39		39		39

Table 4. Indications for tetracosactide in asthma.

Severe asthma
Status asthmaticus
Preparatory treatment prior to administration of disodium cromoglycate
Withdrawal of corticosteroid medication
Readaptation following climatotherapy

this latter preparation—which we, like many other authors, found to be both more effective and easier to handle—was 0.5 to 1 mg., injected once a day until the dyspnoea had abated. The doses were then spaced out, the intervals between injections being each time successively prolonged by 24 hours until the patient was receiving only one injection per week; for prophylactic purposes, these weekly injections can be continued for two to three months or more.

On the whole, the results obtained were excellent, and only three of the 39 children failed to respond. Synacthen, particularly when employed in its depot form, seems to be preferable to corticosteroids in the treatment of asthma, because it is highly effective and—as we shall see later—well tolerated, and because it produces fewer side effects and is easy to handle.

Its indications in asthmatic children can be summarised as follows: severe asthma, status asthmaticus, preparatory treatment prior to administration of disodium cromoglycate, withdrawal of corticosteroid medication, and readaptation following climatotherapy (Table 4).

Acute laryngitis

In young children, acute laryngitis is a potentially serious disease, because, if inadequately or ineptly treated at the start, it may result in respiratory distress due to suffocation—in which case resuscitatory measures have to be taken. At this late stage, however, prolonged anoxia is liable to produce irreversible cerebral damage. Hence the importance of recognising these acute forms of laryngitis and treating them properly in good time.

Although it is far from certain that acute laryngitis of infancy is always of viral origin, the disease at least presents a fairly consistent clinical picture, which means that it lends itself more readily to a standardised treatment schedule than does a polymorphous condition such as asthma.

In my experience, an immediate injection of short-acting Synacthen, which, depending on the degree of urgency, can be given either by the intramuscular or by the intravenous route, very quickly counteracts dyspnoea and inspiratory recession of the chest wall due to the laryngeal obstruction, while at the same time rapidly promoting resolution of the accompanying oedema; this avoids the necessity for intubation or tracheotomy, which nowadays in fact is very seldom indicated. In all cases of this type, however, the initial dose of Synacthen should be followed by daily injections of 0.5 to 1 mg. Synacthen Depot for four to six days in order to prevent a relapse (Figure 1).

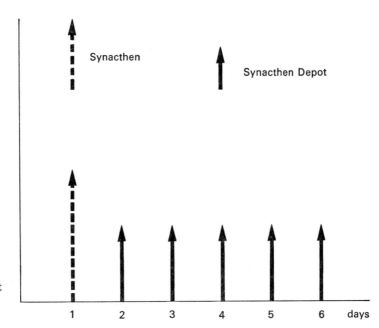

Fig. 1. Recommended dosage schedule for Synacthen and Synacthen Depot in acute laryngitis.

This treatment schedule—naturally, under antibiotic cover—has been successfully employed in 11 infants under three years of age suffering from asphyxiating subglottic laryngitis coupled with very severe dyspnoea. It may indeed be asserted that acute infantile laryngitis is one of the most rewarding indications for tetracosactide and that here this drug yields results at least as good as those obtained with cortisone derivatives.

Dyspnoeic bronchopneumopathy

Tetracosactide has been used in the treatment of 55 patients, consisting of 39 infants with bronchopneumonia and 16 children over two years of age suffering from a severe bronchopneumopathy which in four cases was accompanied by disturbances of ventilation. All of them were cases of severe pulmonary disease associated with high fever and marked dyspnoea. Since in these patients the bronchopneumopathy was of bacterial or viral origin—the cases of viral bronchopneumopathy being quite often complicated by secondary bacterial infection—the antibiotic therapy administered was no doubt the main factor responsible for the 100% success rate; but the rapid improvement in the signs of pulmonary dysfunction and respiratory failure must be credited to the treatment with tetracosactide (Table 5).

I am aware of the fact that, in various recent Anglo-Saxon publications dealing with studies on the use of corticosteroids in infantile bronchopneumopathy of viral origin, the conclusion is reached that corticosteroids exert no effect either on the severity of the dyspnoea or on the length of the illness as compared with controls receiving no hormone therapy. I am also aware of the fact that in this field many authors believe treatment with corticosteroids or A.C.T.H. to be

133

Table 5. Results obtained with tetracosactide in cases of dyspnoeic bronchopneumopathy.

Age groups and number of patients per group		Type of bronchopneumopathy		Good responses
<2 years	39	Bronchopneumonia	39	39
>2 years	16	Severe pneumopathy	12	12
		Disturbances of ventilation	4	4
Total	55		55	55

indicated only in a few restricted conditions characterised by disturbances of ventilation. I personally do not share the view that hormone therapy should be ostracised to this extent, since the presence of severe dyspnoea seems to me to be sufficient reason in itself to warrant recourse to such therapy. The chief advantage of A.C.T.H. in these indications is that it very quickly lowers the patient's temperature and eliminates the dyspnoea, thereby affording—much more promptly than treatment with antibiotics alone—a degree of relief that strikes me as being of indisputable value.

In non-dyspnoeic forms of bronchopneumopathy, however, as well as in the vast majority of bacterial lung diseases, there is of course no need to employ A.C.T.H., because these normally respond very well to antibiotics alone.

Severe infections
Included in this category are infections involving the nervous system (meningo-encephalitis, purulent meningitis, and acute dehydration) as well as other severe forms of infectious disease such as whooping cough, measles, and chickenpox (Table 6).

11 cases of acute meningo-encephalitis of viral origin were treated intravenously with short-acting Synacthen, combined with antibiotics. The causative virus was *Herpesvirus varicellae* in one case, rubella virus in three cases, respiratory syncytial virus in two cases, an adenovirus in three cases, and an E.C.H.O. virus in the remaining two cases.

In all 11 cases the patients effected a rapid and complete recovery which was unattended by sequelae; the fever subsided within two to four days, the disturbances of consciousness disappeared after an average of two to six days, the convulsions observed at the onset of the infection never recurred, the E.E.G. changes regressed within seven to 12 days, and the behavioural disorders abated over a period of three to six weeks.

We all know, of course, that acute meningo-encephalitis may run an astonishing variety of clinical courses and that even the possibility of spontaneous regression cannot be excluded. But we also know only too well that by and large this is a very serious type of infection and one that frequently either proves fatal or gives rise to irreversible sequelae. Though the experience thus far acquired is too limited to permit of any final conclusions, the fact that in these 11 cases of

Table 6. Results obtained with tetracosactide in severe infections.

	Number of cases	Good responses	Failures (exitus or sequelae)
Meningo-encephalitis of viral origin	11	11	
Purulent meningitis:			
meningococcal	7	7	
due to other causative micro-organisms	4	2	2
neonatal	4	2	2
Acute dehydration in infants	6	4	2
Severe forms of infectious disease:			
whooping cough	8	7	1
measles	2	2	
chickenpox*	3	3	
Totals	45	38	7

* In children receiving treatment with corticosteroids or immunosuppressants

meningo-encephalitis the patients made a complete recovery does indicate that the treatment was certainly efficacious. Assuming that A.C.T.H. also has the effect of combating cerebral inflammation, it becomes only logical to conclude that, within the field of virus diseases, meningo-encephalitis (excluding forms due to herpesviruses) constitutes one of the best indications for A.C.T.H.

15 cases of severe purulent meningitis—i.e. seven of meningococcal meningitis (including six septicaemic forms with gangrenous purpura), two of meningitis due to infection with *Haemophilus influenzae,* two caused by pneumococci and staphylococci, respectively, and four cases of neonatal meningitis (in which the causative micro-organisms were pneumococci, Proteus, or *Salmonella typhimurium*)—received treatment with antibiotics and tetracosactide.

Although the treatment proved successful in all the patients suffering from meningococcal meningitis, failures were encountered in four of the other cases (two deaths from neonatal meningitis, one death from staphylococcal meningitis occurring as a complication to acute leukaemia, and one case of hydrocephalus as a sequel to pneumococcal meningitis in an infant aged four months).

In purulent meningitis of infancy, the prognosis evidently depends on the type of micro-organism to which the disease is due, on the child's age, and also on the stage at which treatment with antibiotics is instituted. Here, cases constituting the best indications for A.C.T.H. therapy are those involving severe neonatal forms in which the patient is comatose from the very onset, since in such instances it may prevent states of shock and disturbances affecting the circulation of the C.S.F.

Six infants suffering from acute dehydration associated with cardiovascular shock and coma, which had not responded satisfactorily to rehydration, antibiotic therapy, and correction of the metabolic balance, were given treatment with tetracosactide. Following administration of this drug, four of them effected an unexpected recovery, which was devoid of sequelae. The treatment proved a failure,

135

however, in the other two cases, i.e. in two infants aged four and six months, respectively, who were suffering from hyperacute dehydration and in whom a complicating cerebral syndrome resulted in death within 24 hours.

Eight cases of severe whooping cough in infants (three pulmonary forms with asphyxiating fits of coughing, two apnoeic forms, and three encephalitic forms) deserve mention here inasmuch as A.C.T.H. therapy led to a rapid recovery in seven of these patients. Both in my opinion and in that of the authors from Montpellier to whom I have already referred [4], severe whooping cough in infants is a good indication for treatment with tetracosactide. However, the experience we have thus far gained with tetracosactide in cases of this type is not sufficient to outweigh entirely the verdict of those who hitherto have claimed that neither corticosteroids nor A.C.T.H. of natural origin exert any influence on the clinical course of severe whooping cough.

Two cases of measles which were classified as severe in view of the intensity of the general signs, the marked prostration, and the gravity of the respiratory impairment, were treated with tetracosactide, in response to which both patients soon began to recover. A.C.T.H. may thus possibly be indicated in patients suffering from severe measles, or in cases of measles complicated by encephalitis, even though malignant syndromes are beyond the scope of A.C.T.H. therapy.

Finally, *three cases in which chickenpox occurred* in the course of corticosteroid therapy or treatment with immunosuppressive agents were also given tetracosactide. In all three cases the chickenpox responded well, although one of the children subsequently died from the acute leukaemia from which it was also suffering. These three observations pose the problem as to whether or when tetracosactide is indicated in children contracting chickenpox whilst in receipt of corticosteroid therapy. While it is true that treatment with A.C.T.H. cannot be expected to stimulate an exhausted adrenal cortex, and that in such cases increasing the corticosteroid dosage is therefore a reasonable measure, there are nevertheless grounds for hoping that early injection treatment with tetracosactide, instituted as soon as a child in receipt of corticosteroids has become infected, may reduce the risk of its developing a malignant form of chickenpox.

Primary C.N.S. disorders

This category comprises non-infective forms of neuropathy, i.e. West's syndrome, Lennox's syndrome, and the less well-defined group of convulsive encephalopathies (Table 7).

West's syndrome

It was SOREL and DUSAUCY-BAULOYE[7] who in 1958 first drew attention to the fact that A.C.T.H. and hydrocortisone were the only drugs likely to be at all effective in West's syndrome (infantile spasms with hypsarrhythmia). Their therapeutic efficacy in this disease, however, proved to be only mediocre, since the immediately beneficial effects which they exerted on the spasms and E.E.G. anomalies rarely stood the test of time, and the mental damage sustained—which has a major influence on the prognosis—was found to persist to quite a marked degree in more than 75% of cases.

Table 7. Results obtained with tetracosactide in C.N.S. disorders.

	Number of cases	Good responses	Failures
West's syndrome	18	5	13
Lennox's syndrome	19	8	11
Convulsive encephalopathy	12	2	10
Totals	49	15	34

Table 8. Factors influencing the prognosis in West's syndrome.

	Favourable	Unfavourable
Aetiology of syndrome	Primary	Secondary
Patient's age at onset of syndrome	<3 months	>3 months
Whether convulsive seizures absent or present before onset of syndrome	Absent	Present
Whether A.C.T.H. therapy initiated less than or more than two months after onset of syndrome	<2 months	>2 months
Duration of A.C.T.H. therapy	>1 year (?)	<1 year (?)

Has the advent of synthetic A.C.T.H. done anything to improve this bleak outlook? I do not know exactly how many cases of West's syndrome have been treated with synthetic A.C.T.H. to date, because by no means all the relevant observations have been published. Here I can merely give an account of results obtained in a series of 18 patients in whom treatment with tetracosactide was initiated during the period extending from October 1967 to November 1971; in many of these cases, therefore, the time elapsing since the start of the treatment has not been long enough for us to make a definitive assessment of its value. The results, though still to be regarded as provisional, nevertheless appear to confirm the conclusions reached by THIEFFRY and AICARDI [9] in 1958, i.e. that the patient's response depends upon whether the disease occurs in a primary or secondary form, whether it develops before or after the age of three months, whether or not the child had already previously suffered from convulsive seizures, and whether treatment is initiated less than or more than two months after the onset of the symptoms (Table 8). In my opinion it is also *very important to ensure that the treatment is continued over a sufficiently prolonged period.* In the case of the first patients treated with A.C.T.H. of natural origin, the medication lasted only one month, and it was recommended that it be followed up by one or two one-month courses of hydrocortisone. In the aforementioned series of 18 cases, on the other hand, 17 patients were treated for two months, first with short-acting Synacthen and then with Synacthen Depot, but the results were likewise only mediocre. The 18th patient, by contrast, has now been receiving tetra-cosactide for 16 months, and the response has been excellent. This child had been normal up to the age of nine months, but spasms then set in, accompanied by rapid impairment of psychomotor function, characteristic E.E.G. changes, and encephalographic evidence of ventricular dilatation and subcortical atrophy. The treatment, which was commenced one month after the onset of the spasms and consisted of 0.5 mg. Synacthen Depot injected twice daily, restored the E.E.G. pattern to normal within one week. After one month of treatment, the child was capable of sitting up again and of grasping objects held out to it, in addition to which it was also beginning to smile once more. The dosage of Synacthen Depot was then reduced to one injection daily for two weeks, after which the interval between injections was successively prolonged by one day per week until the child was receiving only one weekly injection. After three months its appearance and behaviour had been completely trans-formed: it was now able to stand upright and was already taking its first steps, it also held out its arms, took a lively interest in everything around it, and indulged in hearty laughter. At the moment it is a splendid 26-month-old baby (Figure 2), and the Synacthen Depot which it has been receiving for the past 16 months is still being perfectly tolerated. Admittedly, this infant has not been under observation long enough for us to claim that it has effected a permanent recovery, nor can we answer the question as to when the treatment should be discontinued or hazard a guess as to whether the child, which has so far proved so responsive to tetracosactide, will ultimately become dependent upon the drug. At all events, if this patient continues to do well, I intend in future to give each case of West's syndrome an intensive course of Synacthen Depot therapy lasting two months and, whenever the child shows a marked improvement, to follow this up with a very prolonged period of maintenance treatment in an attempt to uphold the improvement.

Lennox's syndrome
The 19 children in whom synthetic A.C.T.H. was employed as therapy for this form of petit mal (severe myokinetic epilepsy of early infancy) all consist of cases treated at the *Ecole pédiatrique* in Marseilles (BERNARD et al.[2]). Each child was given either Synacthen or Synacthen Depot for a period of three weeks to one month (together with anti-epileptic medication), followed by a course of treatment with hydrocortisone lasting several months. The results, which were generally assessed one year after the cessation of treatment, proved good in eight of the 19 cases (Table 7), but here two reservations have to be made: firstly, a one-year follow-up period is not sufficiently long and, secondly, the authors who have reported on these cases confine their attention to the seizures, the E.E.G. anomalies, and the behavioural disorders of the patients, but do not mention what effect the treatment had on mental retardation, which—as in West's syndrome—is the cardinal factor as regards the long-term prognosis.

138

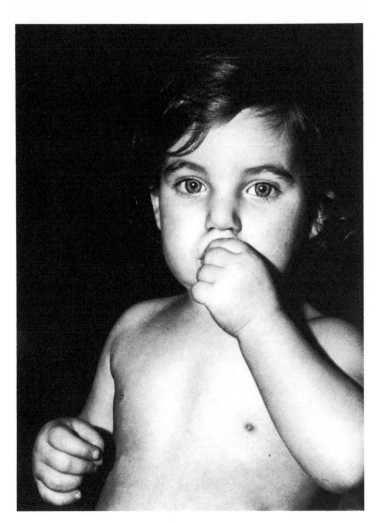

Fig. 2. 26-month-old child after 16 months of Synacthen Depot medication, given as treatment for West's syndrome.

Even when allowance is made for these reservations, however, it can be claimed that the results yielded by synthetic A.C.T.H. appear to be better than those obtained with corticosteroids; moreover, it is also conceivable that, if a much more prolonged course of treatment had been administered, the proportion of good responses might possibly have been higher.

Chronic convulsive forms of encephalopathy
These constitute a heterogeneous group of diseases which can nevertheless be distinguished both from West's and from Lennox's syndrome. They differ from West's syndrome inasmuch as nodding spasms and hypsarrhythmia are not a feature of their clinical picture, and they can be distinguished from Lennox's syndrome by virtue of the fact that they do not involve the occurrence of absences. They also differ from idiopathic epilepsy in that they are associated with an often marked degree of mental retardation and are unresponsive to the standard anti-epileptic drugs.

Unfortunately, treatment with synthetic A.C.T.H. largely failed to improve the prognosis in these intractable forms of encephalopathy: it elicited a good response in only two out of 12 cases (Table 7). These disappointing results confirm once again the extreme gravity of this group of diseases, which have thus far defied all attempts at treatment; and it is quite possible that not even the two good responses to which I have just referred will stand the test of time.

Severe idiopathic epilepsy

In this category I include cases of idiopathic epilepsy which show markedly abnormal E.E.G. tracings and which it proves impossible to control by treatment with the usual anticonvulsant drugs, but which differ from the convulsive forms of encephalopathy in that they entail no mental retardation. I have been treating ten of these patients with Synacthen Depot for the past 18 months—a period which, of course, is not long enough to enable me to express a valid opinion on the effectiveness of the therapy. It is my impression, however, that this may well be a rewarding indication for Synacthen Depot and one in which the drug is likely to exert a better therapeutic effect than in the various types of encephalopathy that I have previously mentioned.

Haemolytic jaundice of the newborn

We have two sets of statistics on infants treated for this disease. The first relates to the use of an A.C.T.H. extract-preparation under antibiotic cover in 36 premature infants suffering from haemolytic jaundice. Here, the treatment

Table 9. Results obtained with an A. C. T. H. extract-preparation and with the short-acting form of Synacthen in premature infants suffering from haemolytic jaundice.

		Number of cases	Mean serum bilirubin levels (%)			Average duration of jaundice	Number of replacement transfusions
			3rd day	6th day	9th day		
1	Untreated infants serving as controls	50	10.4	11.8	8.2	14 days	4
	Infants treated with A.C.T.H. of natural origin	36	9.8	8.0	4.3	9 days	0
2	Infants serving as controls (treated with phenobarbitone or corticosteroids)	15		16.2	16.0	15 days	2
	Infants treated with Synacthen	12		16.8	9.0	8 days	0

1 *Alison* and *Ploussard*[1]
2 *D'Oelsnitz* et al.[6] and the present author

definitely reduced the severity and duration of the jaundice by comparison with an untreated control group of 50 other premature infants with jaundice.

The second set of statistics covers 12 premature infants in whom the short-acting form of Synacthen was employed in a dosage of 0.25 mg. injected twice daily for six to eight days; these cases were compared with a control group of 15 premature infants treated with phenobarbitone or with a corticosteroid. Despite the high serum bilirubin levels recorded in some of them, all the infants receiving Synacthen effected a complete recovery which was unattended by any neurological sequelae (Table 9).

Although replacement transfusion must still be regarded as the *ultima ratio* in infants with hyperbilirubinaemia, A.C.T.H. seems at all events to be more effective in diminishing the severity and duration of the jaundice than do such other forms of treatment as phenobarbitone, phototherapy, infusions of human albumin, or corticosteroid medication. Tetracosactide—possibly in combination with phototherapy—would thus appear to be indicated as a means of minimising the need for replacement transfusions in cases where the serum bilirubin is approaching dangerously high levels.

Chronic rheumatism

Here, I can mention only five cases (four of Still's disease and one of arthritis affecting only a few joints) which were treated by Mozziconacci and Attal [5]. In these five children, the treatment proved remarkably effective in combating fever, improving the patient's general condition, and relieving pain, although its influence on the biological signs was less impressive. Unfortunately, experience with tetracosactide in chronic rheumatic diseases of childhood is too limited and of too recent a date to enable us to assess the long-term results. Moreover, though A.C.T.H. therapy serves to keep the disease under control while the treatment is actually in progress, it must be acknowledged that—like corticosteroid therapy—it cannot effect a cure. In chronic rheumatism, the use of A.C.T.H. also presents certain snags to which reference will be made later.

The main indications for tetracosactide

Besides the indications which have already been discussed, i.e. allergic disorders, respiratory diseases, infections, C.N.S. disorders, rheumatic illnesses, and jaundice, tetracosactide may also profitably be employed in certain blood diseases, in certain collagen diseases and disorders of the reticulo-endothelial system, in severe forms of epidemic hepatitis, in haemorrhagic types of rectocolitis, in certain conditions involving metabolic disturbances (such as nephrotic syndrome, hypervitaminosis D, and neonatal hypoglycaemia), and in some of the more serious skin diseases (Table 10). My own personal experience of these indications, however, is far too restricted to enable me to pronounce on them here. Nevertheless, in this context, I should at least like to emphasise the value of tetracosactide in the treatment of neonatal hypoglycaemia—a condition in which, by markedly accelerating the restoration of normal blood sugar levels, it effectively prevents the grave consequences of hypoglycaemic encephalopathy.   141

Table 10. The main indications for tetracosactide in paediatrics.

Allergic disorders	Rheumatoid diseases, etc.
Asthma	Chronic rheumatism
Eczema	Collagen diseases
Angioneurotic oedema	Disorders of the reticulo-endothelial
Allergy – to penicillin	system
– to cow's milk	
	Blood diseases
Respiratory diseases	Thrombocytopenia
Dyspnoeic forms of bronchopneumopathy	Acute haemolytic anaemia
Disturbances of ventilation	Malignant forms of haemopathy
Acute laryngitis	
	Digestive diseases
Severe infections	Ulcerative and haemorrhagic
Severe forms of measles and whooping	rectocolitis
cough	Severe forms of epidemic hepatitis
Chickenpox in children receiving	Haemolytic jaundice in premature
corticosteroid therapy (?)	infants
Septicaemia	
Rheumatic fever	Metabolic disturbances
Acute meningo-encephalitis of	Anterior-pituitary insufficiency
viral origin	Nephrotic syndrome
	Hypervitaminosis D
C.N.S. disorders	Neonatal and infantile hypoglycaemia
Severe purulent meningitis	
Convulsive forms of encephalopathy	Severe skin diseases
Severe idiopathic epilepsy	Pemphigus malignus
Cerebral oedema	Psoriatic arthropathy
– due to cerebral tumours	Mycosis fungoides
– in cases of neonatal distress	Erythrodermia

Tolerability

Two questions that immediately arise in this connection are: firstly, does treatment with tetracosactide entail the same hazards as corticosteroid therapy, with the added risk that it may possibly also provoke temporary melanoderma and inactivate the pituitary-adrenocortical axis? Secondly, does it on the other hand—thanks to its direct action on the adrenal cortex and to its stimulant effect on production of the entire gamut of adrenocortical hormones—give rise to fewer adverse reactions than treatment with corticosteroids? In the light of observations made in the 224 cases reviewed here, it is possible to provide at least a partial answer to these questions.

Factors conducive to adverse reactions

There are three main factors which tend to affect the tolerability of synthetic A.C.T.H. therapy: the duration of treatment, the size of the doses injected, and the frequency with which the injections are given.

1. *The duration of treatment* plays a fundamentally important role; and, among the 224 patients treated, none of those receiving brief courses of injections (i.e. courses lasting less than one month) ever showed any undesirable reactions. This was the case in a total of 158 patients, all of whom were suffering from

acute conditions which responded rapidly to treatment (i.e. most of the cases of asthma and all the cases of acute laryngitis, bronchopneumopathy, infective disease, and neonatal jaundice).

It was among patients treated for periods of two months or more that complications arose, the 66 patients concerned being made up of 12 cases of asthma, 49 of encephalopathy, and five of chronic rheumatism.

2. *Excessively large doses* such as were sometimes employed in the first of the cases treated, i.e. doses in young children exceeding 1 mg. Synacthen Depot daily, gave rise to cushingoid syndromes which the authors themselves admitted to be quite severe in some instances.

3. *The frequency with which the injections are given* is likewise a point to which great attention must be paid; the majority of the adverse reactions encountered were found to disappear whenever it was possible to reduce the frequency of the injections from once a day to twice or even once a week. In this connection, I should like to emphasise that the young patient aged 26 months to whom I referred earlier has been receiving one injection of 0.5 mg. Synacthen Depot once a week for over a year and has never developed mooning of the face, hypertension, osteoporosis, or muscular atrophy; what is more, this child has also maintained a normal rate of growth.

Complications of A.C.T.H. therapy

It is very difficult to determine the precise incidence of complications in the 66 patients in whom high doses and/or prolonged courses of treatment were given, because, whereas all the authors deal at length with their studies on the therapeutic efficacy of tetracosactide, many of them make no mention of the drug's tolerability. Consequently, I have been able to find references to side effects in only 28 cases—which means that one can neither state that in the remaining cases the drug was well tolerated nor draw up any reliable statistics on its side effects. The fact remains, however, that in this relatively small number of cases quite a few adverse reactions did appear (Table 11).

Table 11. Adverse reactions liable to occur in response to treatment with synthetic A.C.T.H., and extent to which they were or were not observed in 28 children.

Type of reaction	Number of cases
Cushing's syndrome	18
Hypertension	9
Suppression of pituitary-adrenocortical function	3
Melanoderma	2
Osteoporosis	2
Rebound phenomena	2
Muscular atrophy	1
Allergic reactions	0
Dependence on A.C.T.H.	0
Diabetes	0
Inhibition of growth	0
Secondary infection	0

Cushingoid syndrome was by far the commonest side effect; it was encountered in 18 cases, but quickly disappeared again when the doses were reduced or the interval between injections prolonged.

Hypertension in nine cases and suppression of pituitary-adrenocortical function in three cases were observed after two months of treatment with large daily doses of Synacthen Depot in children suffering from West's syndrome. In the event of such side effects, the injections should be spaced out in the hope that this may enable the pituitary-adrenocortical axis to recover and also have the effect of lowering the blood pressure.

Rebound phenomena occurred in two cases in which treatment with tetra-cosactide had been withdrawn too abruptly.

Osteoporosis (two cases), melanoderma (two cases), and muscular atrophy (one case) appeared after treatment with daily injections had been in progress for two months; these side effects, however, abated spontaneously once the interval between injections had been prolonged to one week.

Although neither diabetes, dependence on tetracosactide, nor inhibition of growth were observed, it should be borne in mind that the number of patients treated for periods of more than three months was only six, and that these six received only one injection per week.

Finally, no reference has been made to the occurrence of secondary infection or of allergic reactions in any of the cases—a fact which suggests that tetracos-actide, since it can also be accurately dosed by weight and displays unvarying activity, is infinitely superior to the older A.C.T.H. extract-preparations.

Contra-indications to A.C.T.H. therapy

Like all other forms of treatment, A.C.T.H. therapy, too, has its contra-indications. The majority of these are the same as for corticosteroid therapy, i.e. certain virus diseases, such as poliomyelitis, herpes, and chickenpox (except chickenpox occurring in patients receiving treatment with corticosteroids), reactions to vaccination with live viruses, hypertension, and peptic ulcers. A.C.T.H. is, of course, also contra-indicated in primary forms of hyper-corticism. Since the rationale of A.C.T.H. therapy is based on stimulation of the adrenal cortex, A.C.T.H. proves ineffective in cases of primary hypo-

Table 12. Contra-indications to the use of tetracosactide in paediatrics.

Peptic ulcers
Hypertension
Certain virus diseases: poliomyelitis, herpes, and uncomplicated chickenpox
Reactions to vaccination with live viruses
Primary hypercorticism (Cushing's syndrome, tumours)
Primary hypocorticism (Addison's disease, acute adrenocortical insufficiency, and congenital adrenal hyperplasia)

corticism, because it cannot stimulate adrenals that have been destroyed or that are already aplastic. Finally, A.C.T.H. is likewise contra-indicated in the presence of adrenocortical hyperplasia (Debré-Fibiger syndrome)—a condition in which its effect would be to increase sodium excretion and thus to aggravate the risk of sodium depletion (Table 12).

The highly encouraging results thus far obtained with synthetic A.C.T.H. indicate that, provided its indications are carefully selected, its contra-indications observed, and its dosage appropriately adapted from case to case, tetracosactide can justifiably be employed on a broad scale in paediatrics.

References

1 ALISON, F., PLOUSSARD, J.P.: L'ictère néo-natal par immaturité. Traitement. Journées paris. Pédiat. *1970*, 113
2 BERNARD, R., PINSARD, N., LAFON, S., SOULAYROL, R., ROGER, J., LOUBIER, D., DRAVET, C.: Synacthène-thérapie dans les épilepsies infantiles en dehors du syndrome de West. In: A.C.T.H.-thérapie moderne en pédiatrie, Coll. thér. CIBA, Paris 1971, p. 97 (Soc. Annonces et Publicité, Paris 1972)
3 BRISSAUD, H.-E., GIRARD, F., VAUDOUR, G.: Synacthène-thérapie des encéphalopathies épileptiques, loc. cit.[2], p. 87
4 JANBON, M., BRUNEL, D., JEAN, R., BONNET, H., ASTRUC, J.: A.C.T.H.-thérapie et maladies infectieuses de l'enfant, loc. cit.[2], p. 41
5 MOZZICONACCI, P., ATTAL, C.: Synacthène-thérapie et rhumatologie infantile, loc. cit.[2], p. 21
6 D'OELSNITZ, M., DESWARTE, M., BOURRIER-REYNAND, C., MAISSA, S.: A.C.T.H.-thérapie et ictères néo-nataux, loc. cit.[2], p. 127
7 SOREL, L., DUSAUCY-BAULOYE, A.: A propos de 21 cas d'hypsarythmia de Gibbs. Traitement spectaculaire par l'A.C.T.H. Rev. neurol. *99*, 136 (1958)
8 SOULAYROL, R., ROGER, J., ROMAGNAN, G., GASTAUT, H., PINSARD, N., BERNARD, R.: Essai du Synacthène dans les encéphalopathies épileptiques diffuses de l'enfant (syndrome de West – syndrome de Lennox). In: A.C.T.H.-thérapie moderne, Coll. thér. CIBA, Marseilles 1969, p. 171 (Kapp & Lahure, Vanves 1970)
9 THIEFFRY, S., AICARDI, J.: Les spasmes en flexion du nourrisson. 36 observations. Etude clinique. Ann. Pédiat. *34*, 187 (1958)
10 VIALATTE, J., PAUPE, J.: Le Synacthène dans le traitement de l'asthme infantile, loc. cit.[2], p. 31

A.C.T.H. and hydrocortisone in the prophylaxis of the neonatal respiratory distress syndrome

by H. V. PRICE*, H. CAMPBELL**, and E. CAMERON***

The cause of the onset of labour is not known. GALEN suggested that the foetus kicked its way out of the womb when the time was ripe. While we cannot accept this simple explanation, it does introduce the concept that it is the foetus which initiates labour. The modern view is that the foetal adrenal may well contain the operative trigger mechanism.

LIGGINS[1] reported that injection of A.C.T.H. or corticosteroids into the foetal lamb tended to initiate labour. Unexpectedly, he found that surfactant production was also induced, enabling prematurely born lambs to survive at a period of gestation when they would normally die of respiratory distress. Our investigations were undertaken to see if the findings in sheep also apply in man.

Methodological studies

In a first study, tests with short-acting ®Synacthen (tetracosactrin) were performed on 43 infants admitted to a special-care baby unit. The infants were of varying gestational ages. Venous samples were taken before and 30 minutes after intramuscular injection of Synacthen. They were analysed by the MATTINGLY[3] sulphuric acid fluorescence method (Figure 1).

In Figure 1, each vertical line represents the rise in plasma cortisol in one baby following the injection of Synacthen. The results varied widely from one baby to another. Thus, some, but not all, babies born prematurely do show evidence of adrenal hyperactivity. However, the technical difficulties encountered in performing the tests were considerable.

We therefore attempted to miniaturise the method, but could not obtain reproducible results with plasma samples of less than 50 mcl. Consequently, the MURPHY[4] method of competitive protein binding radioassay was used, and reproducible results were achieved with 10 mcl. plasma samples. Samples were taken from a variety of newborn infants, and the results obtained by both methods showed a very good correlation, although the Mattingly values were higher. This finding was unexpected, since the two methods measure different steroids. However, this enabled us subsequently to carry out the tests on capillary blood samples.

Tests with short-acting Synacthen were then performed on normal full-term healthy babies, in order to obtain normal values. Ten babies were tested one

---

* Department of Child Health, Welsh National School of Medicine, Cardiff, Wales.
** Department of Medical Statistics, Welsh National School of Medicine, Cardiff.
*** Tenovus Institute for Cancer Research, Cardiff.

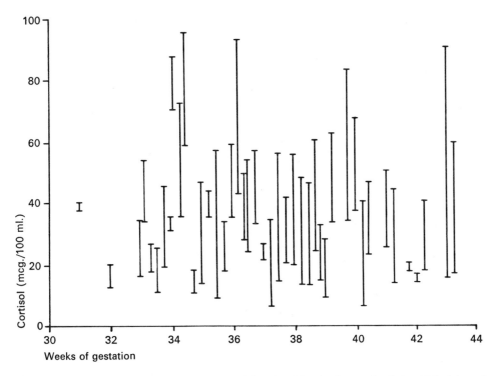

Fig. 1. Plasma cortisol levels, determined by the Mattingly method, in 43 babies of varying gestational ages 30 minutes after an intramuscular injection of Synacthen.

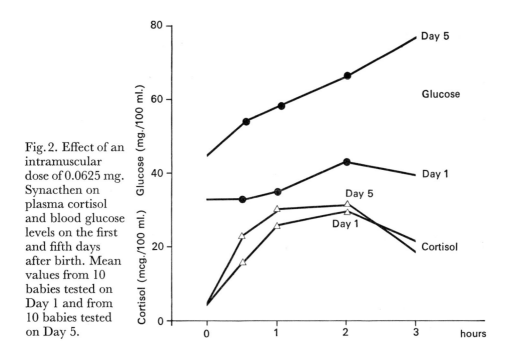

Fig. 2. Effect of an intramuscular dose of 0.0625 mg. Synacthen on plasma cortisol and blood glucose levels on the first and fifth days after birth. Mean values from 10 babies tested on Day 1 and from 10 babies tested on Day 5.

147

day after birth, and ten babies five days after birth. The dose of Synacthen administered was 0.0625 mg. by the intramuscular route. In view of the enormous changes occurring in the adrenal during this period of life owing to the involution of the foetal zone and the growth of the adult cortex, it seemed possible that differing results would be obtained at these two times.

The blood glucose was measured concurrently. Samples were taken before the injection of Synacthen, as well as 30, 60, 120, and 180 minutes afterwards.

A good plasma cortisol response occurred after 30 minutes, reaching a maximum at 120 minutes. The blood glucose varied between individual babies, but was little affected by Synacthen.

In Figure 2 the results on Day 1 and Day 5 have been superimposed on one another. The plasma cortisol response was very similar, but the blood glucose response was greater on Day 5 than on Day 1.

Although there was a good correlation between the results obtained by the Mattingly fluorescence and Murphy competitive protein binding methods, these methods do not indicate what is happening to the true cortisol, cortisone, and corticosterone levels.

These steroids were separated by ®Sephadex LH-20 column chromatography and measured by competitive protein binding radioassay (MURPHY[5]). Table 1 shows the response of these steroids to tetracosactrin.

When serial samples were compared, there was an overall difference of only 2.2 mcg./100 ml. in the plasma cortisol results obtained before and after column chromatography. This indicates that the levels recorded in capillary blood samples by competitive protein binding correlate closely with the actual plasma cortisol concentrations.

Table 1. Plasma corticosterone, cortisone, and cortisol levels before and after tetracosactrin stimulation in newborn infants.

Baby	Sample	Cortico-sterone	Cortisone	Cortisol	"Normal" C.P.B.	Difference
A	Before	<1	5.2	1.4	4.8	+3.4
A	After	1.8	1.7	20.2	22.2	+2.0
B	Before	<1	7.7	18.0	15.7	−2.3
B	After	1.9	4.9	33.1	29.4	−3.7
C	Before	<1	9.0	8.3	8.2	−0.1
C	After	4.2	4.7	40.4	31.6	−8.8
D	Before	<1	1.1	2.5	2.2	−0.3
D	After	1.5	2.5	28.8	20.1	−8.7
E	Before	<1	10.4	5.5	9.0	+3.5
E	After	2.5	3.8	24.3	27.2	+2.9
F	Before	<1	1.2	5.2	4.9	−0.3
F	After	1.4	2.8	19.8	20.2	+0.4

Values expressed in mcg./100 ml.
The stimulus used was 0.0625 mg. of short-acting Synacthen administered by the intramuscular route.
C.P.B. = competitive protein binding

Clinical trial

If the findings obtained by LIGGINS[1] in sheep applied to man, then overactivity of the adrenal cortex would, firstly, stimulate premature labour and, secondly, diminish the incidence of respiratory distress syndrome.

In mammals, Type I surfactant production is normally sufficient to sustain respiration and life after approximately 87% of the normal length of gestation, which in man is equivalent to 35 weeks. Full term is, of course, 40 weeks in man. In man and higher primates only, the less efficient Type 2 surfactant production is also present after approximately 55% of the normal period of gestation. This enables many premature human infants to survive when born before 35 weeks' gestation; however, this inefficient Type 2 pathway of surfactant production is easily overwhelmed, and respiratory distress is the commonest cause of death in these infants.

Data from the Cardiff birth survey show that the incidence of respiratory distress falls from over 30% at 30 weeks' gestation to under 5% at 37 weeks.

LIGGINS and HOWIE[2] have demonstrated that a significant improvement in neonatal survival, as well as a diminution in respiratory distress, occurs when corticosteroids are administered to mothers who are in premature labour. One-quarter of the patients were excluded from these authors' trial because labour progressed rapidly in spite of efforts to delay it.

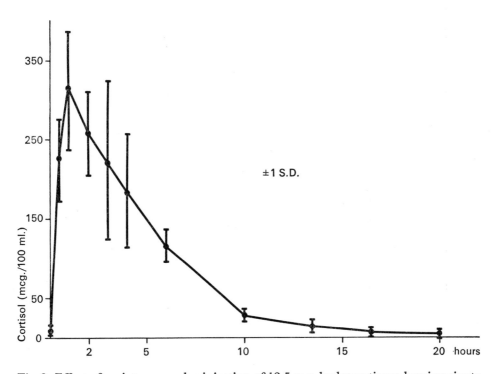

Fig. 3. Effect of an intramuscular injection of 12.5 mg. hydrocortisone hemisuccinate on the plasma cortisol in newborn infants.

We carried out a controlled clinical trial in 100 premature infants to see if similar results could be produced by corticosteroid and corticotrophin therapy given immediately after birth. Infants born before 35 weeks' gestation were randomly allocated to a treatment or a control group.

The 49 treated infants were given intramuscular injections of 12.5 mg. hydrocortisone hemisuccinate and 0.05 mg. Synacthen Depot immediately after birth. This regime was chosen in order to produce a rapid rise in plasma cortisol at birth and to maintain high levels for 72 hours without suppressing the infants' own adrenal function. This period of 72 hours is the normal time required for resolution of the respiratory distress syndrome.

Figure 3 shows the effect of an intramuscular injection of 12.5 mg. hydrocortisone hemisuccinate in newborn infants. There was a rapid rise in plasma cortisol which reached a peak of around 300 mcg./100 ml. after 60 minutes. The half-life was very prolonged in newborn infants, and significant levels were still present after 12 hours. When larger doses are injected, the cortisol peak is higher and the effect is somewhat more prolonged.

Indicated in Figure 4 is the plasma cortisol response to an intramuscular injection of 0.05 mg. Synacthen Depot. There is a very wide scatter of response, as shown by the large standard deviations. This is an important finding, and is also encountered when standard tests with short-acting tetracosactrin are

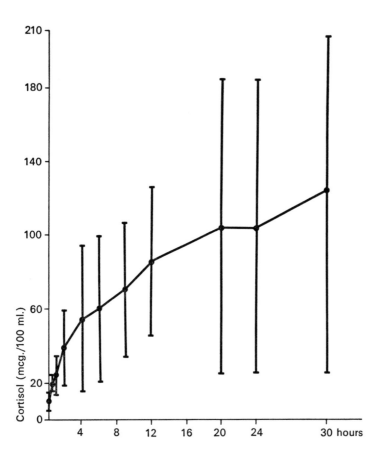

Fig. 4. Effect of an intramuscular injection of 0.05 mg. Synacthen Depot on the plasma cortisol in newborn infants.

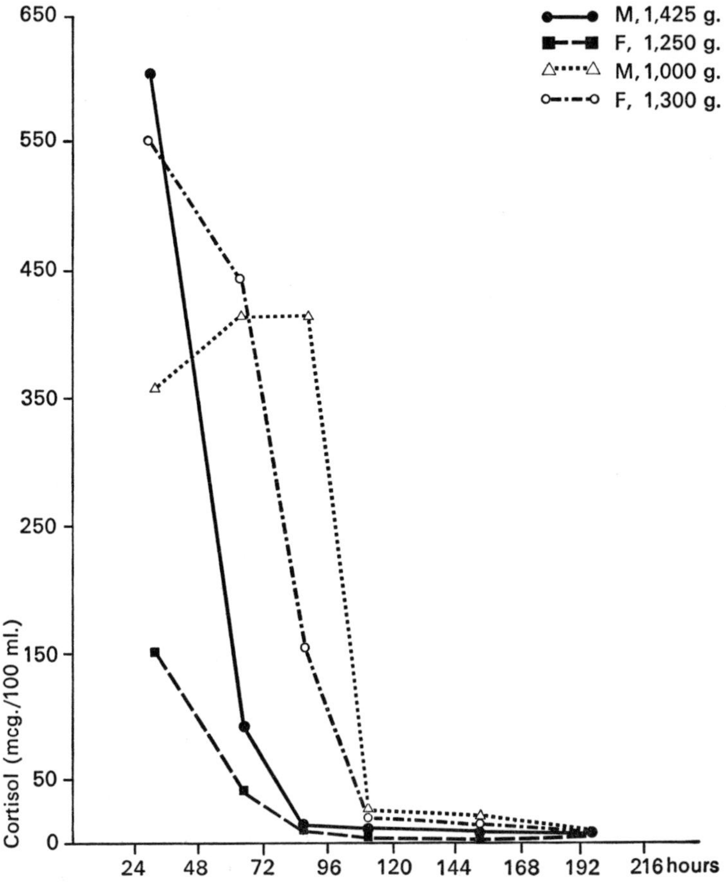
M, 1,425 g.
F, 1,250 g.
M, 1,000 g.
F, 1,300 g.
650
550
450
350
250
150
50
0
Cortisol (mcg./100 ml.)
24
48
72
96
120
144
168
192
216 hours

Fig. 5. Effect of Synacthen Depot (0.05 mg. i.m.) and hydrocortisone hemisuccinate (12.5 mg. i.m.) on the plasma cortisol levels in quadruplets.

performed on a variety of prematurely born infants. It suggests that overactivity of the adrenal cortex may play a significant role in initiating premature labour in many, but not all, babies who are born early.

Figure 5 shows the variability in plasma cortisol response obtained in a set of quadruplets studied prior to the trial. Two of the infants were given subsidiary injections of hydrocortisone hemisuccinate in the first 12 hours after birth; in these infants, the cortisol peaks were higher, but in retrospect it seems unlikely that these additional injections provided any therapeutic benefit. In the actual trial only one dose of hydrocortisone hemisuccinate and one dose of Synacthen Depot were given to each baby.

The results obtained in this trial are outlined in Table 2. The survival rate among infants born after more than 27 weeks' gestation was significantly higher in the treated group (P = 0.01, Fisher exact test). All the five deaths that did occur in this group were accounted for by two pregnancies, in which the infants were born after a gestation of 27 weeks or less: firstly, a singleton baby of 27 weeks' gestation and weighing 1,170 g. died of probable intracranial haemorrhage and respiratory distress syndrome; secondly, a set of quintuplets

Table 2. Survival rates in infants given combined prophylactic treatment with Synacthen Depot + hydrocortisone hemisuccinate, as compared with a control group.

Gestation period (weeks)	N	Alive				Dead			
		Treated group		Control group		Treated group		Control group	
		Male	Female	Male	Female	Male	Female	Male	Female
<27	7	–	–	–	–	4	1	1	1
<32	31	9	2	8	5	–	–	3	4
<36	62	24	9	16	10	–	–	2	1
	100	33	11	24	15	4	1	6	6

(one anencephalic) died soon after birth at 25 weeks' gestation. Fertility drugs had been used for their conception.

In the control group, nine of the 12 deaths were associated with the respiratory distress syndrome. Two female infants died of congenital heart disease and haemolytic disease of the newborn, respectively. One male infant had adrenal haemorrhage with mild respiratory distress.

All infants received appropriate supportive measures, which in some cases included continuous positive airway pressure (Gregory headbox) and intermittent positive-pressure ventilation. None of the surviving infants in the treated group needed these two aids, whereas three control infants survived with their help.

Hypoglycaemia was not a significant problem either in the treated or in the control group, since particular care was taken to prevent hypothermia and to initiate early feeding.

Conclusions

It is suggested that the therapeutic results obtained with this Synacthen Depot + corticosteroid regime are encouraging. The main potential danger is that of reducing resistance to infection.

All the infants will be assessed at the age of one year. No differences between treated and control infants have yet been detected in the four completed months of the follow-up period. Whether or not more subtle long-term effects may occur, is not known.

It is stressed that combined treatment with Synacthen Depot and a corticosteroid is of no use in established cases of respiratory distress syndrome and, in our experience, may even produce a deterioration. The regime described is therefore a prophylactic measure. Further clinical trials are required before its use in clinical practice can be confidently recommended.

References

1 LIGGINS, G.C.: The foetal role in the initiation of parturition in the ewe. In Wolstenholme, G.E.W., O'Connor, M. (Editors): Foetal autonomy, Ciba Found. Symp., p. 218 (Churchill, London 1969)

2 LIGGINS, G.C., HOWIE, R.N.: A controlled trial of antepartum glucocorticoid treatment for prevention of the respiratory distress syndrome in premature infants. Pediatrics *50*, 515 (1972)

3 MATTINGLY, D.: A simple fluorimetric method for the estimation of free 11-hydroxycorticoids in human plasma. J. clin. Path. *15*, 374 (1962)

4 MURPHY, B.E.P.: Some studies of the protein-binding of steroids and their application to the routine micro and ultramicro measurement of various steroids in body fluids by competitive protein-binding radioassay. J. clin. Endocr. *27*, 973 (1967)

5 MURPHY, B.E.P.: "Sephadex" column chromatography as an adjunct to competitive protein binding assays of steroids. Nature new Biol. (Lond.) *232*, 21 (1971)

Aspects of linear growth and skeletal maturation in asthmatic children treated with synthetic corticotrophin

by J. Taranger, K. L. Möller, and B. Bruning*

Since 1967 we have been employing intermittent treatment with a synthetic corticotrophin, tetracosactide (®Synacthen Depot), in children with severe asthma. These children have been regularly examined at the Allergy Out-Patient Department of the Children's Hospital in Gothenburg. At certain intervals their physical growth has been measured and tests of respiratory function performed, in addition to which some endocrinological studies have also been carried out. In the following report, however, only linear growth and skeletal maturation will be discussed.

Material and methods

Growth data on nine girls and 11 boys have been analysed. At the beginning of treatment with tetracosactide, the age of the girls ranged from 1.1 to 12.3 years, and that of the boys from 1.6 to 12.6 years. All the patients had shown signs and symptoms of a severe obstructive pulmonary disease before the age of three, and nine of them before the age of one year. In 1967 and 1968, only patients who had already undergone prolonged and repeated periods of corticoid therapy for at least one year were given intermittent treatment with tetra-cosactide, whereas since 1969 all children with life-threatening attacks of asthma have received such treatment. The dosage of tetracosactide has consistently been adjusted to the lowest level required to control the signs and symptoms of asthma, and the preparation has been administered at various intervals, ranging from once every three to once every ten days. Since the introduction of this tetracosactide therapy, the attacks of asthma have run a less severe clinical course, and no asthmatic child born after 1967 has yet developed a severe chronic disease. Among these children, there were in January 1973 seven who had required no further treatment with tetracosactide for at least six months; at the time they received their last dose of tetracosactide, these seven had been undergoing tetracosactide therapy for periods of one to four years.

In most of the children, height has been measured every month. The hand and wrist have been X-rayed every six months. The height of the patients has been analysed in comparison with data from a prospective longitudinal-growth study undertaken in Sweden by Karlberg et al.[1]. The velocity of linear growth in our children ("height velocity") has been calculated for periods of three, six, and 12 months. Skeletal maturation has been assessed according to the methods published by Tanner et al.[3,4] and a comparison made with the results which

---

*Department of Paediatrics, University Children's Hospital, Gothenburg, Sweden.

TARANGER et al.[5, 6] obtained when they applied these same methods to the data yielded by the above-mentioned Swedish growth study.

Results

When analysing physical development, the seasonal variation in the growth rate is a factor that also has to be taken into consideration where periods of less than 12 months are being studied (MARSHALL[2]). This point is illustrated in Figure 1, in which the growth rate before and during tetracosactide medication is compared in two girls, one of whom commenced treatment in March and the other in September. When a comparison is made between the last 12 months before treatment and the first 12 months during treatment, it can be seen that height velocity increased in both girls. But when periods of six months are compared in the same way, it becomes apparent that the seasonal variation resulted in a diminished height velocity in the girl who had started treatment in September. On the other hand, a comparison of her growth rate during the first six months of treatment with her growth rate in the corresponding six months of the preceding year reveals a substantial increase. Listed in Table 1 are the mean height velocities recorded during different periods.

In Figure 2 the heights of the children are expressed in standard deviation scores derived from the study by KARLBERG et al.[1], in which "0" in the adjacent scale represents the mean value. The children were divided into two groups of ten each: those in Group A received their first treatment with corticoids more than two years before, and those in Group B less than two years before, the start of tetracosactide therapy (also included in Group A was one

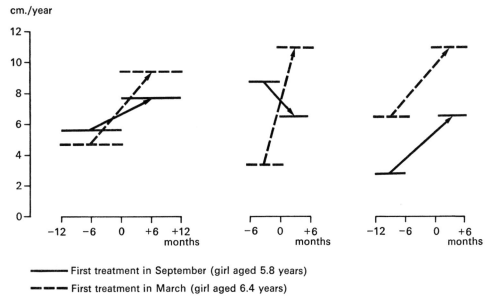

cm./year

——— First treatment in September (girl aged 5.8 years)

--- First treatment in March (girl aged 6.4 years)

Fig. 1. Influence of season on height velocity before and during treatment with tetracosactide, illustrated by reference to two girls of roughly the same age.

girl, aged only 24 months at the beginning of treatment with tetracosactide, who had been in receipt of corticoid medication almost continuously from the age of seven months). After the commencement of tetracosactide therapy, the increasingly marked corticoid-induced retardation of growth in height ceased, and a catch-up growth spurt was observed in Group B.

Table 1. Mean height velocities recorded during different periods in children treated with tetracosactide.

Period		Height velocity (cm./year)	
Last six months before treatment		6.9 (± 3.4)	
	N = 15		t = 0.62; P <0.80
First six months during treatment		7.5 (± 2.5)	
From 12th to 6th month before treatment		5.2 (± 2.4)	
	N = 13		t = 2.68; P <0.02
First six months during treatment		7.2 (± 2.6)	
Last 12 months before treatment		5.8 (± 2.2)	
	N = 14		t = 3.95; P <0.002
First 12 months during treatment		7.7 (± 2.5)	

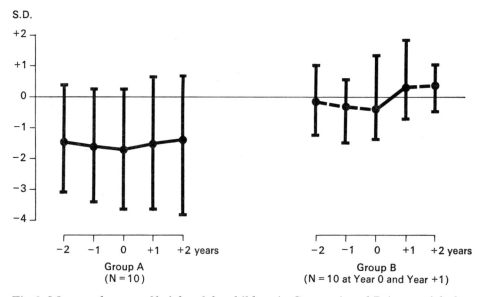

Fig. 2. Mean and range of height of the children in Groups A and B (see text) before and during treatment with tetracosactide.

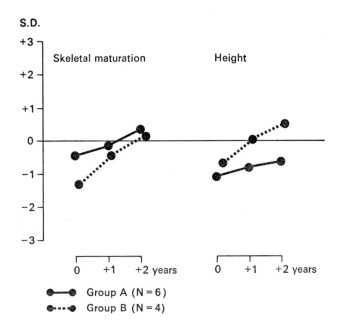

Fig. 3. Mean height and skeletal maturation in ten children from Groups A and B (see text) during treatment with tetracosactide for two years.

Presented in Figure 3 are the growth data on ten children from Groups A and B who had been receiving treatment with tetracosactide for two years (in all, 13 patients from the two groups had been given tetracosactide therapy for two years, but the data on the three oldest children in Group A are not included here, because it was not possible to make comparisons with skeletal maturation in the Swedish growth study after 13 years of age). A significant catch-up growth in height was found in Group B. In Group A, on the other hand, no catch-up growth was observed, but the increasingly marked retardation of growth ceased. At the same time, however, skeletal maturation was also accelerated: a significant increase in skeletal maturation occurred during both years in Group B, but not until the second year in Group A. The increase in skeletal maturation was greater than the increase in height. This may ultimately have the effect of reducing final adult height owing to premature closure of the epiphyses, but this is a point upon which no definite conclusions can yet be drawn from our study. When considering the importance of this possible side effect of treatment with tetracosactide, it also has to be borne in mind that growth would at all events have been retarded by the corticoid therapy which would otherwise have been necessary. Furthermore, since our children have been receiving tetracosactide their asthma attacks have become less severe and less frequent than before, and their growth has thus also been less disturbed. It has in fact been demonstrated that, if uncontrolled, asthma *per se* reduces growth in height.

Summary

Linear growth and skeletal maturation have been studied in 20 children with severe asthma both before and during treatment with the synthetic corticotrophin preparation tetracosactide. During the treatment an increase was observed

157

in their growth rate in terms of height as well as skeletal maturation. The increase in skeletal maturation was greater than the increase in height, but no final conclusions can yet be drawn as to whether this will have any influence on the patients' adult height. The children enjoyed better health than when they had been receiving corticoid therapy, which had also definitely inhibited their growth.

References

1 KARLBERG, P., KLACKENBERG, G., ENGSTRÖM, I., KLACKENBERG-LARSSON, I., LICHTENSTEIN, H., STENSSON, J., SVENNBERG, I.: The development of children in a Swedish urban community. A prospective longitudinal study. Acta paed. scand. Suppl. 187 (1968)
2 MARSHALL, W.A.: Evaluation of growth rate in height over periods of less than one year. Arch. Dis. Childh. 46, 414 (1971)
3 TANNER, J.M., WHITEHOUSE, R.H.: Standards for skeletal maturation, Part 1 (Int. Children's Centre, Paris 1959)
4 TANNER, J.M., WHITEHOUSE, R.H., HEALY, M.J.R.: A new system for estimating the maturity of the hand and wrist with standards derived from 2,600 healthy British children (Int. Children's Centre, Paris 1962)
5 TARANGER, J., KARLBERG, P., LICHTENSTEIN, H., BRUNING, B.: Some aspects on methods for evaluation of skeletal maturation (Int. Children's Centre, Paris 1970)
6 TARANGER, J., KARLBERG, P., LICHTENSTEIN, H., BRUNING, B.: Estimation of skeletal maturity (Int. Children's Centre, Paris 1972)

Discussion

K. F. WEINGES: What advantages do you, Dr. BOISSIÈRE, consider that Synacthen offers as compared with intravenous hydrocortisone therapy in the treatment of acute diseases such as pneumonia or laryngitis?

H. BOISSIÈRE: This is not an easy question to answer. In certain circumstances it is, of course, debatable whether tetracosactide does in fact offer any advantages over corticosteroid therapy. While it seems to me reasonable to give preference to tetra-cosactide in cases requiring prolonged treatment, it is difficult to choose between corticosteroids and tetracosactide in acute conditions. In very severe asthmatic crises, however, I have the impression—an impression which is also shared by my friends VIALATTE and PAUPE—that water-soluble Synacthen, administered intravenously, produces a more rapid improvement than treatment with corticosteroids. But I have no statistical data on which to base a more precise answer.

K. F. WEINGES: But isn't there reason to suppose that, in the acute conditions you have mentioned, endogenous A.C.T.H. secretion will already be sufficient to ensure an optimal degree of adrenocortical stimulation—or is the situation different in children?

H. BOISSIÈRE: I'm afraid this question raises biological problems with which I was not directly concerned in the clinical report that I have presented here. I'm sorry that I cannot shed any light on these problems, because the children we treated were not subjected to biochemical examinations. I think it possible, however, that you may be right, Dr. WEINGES.

H. J. BAUER: I should like to ask Dr. BOISSIÈRE one or two questions about encephalitis and meningo-encephalitis in children. It's still a very controversial problem as to whether differences have to be made in the treatment of the various infections of viral origin. Some years ago, for example, steroids were considered to be absolutely contra-indicated in chickenpox, and this ban was also applied to A.C.T.H. Nowadays, on the other hand, this contra-indication is no longer so strictly observed. Encephalitis due to herpesvirus was first treated with steroids, as well as with A.C.T.H.; later it became the practice to employ antiviral agents instead, and A.C.T.H. was then supposed to be contra-indicated. Finally, it was discovered that these antiviral agents were ineffective, with the result that A.C.T.H. and steroids are now once again being administered. Can you tell me, Dr. BOISSIÈRE, whether you treat viral encephalitis and meningo-encephalitis differently from para-infectious encephalitis, in which an auto-immune reaction is known to be strongly involved? One classic example illustrating this whole problem is that of subacute sclerosing panencephalitis, in which corticosteroids or A.C.T.H. are known to be capable of prolonging survival, although they cannot actually cure the disease.

H. BOISSIÈRE: As regards the question of encephalitis due to herpesvirus, Dr. BAUER, I regret that I have had no personal experience of this problem. As for chickenpox, I am not suggesting for one moment that ordinary cases of chickenpox should be treated with corticosteroids or A.C.T.H. In my paper I made it clear that, in our three children with chickenpox, the infection had occurred in the course of medication with corticosteroids or immunosuppressive drugs, which were being given as treatment for malignant blood diseases. It is now a generally accepted rule that under such circumstances treatment with corticosteroids should never be interrupted, but should be continued and, preferably, even intensified. Moreover, I have advanced the hypothesis that, in a case where a child already in receipt of corticosteroid therapy contracts chickenpox, one should consider the possibility of administering treatment with Synacthen Depot in the hope of preventing the chickenpox from assuming a malignant form. But I'm afraid I cannot quote any personal observations in support of this notion, which at present is purely an hypothesis.

159

With regard to viral encephalitis, I am aware that some authors are still hesitant about using corticosteroids or A.C.T.H. as treatment in such cases, because they fear that this might encourage diffusion of the virus responsible for the disease. In my opinion, however, this fear is unjustified, since viral encephalitis—like all forms of virus infection—is from the very beginning associated with viraemia, as a result of which the virus will already have become distributed throughout the body; and I do not think that either corticosteroids or A.C.T.H. can aggravate a viraemia that is already present.

Finally, just a word about the mode of action of A.C.T.H. in these virus diseases. I believe that in such conditions the anti-inflammatory effect of corticotrophin serves to combat the cerebral oedema which frequently occurs in the course of these types of infection.

You also mentioned subacute sclerosing panencephalitis, Dr. BAUER, but this is a disease of which I have had no personal experience.

J. GIRARD: I should like to revert to a few of the points you raised in your paper, Dr. BOISSIÈRE. You mentioned as indications for Synacthen certain diseases in which I should have thought it would be dangerous to employ the drug; here I am thinking in particular of acute laryngitis, purulent meningococcal meningitis, and, thirdly, dehydration. As for laryngitis—where even the use of corticosteroids is still a controversial topic—the patients in question are emergency cases in which the aim surely is to achieve an immediate increase in the plasma cortisol levels; but a certain amount of time elapses before Synacthen can do this. Now let us turn to purulent meningococcal meningitis: if one is dealing with a Waterhouse-Friderichsen syndrome, i.e. with septicaemia accompanied by massive adrenal haemorrhage, Synacthen will no longer be capable of acting, because its target gland will be unable to respond. Finally, dehydration in infants is almost invariably associated with quite severe disturbances in the electrolyte balance which prove difficult to rectify. Treatment therefore consists in the administration of infusions; if it is also felt necessary to resort to hormone therapy, the hormone selected should be aldosterone rather than A.C.T.H.

H. BOISSIÈRE: Your comments, Dr. GIRARD, relate to three problems: firstly, is there really anything to be gained from using Synacthen in young children with acute laryngitis? Secondly, the question of Waterhouse-Friderichsen syndrome and, thirdly, the treatment of dehydration.

Allow me to point out first of all that none of the children upon whom I reported was suffering from Waterhouse-Friderichsen syndrome. Among the seven children with purulent meningococcal meningitis, six were cases involving septicaemic forms accompanied by gangrenous purpura; none of the patients had acute fulminating meningococcaemia. It is of course true that, once a Waterhouse-Friderichsen syndrome has been diagnosed, intensive resuscitation measures have to be taken immediately—and in such a grave emergency A.C.T.H. has no part to play; on the contrary, here large doses of corticosteroids are indicated. I have never claimed that states of shock due to fulminating meningococcal septicaemia can be effectively treated with tetracosactide. The cases to which I referred were ones of severe septicaemic meningitis associated with gangrenous purpura.

As regards the six cases of dehydration treated with A.C.T.H., these were extremely severe, hyperacute forms in which the infants were comatose and in which intravenous rehydration, antibiotic therapy, and attempts to correct the accompanying metabolic disorders—the three major therapeutic measures applicable whenever a child is suffering from acute dehydration—had failed to control the condition satisfactorily. These were, in fact, desperate cases in which A.C.T.H. was given as a last resort. In other words, A.C.T.H. can certainly not be regarded as an essential drug for use in the treatment of ordinary forms of dehydration as encountered in young children. In my own hospital department, as in all other paediatric departments, acute dehydration in infants is treated, not with A.C.T.H., but with intravenous fluid and electrolyte infusions plus an antibiotic.

Now for a few words about the problems of laryngitis. I admit that, from the didactic point of view, what you have said, Dr. GIRARD, may be quite true. The fact remains, however, that what I have done and what others have done along the same lines has always been justified in practice by the successful therapeutic results obtained. In each of the 11 infants treated with Synacthen Depot, the dyspnoea, fever, and signs of discomfort disappeared immediately. I agree that in acute laryngitis A.C.T.H. may not perhaps be superior to corticosteroids, but it does at all events prove effective—its mechanism of action in these cases being the same as in viral encephalitis, except that the affected site is quite a different one: whereas in viral encephalitis, A.C.T.H. helps to resolve cerebral oedema, in acute laryngitis the purpose in administering A.C.T.H. is to combat the oedema invading the lower pharynx, the glottis, and the subglottis, and for this purpose it is once again the drug's anti-inflammatory action that is all-important. The results it yielded in the 11 cases to which I have referred were consistently excellent and certainly came up to expectations.

W.J.IRVINE: Dr. BOISSIÈRE's comment that he observed hypertension in nine children after two months' treatment with Synacthen Depot prompts me to add a word or two on the question of hypertension. We now know quite a lot more about the physiology of aldosterone secretion. Under normal circumstances, the secretion of aldosterone is largely independent of the pituitary but is under the control of the renin-angiotensin system. However, there are two sets of circumstances under which it is influenced by A.C.T.H.: firstly, when pharmacological doses of A.C.T.H. are given; and, secondly, as RAYFIELD et al.* recently reported, when physiological or near-physiological doses of A.C.T.H. are administered to subjects who are sodium-depleted. In these latter cases, the aldosterone secretion rate was shown to be increased. This might well prove a relevant factor in instances where a child or an adult is being given fairly enthusiastic diuretic therapy in order to counteract fluid retention. Now, it is known that increasing the dose of Synacthen Depot from, say, 0.5 to 1.0 mg. does not produce much further increase in the plasma cortisol concentration after a certain level has been reached. On the other hand, it is not known whether the aldosterone response may not continue to be dose-dependent. The cortisol and the aldosterone responses don't necessarily run parallel with each other. Until we have more information on the way in which aldosterone levels are affected by changes in the dose of tetracosactrin, I fear that by increasing the dose of Synacthen Depot we may be proportionately increasing aldosterone secretion without at the same time deriving any additional benefit in the form of a further rise in the plasma cortisol levels. Hypertension might therefore well be quite a serious complication of treatment with Synacthen Depot, particularly if the drug were used in excessive dosage. Other side effects, such as acne and hyperpigmentation, are obvious enough, and the same applies to amenorrhoea in women. But, unless one is aware of and on the look-out for hypertension, it may pass unnoticed; it might also resemble osteoporosis as a complication insofar as it could possibly prove difficult to reverse once it had become established.

J.GELZER: I was struck by the fact that in his paper Dr. BOISSIÈRE made no reference at all to any cases of skin disease in children. In this connection I am thinking not only of the more trivial skin disorders of childhood, but also of the rarer types of skin condition, such as hereditary epidermolysis bullosa. Are there any relevant data in the literature?

R.SCHUPPLI: Since these dermatological diseases of childhood don't really constitute indications for A.C.T.H., we have never used Synacthen to treat skin conditions in children. The chronic form of eczema that the Americans refer to as atopic dermatitis would, it is true, be a suitable indication, but this can be kept under satisfactory

*RAYFIELD, E.J., ROSE, L.I., DLUHY, R.G., WILLIAMS, G.H.: Aldosterone secretory and glucocorticoid excretory responses to alpha 1–24 ACTH (Cortrosyn) in sodium-depleted normal man. J. clin. Endocr. 36, 30 (1973)

control by means of external treatment. Hereditary epidermolysis bullosa is definitely not a good indication for corticosteroids, because sudden deaths have been known to occur under such treatment; for this reason we have so far refrained from using Synacthen in this disease. Pemphigus does not occur during childhood, and dermatitis herpetiformis in children often shows a better response to sulphones. For the more trivial skin disorders encountered in children, the main form of treatment used by us consists in the application of topical corticoids, supplemented if necessary by systemic therapy.

T.B.BINNS: To add to the figures presented by Dr. PRICE, some useful information on the cortisol response of newborn babies to ordinary Synacthen (50 mcg. intramuscularly) was recently included in a paper by SHARP et al.*. This information probably escaped attention because it was buried in a case report on bronchial carcinoma in a mother. Dr. LOGAN has kindly provided the original data, from which the results in Table 1 are derived. Although there is wide variation between subjects, the mean plasma cortisol levels before and after Synacthen are higher in the newborn than was originally found in adults.

Table 1. Plasma cortisol levels in neonates before and one hour after intramuscular injection of 50 mcg. Synacthen. (Data from SHARP et al.)

Age (days)	Number of babies	Plasma cortisol (mcg./100 ml.). Mean values ± S.E.M.		
		Basal	1 hr after 50 mcg. Synacthen	Increment
1	25	29.7±3.3	79.9±5.0	47.3±3.9
3	25	15.6±1.5	62.5±4.0	46.8±3.9
5–7	20	13.5±1.5	57.5±5.9	44.1±5.0

Table 2. Plasma cortisol levels before and 30 minutes after the intramuscular administration of Synacthen in children aged between two months and 14 years. (Data from BARNES et al.)

	N	Plasma cortisol (mcg./100 ml.). Mean values ± S.E.M.		
		Resting	30 min. after Synacthen (0.25 mg./70 kg.)	Increment
Normal children	38	18.2±1.4	39.6±1.7	21.1±1.1
Children with adrenal hypofunction	8	13.6±2.0	13.3±2.3	−0.3±0.7
Children with pituitary hypofunction	9	8.7±1.8	20.3±2.2	11.6±1.2

*SHARP, J.C., CARTY, M.J., LOGAN, R.W.: Maternal bronchial carcinoma and its possible relation to neonatal hypoglycaemia. Postgrad. med. J. *48*, 682 (1972)

Since, until recently, there has been very little information on the response of children of any age to Synacthen, I should also like to draw attention to a paper by Prof. BARBARA CLAYTON and her colleagues at The Hospital for Sick Children, Great Ormond St., London*. They studied normal children between the ages of two months and 14 years, as well as small groups with adrenal or pituitary hypofunction, and obtained the results shown in Table 2.

*BARNES, N.D., JOSEPH, J.M., ATHERDEN, S.M., CLAYTON, B.E.: Functional tests of adrenal axis in children with measurement of plasma cortisol by competitive protein binding. Arch. Dis. Childh. 47, 66 (1972)

A.C.T.H. in the treatment of rheumatoid arthritis

by H. Jesserer*

Methods of treatment for rheumatoid arthritis have in the course of the years undergone various modifications in the light both of changing views on the pathogenesis of the disease and of progress in the therapeutic possibilities available. It is still upon these two determinant factors that recommendations concerning the management of rheumatoid arthritis are essentially based. Briefly recapitulated, the current status of our knowledge as to what happens in rheumatoid arthritis can be outlined as follows:

The cause of the disease is still unknown. Apparently, however, it requires particular predisposing features to induce the body to react to certain noxae in a manner characteristic of rheumatoid arthritis and involving an auto-immunogenic process of self-perpetuation. The first anatomically detectable changes take the form of fibrin exudation in the region of the diseased joints, which is due to some type of capillary damage that has yet to be precisely defined and which strongly stimulates proliferation of synovial connective-tissue cells. These cells multiply to excess and give rise to inflammatory granulation tissue which spreads over the cartilage. At the same time, from the recess of the joint this granulation tissue acts upon the cortex of the adjacent bone and also invades the subchondral marrow-space. This two-pronged attack leads to progressive destruction of the cartilage and impairment of articular function.

In the course of these destructive processes, however, products resulting from the breakdown of tissue also occur, and—owing to the peculiar mode of reaction which, as already mentioned, is displayed by patients susceptible to rheumatoid arthritis—the body treats these products as antigens, to which it shows a specific immune response. The latter involves the entry into play of so-called immunologically competent lymphocytes and plasma cells which become recognisable as discrete infiltrates within the villi of the proliferating synovial membrane and which participate in the subsequent antigen-antibody reaction either directly or by producing the corresponding immunoglobulins. The purpose of this reaction is to destroy what to the body appears to be a foreign substrate. The reaction manifests itself morphologically in the form of necrosis in the joint capsule as well as in other structurally related mesenchymal tissues. Such necrosis results in the shedding of further fragments of tissue which likewise act not only as antigens, but also as non-specific inflammatory substances, and thus serve to perpetuate the insidious pathogenic reaction.

In this complex chain of events there is of course still much that has yet to be clarified. However, when one studies the histological material which can

*II. Medizinische Abteilung des Kaiser-Franz-Joseph-Spitals, Vienna, Austria.

nowadays be obtained by synovectomy, the chief feature that impresses one is the variety of forms assumed by the tissue proliferations, some of which are even reminiscent of tumorous growths. When one bears in mind, too, that the "rheumatoid factors" which appear in the course of the disease, and which are generally regarded as indicative of a progressive worsening, are also products of an abnormal cell activity, then it seems only logical that antiproliferative agents should be resorted to as a means of combating these processes.

It was to this end that cortisone and other hormone preparations related to cortisone were first employed. But the fact that they have to be administered at brief and regular intervals in order to ensure a sustained therapeutic effect, and that the unphysiologically high doses required produce undesirable consequences, soon damped the enthusiasm which they had initially aroused and led finally to attempts at treatment with other cell-inhibiting substances. Hence the efforts made to treat rheumatoid arthritis with cytotoxic agents, which it was hoped would—by inhibiting specific lymphocyte and plasma-cell proliferation—exert a primarily "immunosuppressive" action and thus serve to arrest the mechanism of self-perpetuation responsible for the progress of the disease.

It has meanwhile been discovered that cytotoxic agents have a far less specific action than was at first supposed, but that, thanks to their antireproductive effect on rapidly regenerating or vigorously proliferating cell systems of various types, they are nevertheless quite capable of eliciting the desired response. The results obtained with these substances in cases where they were appropriately employed did in fact prove remarkable, and, provided these drugs were not administered over too long a time, they were also found to produce hardly any serious "side effects". The therapeutic response—once again, in appropriately selected cases—also persisted for a more or less prolonged period after the treatment had been stopped, and in many cases it was found possible, by prescribing cytotoxic agents in combination with other non-steroid antirheumatic drugs, either to replace corticoid medication which had provoked excessive side effects or even to manage without such medication from the outset.

But treatment with cytotoxic agents, too, was not devoid of snags. For example, to ensure that they would be as effective as possible and to avoid recourse to long-term oral medication such as had proved so problematical in the case of corticoid therapy, these drugs had to be given by intravenous drip infusion—which in turn, of course, entailed a certain technical outlay and usually also required the patient's admission to hospital. Another complication was that, owing to the effect exerted by such drugs on leucocytopoiesis, a watch had to be kept on the patient's blood picture. Finally, the treatment always involved a certain risk—at least in women of child-bearing age—and it was thus often only after some hesitation that the decision to resort to it was taken.

Despite this, the use of cytotoxic agents was the first form of treatment based on clear concepts of the pathogenesis of rheumatoid arthritis and aimed at influencing certain precise phases of the pathological process, i.e. phases characterised clinically by marked inflammatory activity and anatomically by vigorous cell proliferation both of a non-specific and of a specific (immunopathogenic) nature. Where these acute phases can be brought under control and converted into less active phases, it is then possible to maintain the therapeutic response with doses of relatively harmless anti-inflammatory agents until such time as the next acute exacerbation occurs, and in this way to avoid the hazards of long-term corticoid therapy.

Apart from certain special forms of damage which corticoids are liable to inflict, the hazards of such medication lie chiefly in the fact that it may lead to an organically induced impairment of adrenocortical function, which compels one to continue administering glucocorticoids despite all the undesirable repercussions which this may entail. The danger can be circumvented, however, by resorting to A.C.T.H. in lieu of cortisone or cortisone-like preparations. The chief reason why A.C.T.H. has hitherto seldom been used for this purpose is that it has to be given by the parenteral route—which is certainly a disadvantage. But, when one examines the problem in the light of the concept underlying the use of cytotoxic agents in rheumatoid arthritis, one is bound to ask oneself why A.C.T.H. too should not be employed in the same manner, particularly now that the new synthetic corticotrophins have eliminated some of the drawbacks encountered with the older A.C.T.H. extract-preparations. Thanks to the intensive stimulant action which they exert on the adrenal cortex, these A.C.T.H. preparations are capable of stepping up cortisol production to such an extent that the full anti-inflammatory, antiproliferative, and immunosuppressive effect of quite large quantities of glucocorticoids is thus achieved. Moreover, this activating influence on the adrenal cortex disposes of all the problems that are liable to arise in cases where high doses of corticoids are either withdrawn or drastically reduced. Finally, the disadvantages of intramuscular injection are but minor ones in comparison with the expense and inconvenience of having to administer and supervise intravenous infusions.

This, of course, does not mean that cytotoxic agents have become obsolete in the treatment of rheumatoid arthritis; on the contrary, they still have their justified uses in this field and, when employed under the right circumstances, they can and do still yield good results. But in all instances where this form of therapy poses problems—even if the problems are only of a psychological or emotional nature—a daily dose of ®Synacthen offers a good alternative, provided one adheres within the overall plan of treatment to the rule that the medication should be tailored to fit the phases of the illness.

In practical terms, this means that, having established a diagnosis, one should first determine the degree of acuteness of the process. This can be done by reference to the clinical signs, the E.S.R., or C-reactive protein determinations or also, if material from a synovectomy is available, by studying the histological picture. Another important factor is whether or not the patient is already receiving corticoid medication; if this is the case, an attempt should first be made to replace it by doses of A.C.T.H. This, as we all know, is a laborious undertaking, because the corticoid dosage can usually be reduced only slowly and because it is only in exceptional cases—i.e. where the patient has not been taking corticoids for too long a time—that a direct switch can be made to A.C.T.H. medication. On the whole, treatment either with A.C.T.H. or with cytotoxic agents is likely to prove all the more promising the less advanced and the more active the process of mesenchymal proliferation. On the other hand, where relatively severe destruction of the joint has occurred, or where the disease process has already "burnt itself out", the chances of attaining a significant improvement are understandably slight. The same also applies to patients displaying marked "cortisonism", who pose special problems, a discussion of which would exceed the scope of the present paper.

Treatment with A.C.T.H. should be continued until such time as the clinical signs indicative of an acute process have disappeared and the E.S.R. has declined. In patients not previously treated with corticoids, this effect can as a rule be achieved within about three weeks. In contrast to cytotoxic medication, however, the improvement resulting from A.C.T.H. therapy does not persist after the drug has been withdrawn; it is therefore advisable to continue administering the A.C.T.H. for a while, with progressively longer intervals between doses, and at the same time to build up a basic treatment schedule involving the use of other drugs such as D-penicillamine, gold salts, or a preparation from the group of the non-steroid antirheumatic agents. Ultimately, however, the A.C.T.H. therapy should be completely withdrawn, so as to avoid the development of a drug-induced Cushing syndrome. Incidentally, it should be noted that the type of Cushing syndrome liable to occur in response to A.C.T.H. differs from that provoked by corticoid medication inasmuch as it soon disappears once the treatment has been discontinued. Following corticoid therapy, by contrast, adrenocortical function is likely to remain impaired over a more or less prolonged period—so that in certain cases troublesome incidents may still occur some time after the medication has been withdrawn.

To sum up, it may thus be said that in rheumatoid arthritis administration of cytotoxic agents constitutes at present the soundest and most effective method of treating phases during which the disease process is highly active. Where such medication presents difficulties, however, a genuine therapeutic alternative is now available in the shape of treatment with A.C.T.H., which—since it is easy to administer—also lends itself to use in general practice.

References

1 BEICKERT, A.: Glukokortikoid-Entzugssyndrome. Dtsch. Gesundh.-Wes. *24*, 433 (1969)

2 BETHGE, H.: Die steroidinduzierte Nebennierenrindenunterfunktion. Klin. Wschr. *48*, 317 (1970)

3 CHLUD, K.: Die medikamentöse Behandlung der rheumatoiden Arthritis. Therapiewoche *21*, 762 (1971)

4 FASSBENDER, H.G.: Morphologische Beurteilung und Klassifikation von Synovialgewebe. Z. Rheumaforsch. *31*, Suppl. 2: 47 (1972)

5 FASSBENDER, H.G.: Konzept einer Pathosystematik der chronischen Polyarthritis. Z. Rheumaforsch. *31*, 129 (1972)

6 JESSERER, H.: Antiphlogistika-Immunsuppressiva-Zytostatika. Therapiewoche *21*, 820 (1971)

7 JESSERER, H.: Probleme des Cortisonismus. Therapiewoche *21*, 1884 (1971)

8 MÜLLER, W.: Zur Immunpathogenese der chronischen Polyarthritis. Therapiewoche *21*, 721 (1971)

Indications for depot tetracosactide in rheumatology

by P.MASSIAS*

Although eight years have meanwhile elapsed since tetracosactide (β1–24 corticotrophin) was first introduced for therapeutic use, it is still difficult to define the indications for this synthetic A.C.T.H. preparation in rheumatology. That it exerts a prompt and potent anti-inflammatory effect is a fact which all acknowledge; despite this, however, many rheumatologists remain in doubt as to the role which tetracosactide, as compared with corticosteroids, deserves to play in the long-term treatment that so often proves necessary in patients suffering from rheumatic disorders.

The indications for A.C.T.H. therapy do in fact differ very sharply, depending on whether the case to be treated involves an acute or subacute inflammatory condition or a chronic form of rheumatic inflammation.

1. Acute and subacute inflammatory conditions

Included under this heading are various affections which, in spite of their wide differences, all have one feature in common, i.e. the fact that—in addition to their inflammatory component—they are self-limiting and can be expected to respond to treatment lasting only a few days or a few weeks. Disorders falling within this category are rheumatic fever, rheumatism of infective or allergic origin in adults, hyperalgesic forms of neuralgia, bouts of inflammation oc- curring in association with osteoarthritis and certain non-articular types of rheumatism.

1.2. Acute rheumatic inflammation

1.2.1. Rheumatic fever

It was in 1967 that attention was first drawn to the effectiveness of β1–24 corticotrophin in rheumatic fever. Several other investigators subsequently also referred to the drug's use in this indication, but the scattered reports that have thus far appeared chiefly emphasise the rapidity with which this synthetic A.C.T.H. derivative acts on signs and symptoms referable to the joints. In a paper presented in 1971, MOZZICONACCI and ATTAL[15] state that they reserve tetracosactide for the treatment of forms of rheumatic fever complicated by pancarditis and of such gravity as to warrant emergency measures from the very outset. But such forms of the disease have of course nowadays become excep- tional.

*Hôpital Antoine Béclère, Clamart, France.

1.2.2. Acute or subacute rheumatic inflammation in adults

The relevant literature features also a limited number of observations relating to acute or subacute rheumatic inflammation in adults. Among our own patients, four suffering from rheumatic conditions of this type (two cases of streptococcal rheumatism, one of rheumatism of allergic origin, and one of acute arthritis of indeterminate aetiology affecting only a few joints) have received treatment with depot tetracosactide.

During the first three to seven days, these patients were given doses of 0.5 to 1 mg. per 24 hours, the interval between injections then being successively prolonged to two, three, and four days; the total duration of the treatment ranged from 20 to 45 days.

The injections elicited a prompt response in all four cases, three of which steadily improved. In the one patient in whom an inflammatory rebound reaction set in upon withdrawal of the medication, this reaction abated when treatment with intermittent doses was resumed for an additional two weeks; no further relapses occurred. In these four patients the effect of the A.C.T.H. therapy was comparable with that normally observed in cases treated with corticosteroids.

1.3. Radiculalgia and neuralgia

In radiculalgia and neuralgia we have a clearer impression of the indications for tetracosactide, because here more extensive documentation is available.

In 1970 I was able to report on 28 cases of hyperalgesic neuralgia (cervico-brachialgia, lumbago and sciatica, and leg pain)[12] which had failed to respond to corticosteroid therapy, but in which 50 % of the patients completely recovered following treatment with depot tetracosactide (Table 1). In the cases where this treatment proved unsuccessful, the main reason was the presence of organic lesions (prolapsed discs, spinal metastases) refractory to anti-inflammatory therapy. Comparable results were presented in 1971 by LIÈVRE et al.[8], who had employed tetracosactide in patients with more or less severe forms of neuralgia, included among whom were several long-standing cases. Finally, in 1972

Table 1. Results obtained with depot tetracosactide in 28 cases of hyperalgesic neuralgia which had failed to respond to corticosteroid therapy.

	Results of treatment			
	Good or very good	Fairly good	Mediocre or poor	Totals
Cervicobrachialgia	6	2	3	11
Lumbago and sciatica	7	3	3	13
Leg pain	2	1	1	4
Totals	15	6	7	28

GALIBERT et al.[6] published an account of 125 cases of sciatica encountered among candidates for neurosurgery, of whom 50 to 60 % showed an improvement in response to tetracosactide; these authors consider recourse to tetracosactide to be justified as a last resort whenever surgery would otherwise have to be contemplated. Particularly interesting are the findings they obtained when patients who had received tetracosactide were afterwards nevertheless obliged to undergo an operation: in a number of cases, the relief from pain which these patients had experienced seems to have been due, not to a decrease in inflammation affecting the sheath of the nerve root, but to a direct action on oedema of the root itself—an observation which suggests that in this type of case A.C.T.H. may exert an effect similar to that reported in other neurological disorders.

Tetracosactide would thus appear to be eminently suitable for use in severe forms of neuralgia. In such indications its rapidity of action quite often makes it preferable to corticosteroid therapy, and the fact that the treatment is as a rule of relatively brief duration enables one to avoid the undesirable side effects which prolonged medication with high doses of A.C.T.H. is liable to provoke.

1.4. Other acute or subacute inflammatory conditions

1.4.1. Attacks of hyperalgesia occurring in the presence of osteoarthritis

A short course of treatment with corticosteroids or A.C.T.H. may also be justified in certain forms of osteoarthritis (e.g. osteoarthritis of the knee or hip joint) if and when a bout of hyperalgesia sets in. In these acute episodes, which are sometimes accompanied by an overt local inflammatory reaction, such treatment usually yields results that are both spectacular and lasting—as confirmed by several very conclusive examples which we have recorded. On the other hand, however, episodes of this kind rarely occur in the course of degenerative rheumatic diseases, and it should therefore be pointed out that adrenocortical hormone therapy is normally not indicated in cases of osteoarthritis.

1.4.2. Non-articular rheumatism

According to certain authors, patients suffering from non-articular forms of rheumatism (tendinitis, tenosynovitis, periarthritis, bursitis, apophysitis) have likewise derived benefit from intramuscular injections of synthetic corticotrophin. But such benign disorders, which as a rule are only mildly incapacitating, generally respond very well to non-steroid anti-inflammatory agents or to local treatment with corticosteroids. It is thus only in very exceptional cases that A.C.T.H. therapy would be indicated in these non-articular rheumatic disorders.

2. Chronic forms of rheumatic inflammation

When tetracosactide is employed in the treatment of chronic forms of rheumatic inflammation, several difficulties are liable to be encountered, chief among them being the persistent nature of the inflammatory syndrome and the fact that in these cases such hormone therapy merely exerts a symptomatic effect from which the patient derives relief only for as long as the medication is actually in progress.

The clinical course of these chronic rheumatic diseases and the way in which they respond to the various types of anti-inflammatory treatment differ widely from one form to another; and rheumatoid arthritis in particular tends to prove so tenacious that it would appear logical *a priori* to separate it from the other chronic forms of rheumatic inflammation.

2.1. Dosage

High dosages of β1–24 corticotrophin administered over prolonged periods involve the risk of provoking a variety of side effects, which also include the well-known manifestations of hypercorticism. When resorting to long-term therapy one should therefore endeavour to adhere to a dosage schedule calculated to obviate these dangers while at the same time keeping the inflammation under adequate control. The difficulties met with in trying to achieve this goal remain one of the chief stumbling-blocks that arise both with A.C.T.H. and with corticosteroid therapy.

The ideal dosage schedule for depot tetracosactide in chronic cases of rheumatic inflammation would seem to be roughly as follows (Figure 1):

1) Daily injections of 0.5 to 1 mg. tetracosactide for approximately one week.
2) At the beginning of the second week, the interval between the injections of 0.5 to 1 mg. should be extended to 48 hours, and this alternate-day dosage continued for about two weeks.
3) From the third or fourth week onwards, one injection should be given every three days; these injections separated by a three-day interval, which it may later be possible to extend even further, represent a maintenance dosage that can safely be administered for a period of several weeks or months.

The two main obstacles likely to be encountered in implementing this dosage schedule are, firstly, that of spacing out the injections to an extent sufficient to avoid hypercorticism and, secondly, that of maintaining the desired interval between doses despite fluctuations in the course of the chronic inflammatory syndrome.

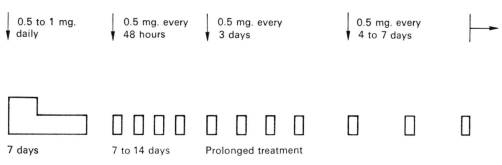

Fig. 1. Suggested dosage schedule for treatment with depot tetracosactide in chronic forms of rheumatic inflammation.

I propose now to give a brief account of the results obtained when an attempt was made to employ the type of dosage schedule outlined above in two groups of patients, one suffering from chronic forms of rheumatic inflammation and the other from rheumatoid arthritis, which, as already explained, we classify as a separate category of chronic rheumatic inflammation.

2.2. Group I: chronic forms of rheumatic inflammation

This group comprised 26 patients, i.e. eight cases of spondylarthritis, six of Reiter's disease, three of rhizomelic pseudo-polyarthritis, five of psoriatic arthropathy, and four of chronic idiopathic monarthritis (Table 2).

In all these cases the decision to administer tetracosactide was taken in view of the patient's failure to respond to non-steroid anti-inflammatory agents in the course of a particularly painful and incapacitating bout of severe inflammation. In five of the patients, corticosteroid therapy (in daily doses equivalent to 30 or 40 mg. prednisone) had likewise proved of no avail.

Tetracosactide exerted an immediate effect on the clinical and biological signs of inflammation—an effect which elicited excellent responses in almost all of the 26 cases. Only in one atheromatous patient suffering from spondylarthritis did it prove necessary to interrupt the treatment owing to a sharp rise in blood pressure. In four other patients (two cases of Reiter's disease, one of psoriatic arthropathy, and one of chronic monarthritis), it was found impossible—even after several weeks—to extend the interval between injections, with the result that the dosage required (0.5 or 1 mg. every 24 or 48 hours) led to frank A.C.T.H.-dependence and to side effects which necessitated the withdrawal of tetracosactide. In the remaining 21 patients, by contrast, the results obtained were very favourable—so favourable, in fact, that in 13 cases we were able after

Table 2. Results obtained with depot tetracosactide in 26 patients suffering from chronic forms of rheumatic inflammation. Average duration of treatment: 128 days; average dosage: 0.34 mg. per 24 hours.

	Results of treatment				
	Failure	A.C.T.H.-dependence	Satisfactory intermittent dosage schedule established	Patient weaned from A.C.T.H.	Totals
Spondylarthritis	1*	0	2	5	8
Reiter's disease	0	2	1	3	6
Rhizomelic pseudo-polyarthritis	0	0	1	2	3
Psoriatic arthropathy	0	1	3	1	5
Chronic monarthritis	0	1	1	2	4
Totals	1	4	8	13	26

*Treatment discontinued owing to intolerance

several weeks to wean the patient from tetracosactide under cover of another anti-inflammatory agent, while the other eight cases were maintained on tetracosactide injections separated by intervals sufficiently long to prevent the occurrence of undesirable side effects. These results were achieved after an average duration of treatment of 128 days and with an average dosage of 0.34 mg. per 24 hours.

Some of the cases appeared to us to provide particularly convincing testimony to the effectiveness of treatment with tetracosactide; this applies especially to three patients who had failed to respond to corticosteroid therapy, but who showed a sustained improvement after having received tetracosactide. In this group of diseases we nevertheless still find it difficult to codify the indications for A.C.T.H. therapy. Relatively short-term treatment with large doses of corticosteroids often also yields results comparable with those we obtained using tetracosactide, and the failures met with in patients receiving corticosteroids are no doubt quite often due simply to the fact that an inadequate dosage has been employed. Moreover, it should be emphasised that acute flare-ups occurring in the course of these chronic forms of rheumatic inflammation generally prove less prolonged and refractory to treatment than those encountered in cases of rheumatoid arthritis.

In such chronic rheumatic diseases, however, there are certain indications in which tetracosactide—by virtue of its rapid action, its good gastro-intestinal tolerability, and the relative ease with which it can be withdrawn—is undoubtedly the form of hormone therapy that deserves preference.

2.3. Group II: rheumatoid arthritis

Treatment with tetracosactide was administered to 46 of our patients suffering from rheumatoid arthritis (35 women and 11 men, whose ages ranged from 21 to 71 years). Of these 46 patients, 16 had never previously received any form of hormone therapy, whereas the remaining 30 had undergone prolonged treatment with corticosteroids which either had ceased to produce an adequate response or had sometimes given rise to troublesome side effects. Serological examinations had confirmed the presence of rheumatoid factor in 75 % of these cases. The diagnosis was established in accordance with the criteria of the American Rheumatism Association. In 80 % of the cases, extensive lesions of the cartilage and bone were observed, and 25 % of the patients were either bedridden or severely incapacitated.

The doses employed closely resembled those stipulated in the schedule already outlined, but in the first 16 cases a higher dosage was given, i.e. the daily injections were continued for a longer period, amounting sometimes to over two months.

The short-term results obtained were consistently very good: the signs and symptoms of joint involvement were rapidly brought under control, and the E.S.R. decreased within a few days in the patients who had received no previous corticosteroid therapy and within one to two weeks in the steroid-dependent cases.

Maintenance treatment with tetracosactide was then administered regularly, the medium-term response being assessed after four to six months, and the long-term response after 12 to 44 months.

2.3.1. Medium-term response (Table 3)
1) Poor results
In 12 of the 46 cases treated, the results proved disappointing for the following reasons:
– In four steroid-dependent cases, tetracosactide failed to elicit the desired response: one patient was evidently resistant to the drug despite the fact that his adrenal cortices reacted normally to it, two patients showed troublesome side effects early on in the treatment (here, pre-existing atheromatosis and hypertension were complicating factors, to which tetracosactide added by aggravating the hypertension and provoking oedema), and the fourth patient—for reasons unknown—developed signs of adrenocortical hypofunction during the third month of treatment.
– In eight cases, it was found impossible to prolong the interval between injections to more than 48 hours—a fact which indicated A.C.T.H.-dependence and which induced us to break off the treatment before the sixth month.

2) Good results
In the remaining 34 patients, the medium-term results obtained could be regarded as favourable:
– In 11 of them we were able, thanks to various adjuvant measures (treatment with indometacin, immunosuppressants, and injections of a radioactive isotope into the synovial membrane), to withdraw the tetracosactide within four to six months; the drug exerted a sustained effect which was still apparent six months after its withdrawal.
– In the other 23 patients we managed to prolong the interval between injections to three days or more; this regime was sufficiently effective in controlling the signs of inflammation and was also sufficiently well tolerated to enable us to

Table 3. Medium-term results (assessed after four to six months) obtained with depot tetracosactide in 46 cases of rheumatoid arthritis.

Number of cases	Results of treatment			
	Failure	A.C.T.H.- dependence	Satisfactory intermittent dosage schedule established	Patient weaned from A.C.T.H.
Total: 46	4	8	23	11
Corticosteroids −*: 16	0	3	7	6
Corticosteroids +*: 30	4	5	16	5

* Here, as well as in Tables 4, 5, and 8, "Corticosteroids −" = patients not previously treated with corticosteroids, and "Corticosteroids +" = patients who had already undergone prolonged corticosteroid therapy

administer long-term treatment with tetracosactide. Five of the patients subsequently defaulted, however, with the result that the long-term response could be assessed only in 18 of these 23 cases.

– Finally, it should be noted that, of the 30 steroid-dependent patients, 21 were weaned without difficulty from the corticosteroids which they had been receiving, and five of them taken off all hormone therapy by also withdrawing the tetracosactide after a few months.

2.3.2. Long-term response (Table 4)

Of the total of 46 patients, 18 were treated with tetracosactide for periods ranging from 12 to 44 months. All 18 patients were found to derive benefit from additional anti-inflammatory therapy in the form of indometacin or other non-steroid anti-inflammatory drugs, chlorambucil, cyclophosphamide, and radio-isotope injections into the synovial membrane.

1) Poor results

In seven of the 18 cases, in which it had been possible for several months to manage with intermittent doses, a renewed flare-up of the inflammation subsequently made it necessary to increase the dosage of tetracosactide, thereby creating a condition of A.C.T.H.-dependence which duly compelled us to interrupt the treatment and revert to corticosteroid therapy. All these seven patients were suffering from steroid-dependent rheumatoid arthritis, but had initially exhibited adequate adrenocortical reactivity (as confirmed by their positive responses to tests conducted with depot tetracosactide).

2) Good results

In the remaining 11 patients, the long-term effect of the treatment proved to be satisfactory:

– In four of them, the intermittent maintenance dosage was well tolerated and produced an adequate therapeutic effect.

– In the other seven cases, we were able to withdraw the tetracosactide injections after a period of 19 to 29 months without encountering any endocrinological problems and without thereby provoking any recurrence of the signs of inflammation.

Table 4. Long-term results (assessed after 12 to 44 months) obtained with depot tetracosactide in 18 cases of rheumatoid arthritis.

Number of cases	Results of treatment		
	A.C.T.H.-dependence	Satisfactory intermittent dosage schedule established	Patient weaned from A.C.T.H.
Total: 18	7	4	7
Corticosteroids −: 3	0	1	2
Corticosteroids +: 15	7	3	5

2.3.3. Overall results in cases of rheumatoid arthritis (Table 5)

An analysis covering 41 out of the total of 46 patients who received depot tetra-cosactide as treatment for rheumatoid arthritis reveals the following results:
- 4 failures within the first three months
- 15 cases of A.C.T.H.-dependence (eight medium-term and seven long-term)
- 18 successful withdrawals of A.C.T.H. therapy under cover of other forms of anti-inflammatory treatment
- 4 cases successfully maintained on long-term treatment with tetracosactide.

These results, obtained in particularly severe and refractory cases of rheumatoid arthritis which included a large proportion of steroid-dependent patients, are roughly equivalent to a 50% success rate.

2.3.4. Results achieved in steroid-dependent rheumatoid arthritis (Table 6)

When we confine our attention to the 30 steroid-dependent cases in which it was deemed necessary to withdraw corticosteroid therapy, the results yielded by tetracosactide are found to be as follows:
- Provided certain precautions were taken (i.e. provided the two forms of treatment were given in combination for an initial period of one to three weeks, and the tetracosactide administered at the start in a low dosage), no trouble was

Table 5. Overall results obtained with depot tetracosactide in 46 cases of rheumatoid arthritis.

Number of cases	Results of treatment			
	Failure	A.C.T.H.-dependence	Satisfactory intermittent dosage schedule established	Patient weaned from A.C.T.H.
Total: 41*	4	15	4	18
Corticosteroids −: 12	0	3	1	8
Corticosteroids +: 29	4	12	3	10

*Of the original total of 46 patients, five (corticosteroids −: 4; corticosteroids +: 1) defaulted.

Table 6. Results obtained with depot tetracosactide in 30 corticosteroid-dependent cases of rheumatoid arthritis.

Time lapse	Results of treatment			
	Failure	A.C.T.H.-dependence	Satisfactory intermittent dosage schedule established	Patient weaned from A.C.T.H.
4 to 6 months	4	5	16	5
12 to 44 months*	0	7	3	5

*One patient defaulted.

encountered in weaning the patients from corticosteroids by replacing the latter with tetracosactide injections*.

– In nine cases, we ran into difficulties after the treatment with tetracosactide had been in progress for only a fairly short time, i.e. in four cases the therapeutic effect was found to be wearing off and in the other five cases the patients developed A.C.T.H.-dependence.

– Five patients were successfully weaned from tetracosactide within the space of a few months.

– Of the remaining 16 cases receiving long-term treatment, one subsequently defaulted, five were eventually weaned from tetracosactide, and three managed satisfactorily on intermittent therapy, but seven finally became dependent on A.C.T.H.

Although the failures (16 cases) recorded in this series of steroid-dependent patients outnumbered the successes (13 cases), it must be emphasised that these successes were achieved under extremely unfavourable conditions and for this very reason are therefore all the more encouraging; it would seem in fact that attempts to wean patients from corticosteroids in cases where this is likely to prove difficult constitute one of the best indications for tetracosactide.

3. Observations on the tolerability of tetracosactide

In rheumatology, as in other branches of medicine, the indications for tetracosactide have to be determined within the limits imposed by the drug's side effects.

– Allergic complications, which prove such a frequent problem in patients receiving A.C.T.H. extract-preparations, appear to occur only in exceptional cases in response to tetracosactide. We have never observed any such complications, even in patients undergoing treatment for periods of more than three years.

– Melanoderma, on the other hand, was found to be a very common and early side effect, the severity of which seems to depend to some extent on the size and frequency of the doses of tetracosactide employed. Such pigmentation invariably receded after the drug had been withdrawn or the dosage reduced; and patients receiving injections of 0.5 mg. every three days very rarely suffered from this side effect.

– Side effects due to hypercorticism (e.g. mooning of the face, flushing, hypertension, and signs of salt and water retention) appear to be an ever-present risk and one that, here again, the use of high dosages is liable to encourage. Although side effects of this type were regularly observed in those of our patients who received daily doses of 0.5 to 1 mg. tetracosactide for more than two weeks, the majority of them readily abated after the interval between injections had been prolonged. An increase in body-weight following each injection was also

---

*Steroid-dependent patients with rheumatoid arthritis in whom initial tests of adrenocortical reactivity performed with tetracosactide yielded a negative response were excluded from this study.

frequently noted, and nine of the 18 patients whom we treated with tetra-cosactide for more than one year also showed a slight rise in their blood-pressure levels.

Such side effects impose restrictions on the use of tetracosactide in elderly subjects, in patients suffering from atheromatosis and/or hypertension, as well as in those with suspected heart failure; in all cases of this kind, long-term treatment with tetracosactide is contra-indicated. In view of the risk of these side effects, a careful check should be kept on the cardiovascular status of patients undergoing treatment with tetracosactide, and the utmost caution should be observed when selecting the dosage to be employed—particularly in cases of chronic rheumatic inflammation requiring prolonged therapy.

In a few instances we also encountered hyperglycaemia and phlebitis. Hypo-potassaemia, too, occurred in certain patients treated with high dosages for two to three months, but we now refrain from administering large doses over such prolonged periods.

Apart from a few minor incidents, the gastro-intestinal tolerability of tetra-cosactide has on the whole been very good.

At this point, it should be stressed once again that the incidence of side effects varies depending on the dosage used (Table 7); hence the importance of administering the drug in small, adequately spaced doses.

With regard to the side effects of tetracosactide, one cardinal question remains the subject of controversy, i.e. the problem as to whether, by maintaining elevated plasma cortisol levels, treatment with A.C.T.H. may inhibit hypo-thalamo-pituitary function.

No valid conclusions relevant to this question can be drawn from clinical observations as such. Whereas, for example, some of our patients who had been treated with depot tetracosactide for more than two years had no difficulty in tolerating the drug's withdrawal, there were other cases in which the presence of A.C.T.H.-dependence—occasioned largely by the very persistent character of the inflammatory signs—may well have been due to suppression of the hypo-thalamo-pituitary-adrenocortical axis.

Table 7. Incidence (in %) of side effects in rheumatological cases treated with depot tetracosactide.

	Medium dosage: 0.5 mg./48–72 hours %	High dosage: 0.5 mg./24–48 hours %
Allergic complications	0	0
Mooning of the face	40	64
Increase in body-weight	46	60
Rise in blood pressure	15.5	34
Hyperglycaemia	4.5	20
Gastro-intestinal side effects	2.5	18
Nervous side effects	3	14
Genital side effects	4	12
Pigmentation	48	48

Endocrinological tests* were performed in 14 of our patients after six months of treatment with predominantly high dosages of depot tetracosactide (0.5 mg. every 24 to 48 hours). In six of these patients, both the base-line plasma cortisol levels and the excretion of 17-hydroxycorticosteroids in the 24-hour urine were measured; the results were found to be normal—a finding which suggests that function of the hypothalamo-pituitary-adrenocortical axis was unimpaired. In the other eight cases, a lowering of the base-line plasma cortisol levels was observed; but, as shown in Table 8, the depot tetracosactide test elicited a normal response in seven of them and a strong response in the eighth patient. The results of the ®Metopirone and lysine-vasopressin tests were as follows (Table 8):

1) In three patients who had never previously received corticosteroid therapy:
– Metopirone test:
  one normal response
  two strong responses (clinical and biological hypercorticism in one case).
– Lysine-vasopressin test:
  three normal responses.
2) In five patients who had previously undergone corticosteroid therapy:
– Metopirone test (Patients D–H):
  three weak responses
  one strong response.
– Lysine-vasopressin test (Patients D, E, and F):
  two weak responses
  two normal responses.

Table 8. Results yielded by tests of hypothalamo-pituitary-adrenocortical function in eight patients after six months of treatment with depot tetracosactide (+++ = strong response; + = normal response; − = weak response).

8 patients (designated A–H)	Depot tetracosactide test	Metopirone test	Lysine-vasopressin test
Corticosteroids −: A	+	+	+
B	+++	+++	+
C	+	+++	+
Corticosteroids +: D	+	−	−
E	+	+++	±
F	+		+
G	Before* +	−	
	After* +		+
H	Before +	+	
	After +	−	+

*Before = before treatment with depot tetracosactide; After = after treatment with depot tetracosactide

*We wish to thank H. BRICAIRE, J.-P. LUTON, and P. LAUDAT (Hôpital Cochin, Paris) for having carried out these tests.

When tested after six months of tetracosactide therapy, two of these five patients were found to have base-line plasma cortisol levels lower than before the start of the treatment, but their response to the depot tetracosactide test was still normal. In the same two cases, the Metopirone test—which prior to treatment had yielded a weak response in one patient and a normal response in the other—elicited a weak response in both patients after six months of tetracosactide therapy. The response to lysine-vasopressin, on the other hand, was normal in both cases after six months of treatment.

These findings would tend to suggest that protracted administration of depot tetracosactide does not exert much influence on the hypothalamo-pituitary-adrenocortical axis, provided it is functioning normally at the outset, but that disturbances in hypothalamo-pituitary-adrenocortical function provoked by corticosteroid therapy may be aggravated by prolonged treatment with A.C.T.H.

4. Conclusions

On the basis of rheumatological data recorded during recent years it is possible to postulate certain indications for depot tetracosactide in inflammatory rheumatic conditions, and attempts must now be made to verify these indications in the light of wider experience.

As treatment for acute attacks of inflammation, the use of synthetic corticotrophin is particularly justified in severe cases of rheumatic fever, in certain types of rheumatism of infective origin, and in hyperalgesic neuralgia.

The indications for A.C.T.H. therapy in the course of chronic inflammatory rheumatic conditions have to be selected with considerable care. Though there are a number of conditions of this kind which may benefit from treatment with A.C.T.H., such treatment should essentially be reserved for combating the severe, but usually self-limiting, bouts of inflammation that are characteristic of the clinical course of these chronic illnesses. This involves administering therapy which, since it is of limited duration, is also better tolerated.

Rheumatoid arthritis has to be placed in a special category insofar as treatment with corticotrophin is concerned. A case of rheumatoid arthritis in which no attempt at corticosteroid therapy has yet been made should never be treated with tetracosactide until and unless other forms of anti-inflammatory medication have been tried and found wanting. In such instances, moreover, it is by no means certain that A.C.T.H. therapy will really be preferable to treatment with corticosteroids. On the other hand, in steroid-dependent cases of rheumatoid arthritis, recourse to synthetic corticotrophin may make it considerably easier to withdraw the corticosteroids and to adapt the patient to alternative forms of anti-inflammatory treatment.

Side effects prove a problem mainly in patients undergoing long-term treatment, in whom their occurrence may necessitate a reduction of dosage.

The possible inhibitory effect of synthetic corticotrophin on the hypothalamo-pituitary-adrenocortical axis is still subject to debate; such inhibition of this type as may occur seems to be chiefly confined to cases in which the A.C.T.H. therapy has been preceded by prolonged treatment with corticosteroids.

References

1 BONILLA, R.R., OLIVERA, F.R., CRAVIOTO, M.A., GAYTÁN, G.V.: Synacthen Depot en reumatología. México-méd. *18/3*, No. 15 (1968)

2 BRICAIRE, H., LUTON, J.-P.: Les tests de stimulation de la cortico-surrénale, fonction aldostérone exceptée. In: A.C.T.H.-thérapie moderne, Coll. thér. CIBA, Marseilles 1969, p. 21 (Kapp & Lahure, Vanves 1970)

3 COSTE, F., CAYLA, J., JONCHÈRES, Y.: La place de l'ACTH dans le traitement de la polyarthrite rhumatoïde. Sem. Hôp. Paris *36*, 411 (1960)

4 COSTE, F., MASSIAS, P.: Les hypercorticismes d'origine thérapeutique. Sem. Hôp. Paris *46*, 587 (1970)

5 DEGUILLAUME, R.: Etat actuel du traitement par un peptide corticotrope de synthèse, le tétracosactide-retard. Presse méd. *79*, 233 (1971)

6 GALIBERT, P., DELCOUR, J., GRUNEWALD, P., ROSAT, P., LEGARS, D., BERTOUX, WATTEBLED, R.: L'intérêt de l'ACTH-thérapie au cours du traitement de la sciatique, à propos de 125 observations. Vie méd. *53*, 3769 (1972)

7 LIBERTI, R., LONGO, C.: Sull'impiego della β^{1-24}corticotropina ad azione protratta nella terapia dell'artrite reumatoide. Policlinico, Sez. prat. *77*, 69 (1970)

8 LIÈVRE, J.-A., CAMUS, J.-P., BÉNICHOU, C., GUILLIEN, P.: Le traitement des névralgies par l'A.C.T.H. synthétique (tétracosactide). In: A.C.T.H.-thérapie moderne en rhumatologie, Coll. thér. CIBA, Aix-les-Bains 1971, p. 45 (EDAP, Paris 1972)

9 LUTON, J.-P.: Les accidents de la corticothérapie en neurologie. In: A.C.T.H.-thérapie moderne en neurologie, Coll. thér. CIBA, Strasbourg 1970, p. 13 (Impressions du Val d'Osne, Paris-Evian 1971)

10 LUTON, J.-P., LAUDAT, P., BRICAIRE, H.: L'emploi de la bêta $^{1-24}$corticotrophine retard dans l'exploration fonctionnelle du cortex surrénal. Ann. Endocr. (Paris) *30*, 456 (1969)

11 MASSIAS, P.: A.C.T.H.-thérapie en rhumatologie, loc. cit. [2], p. 41

12 MASSIAS, P.: A.C.T.H.-thérapie des névralgies hyperalgiques, loc. cit. [9], p. 145

13 MASSIAS, P., MARIN, A., DELBARRE, F.: Traitement au long cours de la polyarthrite rhumatoïde par le tétracosactide retard, loc. cit. [8], p. 95

14 MONDRAGÓN Y KALB, M.: Investigación clínica y terapéutica del 42,915-Ba Synacthen Depot en el campo de la reumatología. Sem. méd. Méx. *55*, 149 (1968)

15 MOZZICONACCI, P., ATTAL, C.: Synacthène-thérapie et rhumatologie infantile. In: A.C.T.H.-thérapie moderne en pédiatrie, Coll. thér. CIBA, Paris 1971, p. 21 (Soc. Annonces et Publicité, Paris 1972)

16 NUKI, G., JASANI, M.K., DOWNIE, W.W., WHALEY, K., CARSON DICK, W., WILLIAMSON, J., PATERSON, R.W.W., BOYLE, C., BUCHANAN, W.W.: Clinico-pharmacological studies on depot tetracosactrin in patients with rheumatoid arthritis. Pharmacol. clin. *2*, 99 (1970)

17 SAVAGE, O.: Controversies in the treatment of rheumatoid arthritis. Proc. roy. Soc. Med. *62*, 191 (1969)

Tetracosactide zinc phosphate as a supplement or possible alternative to corticosteroids in rheumatic diseases – a problem requiring further discussion

by M. Giordano*

Introduction

The number of drugs resorted to in the treatment of rheumatic disorders and non-rheumatic diseases of the joints is steadily increasing. In Figure 1 I have outlined the main groups of drugs which I myself am currently employing in the management of these conditions and have tried to indicate in diagrammatic form their relative importance and the scope of their use. Here it can be seen that despite the ever-increasing host of antirheumatic drugs now available, including the non-steroid anti-inflammatory agents in particular, it is my opinion—and also that of many other rheumatologists—that among the antirheumatics the corticosteroids continue, almost a quarter of a century after their introduction, to play a major role, especially from the qualitative aspect.

The position of A.C.T.H., on the other hand, is a very different one. Use of this hormone, which had never enjoyed much popularity with rheumatologists, was almost completely abandoned at the beginning of the 1960s. The advent of tetracosactide and the subsequent introduction of tetracosactide zinc phosphate (®Synacthen Depot) should have prompted rheumatologists to redirect their attention towards treatment with corticotrophin or, rather, with this synthetic derivative of A.C.T.H. In fact, however, such renewed interest as they have shown in A.C.T.H. therapy has been very limited. During these past few years, I myself have often wondered whether, in discussions between rheumatologists, sufficient consideration has been given to the possibility that in some cases tetracosactide might deserve a place as an alternative to the corticosteroids or as a drug serving to complement the latter[13]. This, I fear, is rather a difficult issue on which to pronounce judgment. The verdict should in fact depend not only upon comparisons between the therapeutic activity and side effects of steroids on the one hand and tetracosactide on the other—comparisons which in any case are not easy to make—but, above all, also upon accurate studies of the complex endocrinological problems involved in such treatment. In Figure 1 I have accordingly placed brackets round the A.C.T.H. derivatives, because I feel that this whole question has yet to be clarified.

Cases treated

Before embarking on a brief discussion of the possibility that the A.C.T.H. derivatives may indeed merit a place in the ranks of the antirheumatic agents, I should like to begin by referring to 70 cases of rheumatism treated with

*Istituto di Reumatologia, Università di Napoli, Naples, Italy.

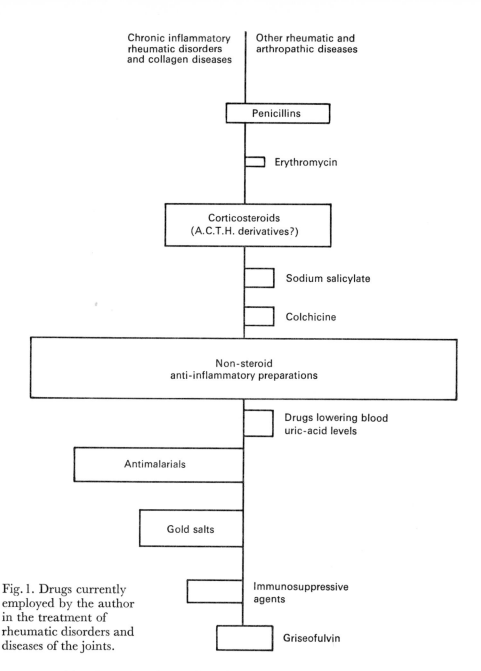

Fig. 1. Drugs currently employed by the author in the treatment of rheumatic disorders and diseases of the joints.

tetracosactide zinc phosphate. The forms of rheumatism from which these patients were suffering are indicated in Table 1.

Doses employed

One method which would certainly prove useful in selecting the dose of tetra-cosactide zinc phosphate appropriate for each patient consists in systematically determining the plasma cortisol levels occurring in response to injections of this polypeptide. Such an approach, however, would obviously pose considerable

183

Table 1. Rheumatic patients treated with tetracosactide zinc phosphate.

Disease	Number of cases
Rheumatoid arthritis	37
Juvenile rheumatoid arthritis	6
Still's disease in an adult	1
Psoriatic arthropathy	2
Sjögren's syndrome	1
Polymyalgia rheumatica	2
Rheumatic fever	4
Chorea minor	1
Unclassifiable subacute rheumatism	1
Systemic lupus erythematosus	6
Diffuse progressive scleroderma	3
Dermatomyositis	2
Unclassifiable collagen disease	1
Arthritis associated with dysgammaglobulinaemia due to a deficit of IgA	1
Corticosteroid-treated gout	2
Total	70

practical difficulties. On the other hand, in clinical rheumatology the patient's response as assessed by reference to the general manifestations of the disease —both objective and subjective—provides a very sensitive guide by which to estimate the intensity and duration of effect of a given dose of tetracosactide zinc phosphate. By taking as a criterion the patient's response to single injections, I have discovered that the optimum dose varies from case to case and that even in one and the same patient it may also vary at different times during the course of treatment. The initial dosage administered was almost invariably 1 mg. every other day; in cases where the patient showed a good response, I then reduced the dose to 0.75 mg. and afterwards to 0.5 mg. In the great majority of cases, injections of 0.5 mg. given on alternate days were found to be adequate, although there were numerous instances in which the benefit derived from an injection ceased after 30–40 hours. In many other cases, by contrast, especially where the course of treatment was continued over a sufficiently prolonged period, it proved possible to lengthen the interval between one injection and the next to 72 hours or more. In certain patients, tetracosactide zinc phosphate elicited a satisfactory response when injected in doses of only 0.33 mg.

These clinical observations would appear to conflict with the results of research indicating that the response of the plasma cortisol levels to single injections of tetracosactide zinc phosphate does not persist for more than 24–36–48 hours[2, 23]. I think it must therefore be postulated that cases occur in which the adreno-cortical response to tetracosactide zinc phosphate is in fact more prolonged than these studies of the plasma cortisol levels would seem to suggest. In this context it should be added that, on the whole, the dosages I employed were the lowest with which it was still possible to obtain a therapeutic effect. Incidentally, it has also been reported[8] that the maximal degree of adrenocortical stimulation apparently cannot be further increased by raising the dose of A.C.T.H.

In the cases to be described here, the duration of treatment with tetracosactide zinc phosphate ranged from a minimum of two weeks to a maximum of 12 months.

Results of treatment

Rheumatoid arthritis

Of the patients whom I treated with Synacthen Depot, 53% were suffering from severe forms of rheumatoid arthritis. It is a well-known fact that, for a number of years now, the vast majority of rheumatologists have been resorting to corticosteroid therapy only in a small percentage of cases of rheumatoid arthritis. A few years ago I came to the conclusion on the basis of my own therapeutic criteria that treatment with corticosteroids is justified in only about 10% of adults with rheumatoid arthritis[13]. Such drugs should in my opinion be reserved for use in those cases where so-called basic therapy—i.e. administration of non-steroid anti-inflammatory agents, antimalarial drugs, or gold salts— has failed either to afford the patient an acceptable measure of relief or to enable him to resume work. In most instances, the failures encountered with these basic preparations are due to the side effects which they provoke in many patients.

In current medical practice, the percentage of patients suffering from rheumatoid arthritis who receive treatment with corticosteroids is far higher than 10%, because the restrictions on their use which I, and almost all other rheumatologists, have advocated are not observed by most physicians. With regard to the expediency of employing tetracosactide in cases of rheumatoid arthritis, I think that here a distinction should be drawn between two different sub-groups. Among my own cases, the first sub-group consisted of 26 patients with rheumatoid arthritis who had already been receiving long-term steroid therapy for some time and in whom, in the light of the criteria to which I have already referred, this therapy was judged to be unnecessary and therefore inopportune. In these cases it was accordingly my aim to wean the patient from the steroid medication. By simply substituting tetracosactide for the steroid I was able to achieve this objective only in three cases in which the patients' dependence upon the steroid had persisted despite the fact that the disease had already passed out of the acute inflammatory phase and was more or less in a state of remission.

In all the other cases (23 patients) in this first sub-group, switching the patient from corticosteroids to tetracosactide merely had the effect of transforming him from a steroid-dependent to a tetracosactide-dependent patient. It was only when I resorted to combined treatment with other drugs (non-steroid anti-inflammatory agents in all cases, plus cyclophosphamide in four cases, antimalarial drugs in 20 cases, and gold salts in one case) that I was able in the majority of these patients to effect a gradual withdrawal of the A.C.T.H. therapy. One important aspect of this problem is the fact that in a number of cases dependence upon A.C.T.H. proves less difficult to overcome than dependence upon corticosteroids; in view of this, I felt that in most of these steroid-dependent patients substitution of the steroid medication by Synacthen Depot would facilitate withdrawal of the steroid.

The second sub-group of patients with rheumatoid arthritis comprised 11 cases which fulfilled the prerequisites for corticosteroid therapy that I have already outlined and in which I therefore considered such therapy to be appropriate. In cases of this type, the "antirheumatic" effects of tetracosactide are of course comparable with those elicited by corticosteroids. Here, however, treatment with tetracosactide can be expected to result in an A.C.T.H.-dependence which it will prove difficult to eliminate, because the patients in question either cannot tolerate the usual run of non-steroid antirheumatic agents or show little response to them; consequently, in contrast to the type of patient in the first sub-group, these cases cannot be weaned from tetracosactide by resorting to combined treatment with non-steroid drugs, and the withdrawal of tetracosactide can therefore only be effected once the acutely active phase of the disease has subsided. In such cases, one is thus confronted with the alternative of either long-term steroid or long-term tetracosactide treatment. The choice between the two possibilities must depend primarily upon the side effects which each form of treatment is liable to involve and to which reference will be made later.

Juvenile rheumatoid arthritis

Here, corticosteroid therapy is indicated under the same conditions as have already been stipulated with regard to rheumatoid arthritis in adults, as well as in clinical pictures in which the general symptoms are more pronounced than those of joint involvement (Still's syndrome in the strict sense of the term[4, 14]) and in the presence of ocular manifestations or myocarditis and pericarditis. But in juvenile rheumatoid arthritis, too, the need sometimes arises to wean the patient from corticosteroid therapy; for this purpose, recourse to treatment with tetracosactide should be regarded as the correct procedure, since under these circumstances the same arguments apply to the drug's use as in adults. As for the problem of choosing between A.C.T.H. and corticosteroids, here again the situation is fundamentally the same as in the case of an adult suffering from rheumatoid arthritis. But it must be borne in mind that, in young patients who are still growing, A.C.T.H. appears to be preferable to corticosteroids. As has been pointed out by BYWATERS[3] and other authors, corticosteroids are known to interfere with growth—possibly because they inhibit somatotrophin[9, 11]. Prolonged treatment with A.C.T.H., on the other hand, seems to be largely or completely devoid of this serious side effect[12, 25], which appears to be closely bound up with inhibition of endogenous A.C.T.H. secretion[25].

Other forms of rheumatism

Among the patients I also treated with tetracosactide were a few cases involving chronic forms of rheumatism that occur less frequently than rheumatoid arthritis or are even decidedly uncommon, but in which the decision as to whether or not corticosteroids or tetracosactide should be employed depends on much the same considerations as are applicable to cases of rheumatoid arthritis in adults and children. Falling within this category were two patients with *psoriatic arthropathy*, one with *Sjögren's syndrome*, one patient who developed *Still's disease* as an adult, and one case of *polyarthritis associated with dysgammaglobulin-aemia characterised by a total deficit of immunoglobulin A*.

In addition, I used tetracosactide to treat two patients suffering from *poly-myalgia rheumatica*. In this disease, in which steroids can probably be regarded as the drugs of choice, Synacthen Depot might well play an important role as an alternative to corticosteroid therapy.

High dosages of corticosteroids are often required during acute phases of *systemic lupus erythematosus* and *dermatomyositis*. But in cases where it is considered advisable to continue the treatment with small doses of corticosteroids or even to suspend steroid therapy altogether, one can give Synacthen Depot either alternately with corticosteroids or in an attempt to withdraw the latter.

Although I rarely prescribe corticosteroids or tetracosactide in cases of *diffuse progressive scleroderma*, I have employed such treatment in two women who had developed pleurisy and in one woman suffering from particularly severe scleroderma which had failed to improve in response to griseofulvin, anti-malarial agents, and non-steroid anti-inflammatory drugs.

It is almost unanimously agreed that large doses of corticosteroids should be given during the initial phase of *rheumatic fever*. After the first four to six weeks of the illness, however, the steroid therapy should be administered in reduced doses; at the same time, various authors (including myself) then add salicylates to the regimen. In this stage of the treatment—especially if the presence of carditis indicates that the hormone therapy, combined possibly with salicylates, should be further prolonged—it may be preferable to resort to tetracosactide as an alternative to corticosteroids. I have done this myself in four cases of rheu-matic fever, in one patient with *chorea minor*, and in another suffering from *unclassifiable subacute rheumatism*.

Finally, my own personal experience also includes two cases of *gout treated with corticosteroids* in which the use of tetracosactide, together with non-steroid anti-inflammatory drugs and allopurinol, made it possible to wean the patient from the corticosteroids which should never have been prescribed in the first place.

Side effects

The side effects I encountered in the 70 rheumatic cases treated with tetra-cosactide zinc phosphate are listed in Table 2, in which the question marks in brackets indicate manifestations that could not be ascribed with certainty to the drug's use.

Only three of these side effects call for comment: salt and water retention, skin pigmentation, and allergic reactions.

Salt and water retention occurred only in patients receiving a dosage of 1 mg. or 0.75 mg. every 48 hours.

The *skin pigmentation* which developed in seven cases manifested itself after medication had been in progress for some time and disappeared again very slowly once the treatment had been completed. In one patient in whom the

187

Table 2. Side effects observed in 70 rheumatic patients treated with tetracosactide zinc phosphate.

Side effect	Number of cases
Shock	1
Angioneurotic oedema	1
Vague feeling of malaise after each injection	1
Oedema	5
Skin pigmentation	7
Mooning of the face	3
Epigastralgia (?)	1
Anxiety (?)	1
Frequency of urination (?)	1

pigmentation became extremely intense, I was obliged to withdraw the tetra-cosactide therapy.

Much more serious in my opinion were the *allergic reactions* which I observed in two patients. In one of these patients—a young woman with rheumatoid arthritis—a cutaneous reaction of the angioneurotic-oedema type set in on the 14th day of treatment, i.e. a few minutes after she had received her seventh injection of 1 mg. This patient was given no further injections. The other case was a woman suffering from severe rheumatoid arthritis who had already previously undergone about two months of treatment with Synacthen Depot; when medication with this drug was resumed after an interval of some three months, the injection of 1 mg. tetracosactide was followed a few minutes later by the appearance of an alarming clinical picture characterised by prostration, profuse sweating, palpitation, and hypotension. When a sensitivity test was performed some time after this shock had occurred, the patient showed a positive skin reaction to a subcutaneous injection of 0.05 ml. Synacthen Depot. It should be added that, during her first course of treatment with the poly-peptide, this patient had complained of a vague feeling of malaise immediately after each injection.

Discussion

From the clinical observations reported here it may be concluded that, thanks to its cortisone-like therapeutic effects, tetracosactide can be employed in the treatment of many rheumatic patients in whom it is not necessary to prescribe particularly high dosages of corticosteroids. Corticosteroids, however, are definitely preferable during the initial phase of rheumatic fever, as well as in particularly active phases of certain systemic collagen diseases and especially of lupus erythematosus and acute dermatomyositis. In other phases of these diseases, and in other chronic rheumatic conditions in which corticosteroid therapy is indicated, the possibility of using tetracosactide instead of cortico-steroids may be considered. Finally, this A.C.T.H. derivative should also be employed in cases where it is desired to wean a patient from corticosteroids, and it likewise deserves preference in young patients with rheumatoid arthritis who have not yet completed their physical growth.

In all diseases in which corticosteroids and A.C.T.H. derivatives may be expected to produce similar therapeutic effects, the choice between them has to be made on the basis of a precise evaluation of their respective side effects. The chief advantage which A.C.T.H. and its synthetic derivatives should offer as compared with corticosteroids lies in the fact that—at any rate in theory—they are likely to cause little interference with the hypothalamo-pituitary-adreno-cortical axis. Several authors have published research findings which at least partially confirm this hypothesis[1, 5, 10, 11, 16, 21, 24]. Moreover, one consequence of the limited degree to which A.C.T.H. interferes with hypothalamo-pituitary-adrenocortical function might well be the clinical impression which certain authors[21, 22, 25] have reported, and which I too have gained in some cases, that the withdrawal of A.C.T.H. treatment is better tolerated by chronic rheumatics than the interruption of corticosteroid therapy. While regarding the papers that have already been published on this topic as worthy of consideration, I nevertheless feel that further endocrinological studies should be undertaken in rheumatic patients treated either with corticosteroids or with A.C.T.H. in order to determine to what extent the two types of drug provoke differing effects in the organism. In this connection, it would be necessary, among other things, to establish whether the limited interference of A.C.T.H. therapy with the hypo-thalamo-pituitary-adrenocortical axis is bound up with the drug's mode of administration, which is usually of the intermittent type[1, 21].

Other advantages as compared with corticosteroids have been ascribed to A.C.T.H. with regard to side effects. It has been alleged that treatment with corticotrophin is equivalent to a form of "polysteroid therapy" since the steroids secreted from the adrenals in response to the stimulus of A.C.T.H. also include certain protein-anabolic hormones. Hence the claim that A.C.T.H. therapy does not provoke osteoporosis[6, 20] or give rise to other manifestations resulting from enhanced protein catabolism, such as atrophy of the skin and muscles. This might also partly account for the finding that A.C.T.H. is less likely to lead to peptic ulceration. Although these claims are interesting, it is difficult to confirm them, and they therefore require more extensive corroboration.

The biggest disadvantage from which A.C.T.H. of natural origin suffered in comparison with corticosteroids was, in my view, the risk of serious allergic reactions which its use entailed. With the advent of the synthetic tetracosactide derivative it was hoped that this problem had been overcome. However, though there seems to be no doubt that tetracosactide is clinically better tolerated than A.C.T.H. extract-preparations[8], reports referring to allergic reactions to tetracosactide—some of them of a serious nature—already began appearing several years ago[17]. I myself have described one reaction of this type in the present paper. On the basis of research in which they studied the occurrence of antibodies directed against A.C.T.H. in patients treated with Synacthen Depot, Glass et al.[15] express the opinion that the antigenic potential of this polypeptide is due to the fact of its being combined with zinc phosphate. If this is indeed the case, then the development of new A.C.T.H. derivatives (such as the octadecapeptide) which are metabolised more slowly[7,18,19] should further reduce the risk of allergic reactions.

Conclusions

Except in conditions calling for the use of very high doses of corticosteroids, the therapeutic effects which it is possible to obtain with A.C.T.H. derivatives in all rheumatic diseases are very similar to those resulting from treatment with corticosteroids.

The possibility that synthetic A.C.T.H. derivatives might be able to play an important role in the management of rheumatic diseases, partly as a substitute for corticosteroids and partly in combination with them, is based mainly upon the following two hypotheses: firstly, that the A.C.T.H. derivatives interfere with the hypothalamo-pituitary-adrenocortical axis to a lesser extent than do the corticosteroids and, secondly, that polypeptide preparations akin to A.C.T.H. do not provoke serious allergic phenomena. Even though these two hypotheses have not yet been adequately confirmed, the data now at our disposal are sufficient to justify legitimate hopes; consequently, the efforts at present being made to develop new A.C.T.H. derivatives deserve wide encouragement.

Summary

An account has been given of clinical observations made in 70 cases of rheumatism treated with tetracosactide zinc phosphate.

In rheumatoid arthritis in both adults and juveniles, in rheumatic fever, in systemic lupus erythematosus, in diffuse scleroderma, and in various other conditions, including chorea minor, psoriatic arthropathy, Sjögren's syndrome, polymyalgia rheumatica, dermatomyositis, arthritis associated with dysgammaglobulinaemia characterised by a deficit of IgA, and corticosteroid-treated gout, tetracosactide was found to yield therapeutic results similar to those obtainable with corticosteroids. Corticosteroids, however, are preferable in cases where a very high dosage is required (i.e. during the initial phase of rheumatic fever, as well as in particularly active phases of systemic lupus erythematosus, dermatomyositis, and other collagen diseases). The A.C.T.H. derivatives deserve preference in juvenile rheumatoid arthritis. Tetracosactide, especially when employed in combination with antimalarial agents, non-steroid anti-inflammatory preparations, gold salts, or immunosuppressive agents, also seems to facilitate the withdrawal of corticosteroids. Its use should therefore be resorted to whenever attempts are being made to wean patients from corticosteroid therapy. At present it is very difficult to determine whether the A.C.T.H. derivatives offer advantages over the corticosteroids such as to render them a preferable alternative to corticosteroid therapy in many cases of rheumatism. It does not yet seem to have been adequately demonstrated that tetracosactide zinc phosphate provokes fewer side effects than the corticosteroids or that it causes less interference with the hypothalamo-pituitary-adrenocortical axis;

nor does the risk of severe allergic reactions appear to have been completely eliminated with the A.C.T.H. preparations currently in use. Research on new polypeptides similar to A.C.T.H. therefore merits encouragement.

References

1 BACON, P.A., DALY, J.R., MYLES, A.B., SAVAGE, O.: Hypothalamo-pituitary-adrenal function in patients on long-term adrenocorticotrophin therapy. Ann. rheum. Dis. *27*, 7 (1968)

2 BESSER, G.N., BUTLER, P.W.P., PLUMPTON, F.S.: Adrenocorticotrophic action of long-acting tetracosactrin compared with corticotrophin-gel. Brit. med. J. *iv*, 391 (1967)

3 BYWATERS, E.G.L.: The present status of steroid treatment in rheumatoid arthritis. Proc. roy. Soc. Med. *58*, 649 (1965)

4 CALABRO, J.J., MARCHESANO, J.M.: The early natural history of juvenile rheumatoid arthritis. A 10-year follow-up study of 100 cases. Med. Clin. N. Amer. *52*, 567 (1968)

5 CARTER, M.E., JAMES, V.H.T.: An attempt at combining corticotrophin with long-term corticosteroid therapy. With a view to preserving hypothalamic-pituitary-adrenal function. Ann. rheum. Dis. *29*, 409 (1970)

6 CODACCIONI, J.-L., BOYER, J.: Indications, possibilités et limites de la cortico-stimulation en pratique courante. Rev. Prat. (Paris) *22*, 30bis: 84 (1972)

7 DESAULLES, P.A., RINIKER, B., RITTEL, W.: High corticotrophic activity of a short-chain synthetic corticotrophin analogue. In Margoulies, M. (Editor): Protein and polypeptide hormones, Proc. Int. Symp., Liège 1968, p. 489 (Excerpta med. Found., Amsterdam 1969)

8 EL SHABOURY, A.H.: Assessment of long-acting synthetic corticotrophin in hypersensitive asthmatics and normal subjects. Brit. med. J. *iii*, 653 (1968)

9 FRANTZ, A.G., RABKIN, M.T.: Human growth hormone. Clinical measurement, response to hypoglycemia and suppression by corticosteroids. New Engl. J. Med. *271*, 1375 (1964)

10 FRIEDMAN, M.: The effect of corticotrophin on hypothalamic-pituitary-adrenal function of children. Proc. roy. Soc. Med. *61*, 291 (1968)

11 FRIEDMAN, M., GREENWOOD, F.C.: The effect of prolonged ACTH or corticosteroid therapy in children on growth and on pituitary-adrenal and pituitary function. Mem. Soc. Endocr. No. 17: 249 (1968)

12 FRIEDMAN, M., STRANG, L.B.: Effect of long-term corticosteroids and corticotrophin on the growth of children. Lancet *ii*, 568 (1966)

13 GIORDANO, M.: Le cure cortisoniche dell'artrite reumatoide. Reumatismo *22*, 65 (1970)

14 GIORDANO, M., ARA, M., CAPELLI, L., TIRRI, G.: Klinische und serologische Betrachtungen über den jugendlichen chronischen Rheumatismus mit besonderer Berücksichtigung der extra-artikulären Erscheinungen. Kassenarzt *12*, 236 (1972)

15 GLASS, D., NUKI, G., DALY, J.R.: Development of antibodies during long-term therapy with corticotrophin in rheumatoid arthritis. II. Zinc tetracosactrin (Depot Synacthen). Ann. rheum. Dis. *30*, 593 (1971)

16 IRVINE, W.J., CULLEN, D.R., KHAN, S.A., RATCLIFFE, J.G.: Hypothalamic-pituitary-adrenal function in patients treated with long-term depot tetracosactrin. Brit. med. J. *i*, 630 (1971)

17 JENSEN, N.E., SNEDDON, I.: Allergic intolerance to tetracosactrin. Brit. med. J. *ii*, 383 (1969); corresp.

18 KEENAN, J., THOMPSON, J.B., CHAMBERLAIN, M.A., BESSER, G.M.: Prolonged corticotrophic action of a synthetic substituted $^{1-18}$ACTH. Brit. med. J. *iii*, 742 (1971)

19 MAIER, R., BARTHE, P., SCHENKEL-HULLIGER, L., DESAULLES, P.A.: The biological activity of (1-D-serine, 17-18-dilysine)-β-corticotrophin-(1-18)-octa-decapeptide-amide. Acta endocr. (Kbh.) *68*, 458 (1971)

20 MALONE, D.N.S., STRONG, J.A.: The present status of corticotrophin therapy. Practitioner *208*, 329 (1972)

21 NELSON, J.K., MACKAY, J.S., SHERIDAN, B., WEAVER, J.A.: Intermittent therapy with corticotrophin. Lancet *ii*, 78 (1966)

22 SAVAGE, O., COPEMAN, W.S.C., CHAPMAN, L., WELLS, M.V., TREADWELL, B.L.J.: Pituitary and adrenal hormones in rheumatoid arthritis. Lancet *i*, 232 (1962)

23 TREADWELL, B.L.J., DENNIS, P.M.: Comparison of depot tetracosactrin and corticotrophin gel. Brit. med. J. *iv*, 720 (1969)

24 WALSER, A., BARTHE, P., SCHÄR, J.: Die Wirkung hoher Dosen von synthetischem ACTH auf die Funktion von Hypothalamus-Hypophyse-Nebennierenrinde. Schweiz. med. Wschr. *98*, 1892 (1968)

25 ZUTSHI, D.W., FRIEDMAN, M., ANSELL, B.M.: Corticotrophin therapy in juvenile chronic polyarthritis (Still's disease) and effect on growth. Arch. Dis. Childh. *46*, 584 (1971)

Discussion

D. Gross: When discussing the numerous types of rheumatic disorder that have been mentioned here, I think we have to draw a fundamental distinction between treatment for the underlying disease itself and treatment for the secondary signs and symptoms of inflammation. This applies both to osteoarthritis, in which the main problem is a mechanical one, as well as to polyarthritis, in which it is a metabolic one. It also applies to rheumatoid arthritis—a condition in which it has been suggested that the pathogenesis of the underlying disease is basically attributable to an immunopathological process. What approach should in principle be adopted when treating these disorders? If the patient develops an acute bout of inflammation affecting one joint only, we can either resort to local treatment with corticosteroids or, alternatively, institute systemic therapy with corticosteroids or Synacthen. Local treatment may take the form of intra-articular injection or infiltration, e.g. into the nerve root in the case of an intervertebral joint. The choice as to the type of treatment to be given will depend not so much on clinical criteria, but rather on considerations relating to the technique of administration itself.

Where, on the other hand, one is dealing with an attack of multi-articular inflammation affecting almost all the joints—such as is liable to occur in cases of polyarthritis or rheumatoid arthritis—the problem becomes a quantitative one. If the inflammatory process is of an extremely acute nature, systemic treatment with corticosteroids, in high daily doses equivalent to 40 mg. prednisone or more, has to be given. In such cases, Synacthen or A.C.T.H. will not always prove adequate, because the quantity of cortisol released into the plasma under their influence may not be sufficient to bring the inflammation fully under control.

In a moderately severe bout of inflammation, however, one is free to choose between either corticosteroids—in a daily dosage equivalent to 20–25 mg. prednisone—or A.C.T.H.

P. Massias: I should like to comment briefly on what Dr. Gross has just said about the inadequacy of treatment with A.C.T.H. in severe bouts of inflammation occurring in rheumatic patients. While I cannot recall any case of rheumatoid arthritis in which such bouts of inflammation failed to respond satisfactorily to a dosage of 40 mg. prednisone per 24 hours, I must add that equally good results can be obtained with injections of 0.5 or 1 mg. A.C.T.H.

R. Deguillaume: The question of dosage has been raised on several occasions during the course of this symposium, and in this connection reference has frequently been made to "high doses". This prompts me to point out that, according to human pharmacological data, an injection of 1 mg. A.C.T.H. provokes maximal stimulation of the adrenal cortices in terms of both intensity and, above all, duration of effect. A dose of 2 mg. does not achieve much more, nor does one of 0.5 mg. achieve much less—which, incidentally, explains why numerous clinicians now prefer to employ doses of only 0.5 mg. I should like to emphasise that, once one exceeds the threshold dose required to produce maximal stimulation, the question of dosage ceases to play a major role. The doses used by Dr. Boissière in children, for example, may perhaps seem enormously high; nevertheless, it cannot be said that he was administering an overdosage, because the adrenal cortex itself limits its secretion of glucocorticoids to its own maximum. Of course, when unnecessarily high dosages are given there is an increased risk of extra-adrenal side effects—including melanoderma in particular—and, according to Dr. Irvine, also an increased risk of hyperaldosteronism. The really important factor, however, is not the absolute size of the doses, but the frequency with which they are injected. The interval between injections should be as long as possible, i.e. as protracted as is still compatible with the attainment of a satisfactory therapeutic response. The decision as to what constitutes an optimal interval between doses can be reached only on the basis of clinical observation. Biological examinations are merely of subordinate value in this connection, because experience has shown that the therapeutic effect of an injection is more prolonged than the rise in the plasma cortisol levels which it provokes.

J. GIRARD: Regarding the problem of dosage, I should like to ask whether any data are available on the plasma concentrations of specific steroids—as opposed to "Mattingly steroids" or "Murphy steroids"—in relation to the dosage of A.C.T.H. administered. It is possible by means of radioimmunoassay to make specific determinations of a whole series of steroids; and, if we were to measure the plasma levels of individual steroids, this might perhaps help us to find an explanation for the fact that A.C.T.H. therapy causes little interference with growth in children. As shown here in Figure 1, radioimmunological determination of the plasma cortisol levels yields values that are only about half as high as those recorded by the Mattingly method.

K. F. WEINGES: I have a basic question I'd like to put to the paediatricians here: how exactly do they account for the growth-inhibiting effect of synthetic glucocorticoids? I have just come across a paper from Hungary* in which it is argued that growth hormone itself cannot play a particularly important role in this connection. In children treated with steroids, the authors of this paper found that the secretion of growth

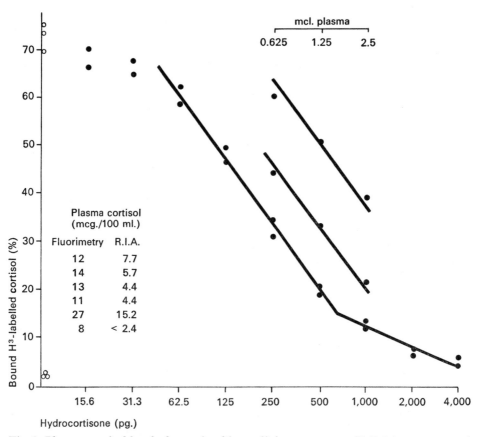

Fig. 1. Plasma cortisol levels determined by radioimmunoassay (R.I.A.) as compared with those obtained by the Mattingly technique (fluorimetry).

* GACS, G., KUN, E., CZIRBESZ, Z.: Growth hormone secretion in children during corticosteroid treatment. Responses to arginine. Horm. metab. Res. 5, 106 (1973)

hormone was either normal or even enhanced. From the paper by TARANGER et al. which has been presented here, it would appear that treatment with A.C.T.H. too —since it also accelerates skeletal maturation—must in the long run likewise have the effect of inhibiting growth. The paediatrician usually sees children only up to the age of about 14 years, but they continue growing till they are 18; the thing I am wondering is whether, in an 18-year-old who had previously received long-term treatment with Synacthen, one might perhaps find evidence that his growth had been inhibited.

J. GIRARD: Prolonged treatment with steroids upsets the regulation of growth hormone secretion, with the result that, for example, the increase in growth hormone

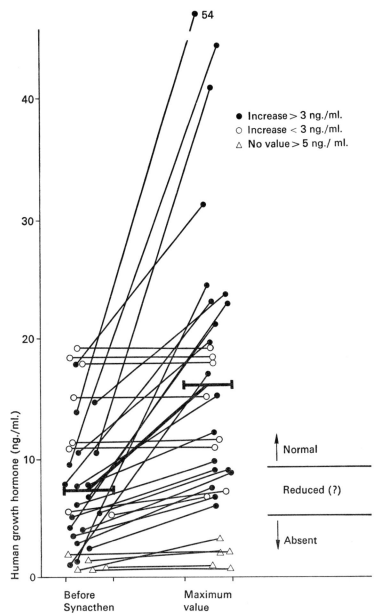

Fig. 2. Plasma levels of human growth hormone in children before and during a Synacthen test of adrenocortical function. Increase assessed by reference to maximum value recorded.

production occurring in response to stress is inhibited. In the periphery, the anabolic effect exerted by growth hormone on the epiphyseal cartilage is antagonised by gluco-corticoids; this in turn has the effect of retarding cartilage and bone growth.

At this point I should like to show you some results illustrating our own experience with regard to the controversial question of the extent to which A.C.T.H. stimulates the secretion of growth hormone. Figure 2 reveals that, after injection of Synacthen, the average growth hormone concentrations were appreciably higher than the initial

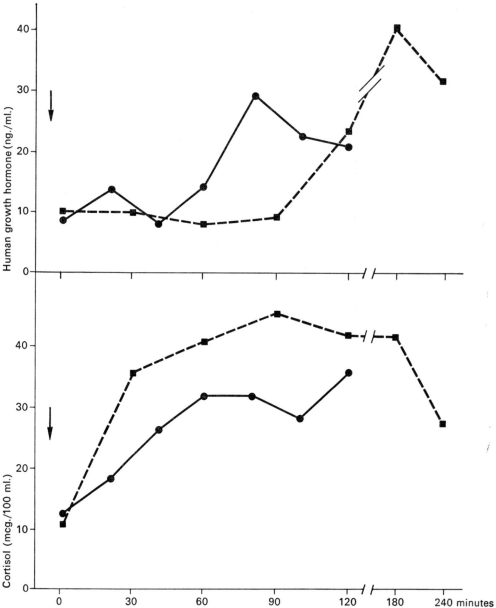

Fig. 3. Approximately parallel increases in plasma growth hormone and cortisol levels in response to insulin-induced hypoglycaemia (●——●) and during a Synacthen test (■———■) in a child with no impairment of hypothalamo-pituitary-adrenocortical function.

levels. As you can see, it is also possible to distinguish between a normal, a reduced, and an absent reaction to Synacthen; and the responses do in fact vary very considerably from one instance to another. Indicated in Figure 3 is a case in which the growth hormone and the cortisol concentrations each underwent roughly parallel increases during a Synacthen test and in response to insulin-induced hypoglycaemia. That the growth hormone and cortisol response may be unrelated to each other is demonstrated by findings obtained in two patients (Figure 4) who, following prolonged steroid

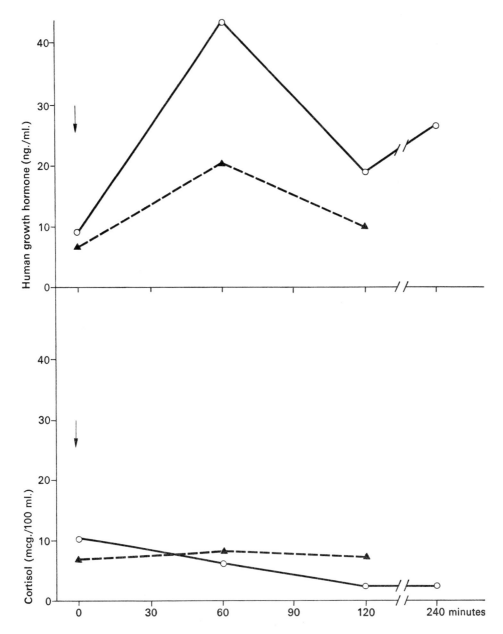

Fig. 4. Increase in growth hormone secretion, but not in plasma cortisol levels, in response to Synacthen in two children following prolonged steroid therapy.

therapy, showed no rise in their plasma cortisol levels in response to Synacthen, but did exhibit an increase in growth hormone secretion. Examples of pathological cases are shown in Figures 5 and 6. A comparison between the results yielded by different types of stimulation test serves to emphasise the value of the A.C.T.H. test as a means by which to investigate growth hormone secretion.

Incidentally, as illustrated in Figure 7, the time at which the growth hormone concentration reaches its maximum during the Synacthen test is subject to variation, and it is impossible on the basis of the concentrations recorded to distinguish any consistent time pattern for the growth hormone response to A.C.T.H.

Finally, although the A.C.T.H. test can provide additional information on growth hormone secretion, the connection between A.C.T.H. and growth hormone is still

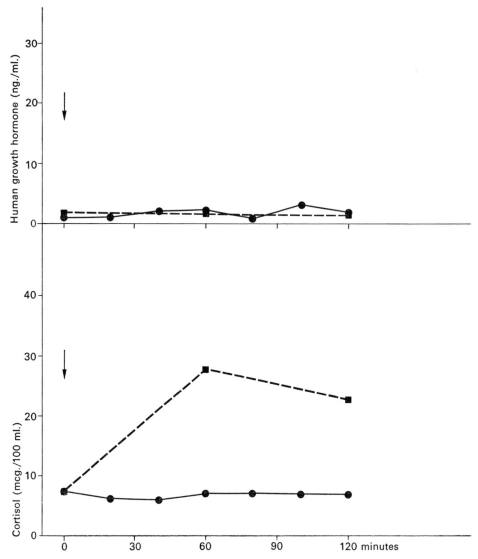

Fig. 5. No increase in plasma growth hormone levels in either the insulin (●——●) or Synacthen (■——■) test, but increase in plasma cortisol in response to Synacthen. The patient was a child suffering from pituitary dwarfism.

198

unclear, and the question as to whether A.C.T.H. is capable of "specifically" provoking the release of growth hormone has yet to be answered.

H. V. PRICE: Just a brief comment on treatment with A.C.T.H. in asthmatic children: it has been mentioned both here and elsewhere that some diminution in growth may

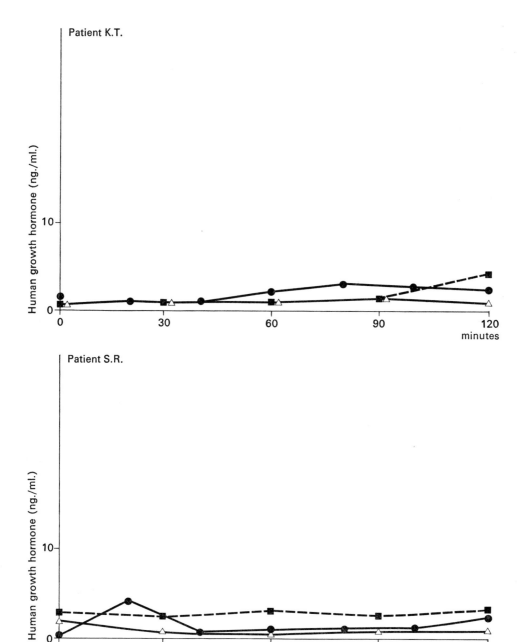

Fig. 6. No increase in plasma growth hormone levels in the Metopirone (△——△), Synacthen (■— —■), and insulin (●——●) tests in two patients.

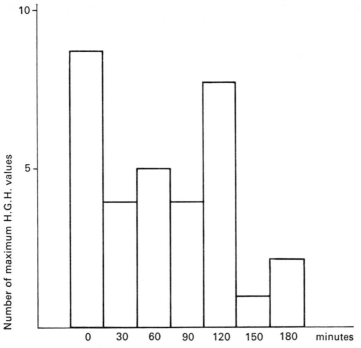

Fig. 7. Times at which human growth hormone (H.G.H.) levels reached their maximum during the Synacthen test. Note that the highest number of maximum values was recorded before and 120 minutes after the injection of Synacthen.

occur in response to treatment with A.C.T.H. preparations and with tetracosactrin, but that this is much less marked than in children receiving corticosteroid therapy; I think it would be incorrect, however, to conclude that there is no suppression of growth at all in asthmatic children treated with A.C.T.H.

W. J. IRVINE: I should like to revert briefly to what has been said about assessing the dose clinically and not by reference to the plasma cortisol levels. I am not sure I agree with this, because there seems to be some evidence indicating that, if you increase the dose of Synacthen Depot, you may get a more prolonged response; this means, not that the absolute plasma cortisol levels increase further to any marked extent, but that the effect of the dose nevertheless lasts longer—and this could well have an important bearing on the question of trying to preserve function of the hypothalamo-pituitary-adrenocortical axis. In other words, if you are administering more depot tetracosactrin than is really required, you may be producing very little increase in the absolute plasma cortisol levels, but you might on the other hand end up by suppressing the hypothalamo-pituitary-adrenocortical axis with the result that you are unable to withdraw the A.C.T.H. therapy afterwards.

H. JESSERER: Although I'm not a paediatrician, I think I am correct in saying that one cannot regard growth and maturation as being solely dependent upon growth hormone. The androgens, too, fulfil a major function here. Consequently, when discussing inhibition of growth and acceleration of maturation, one should first of all decide what age groups the children belong to. If, for example, you administer testosterone to a young child, you will produce a growth spurt; but if you give the same male hormone to a child over ten years of age, the result will be maturation. You have a clinical manifestation of the same sort of thing in children suffering from an adreno-genital syndrome, who are the biggest in the class when they first enter school, but the smallest by the time they have completed their schooling. I feel that this is an extremely important point to bear in mind when talking about growth inhibition and maturation.

In this connection there is a difference between A.C.T.H. therapy and treatment with glucocorticoids, inasmuch as A.C.T.H. also stimulates the production of adrenocortical androgens, whereas glucocorticoids do not.

J. GIRARD: No one, to my knowledge, has ever claimed that only growth hormone is responsible for growth. On the other hand, in the absence of growth hormone secretion, growth undoubtedly is suppressed. Whether or not growth is actually induced by growth hormone, is quite another question. It is conceivable that the metabolic effects of growth hormone serve to promote anabolic processes which are a necessary prerequisite for physical growth, but that the latter is not directly triggered off by growth hormone.

As for the problem of age-dependent differences in the way in which a child responds to androgens, a synergistic relationship exists between growth hormone and the androgens. It is also possible to provoke a growth spurt in a ten-year-old by administering testosterone; but at the same time the child's skeletal maturation is also accelerated, with the result that premature closure of the epiphyses leads to completion of growth at an abnormally early age.

T.B. BINNS: This whole question of the relationships between growth hormone, steroids, and corticotrophin strikes me as being extremely complex, and I must admit that the situation at present is not at all clear to me. If I may, however, I should just like to quote three points from a paper to which Dr. GIORDANO has already referred in his report. In this paper, published by ZUTSHI et al. from the M.R.C. Rheumatism Unit at Taplow in England, it is mentioned that the growth-inhibiting effects of corticosteroids cannot be reversed by administering growth hormone in physiological amounts. That is the first point. Secondly, ZUTSHI et al. quote several authors who claim that long-term A.C.T.H. therapy in children does not suppress the hypothalamo-pituitary-adrenocortical axis to the same extent as treatment with corticosteroids. The third point is that, when children were converted from treatment with steroids to A.C.T.H. therapy, ZUTSHI and his colleagues observed an increase in growth only in cases where there was a recovery of endogenous A.C.T.H. production. It is perhaps precisely in this area that the greatest difficulty arises, and in this connection I should like to remind you of what has already been said earlier in this meeting about the very sensitive physiological test procedure that now exists for measuring the release of growth hormone during sleep. It was recently reported from Edinburgh and London by EVANS and his colleagues* that growth hormone release is suppressed by 1 mg. Synacthen Depot given 16 hours before sleep, but that it is not suppressed by 80 units of A.C.T.H. gel similarly administered. This difference appears simply to reflect the respective durations of action of the two preparations, as indicated by their effects on the plasma cortisol levels. This group of investigators has meanwhile continued along the same lines with the new 1–18 polypeptide (41,795-Ba). They have found that this preparation exerts an intermediate effect between that of Synacthen Depot and A.C.T.H. gel, and they also believe it to be dose-dependent (GLASS et al., personal communication). I think it very likely that this will be an argument in favour of selecting a dose of corticotrophin which—as Dr. IRVINE has already suggested—will ensure that the natural rhythm is preserved.

R. SCHUPPLI: Dr. JESSERER referred in his paper to the use of cytotoxic agents in the treatment of rheumatic conditions. Since it has been our impression that in dermatomyositis both corticosteroids and A.C.T.H. have a poor effect—in fact, among the patients we have treated, the disease almost invariably worsened in response to such therapy—we are now resorting first and foremost to cytotoxic agents and immunosuppressive drugs. For this reason, I should like to ask the rheumatologists here if they have had any experience indicating whether combined treatment with im-

---

* EVANS, J. I., GLASS, D., DALY, J. R., McLEAN, A. W.: The effect of Zn-tetracosactrin on growth hormone release during sleep. J. clin. Endocr. *36*, 36 (1973)

munosuppressants and A.C.T.H. possibly offers an advantage, e.g. by enabling one to reduce the size of the single doses in which the immunosuppressive drug is given.

M. GIORDANO: In four cases of rheumatoid arthritis I administered cyclophosphamide for a time as a supplement to treatment with tetracosactide. In three of these cases this made it possible for me gradually to phase out the A.C.T.H. therapy.

R. SCHUPPLI: In my experience it is sometimes possible to achieve better results in psoriatic arthropathy by employing combined treatment. In cases of lupus erythematosus—i.e. of generalised Libman-Sacks syndrome—one can also obtain an enhanced effect by adding ®Imuran (azathioprine) to the regimen in patients who no longer respond adequately to Synacthen alone.

P. MASSIAS: In the patients referred to in my paper, the majority of the good responses obtained—i.e. cases in which it proved possible either to withdraw A.C.T.H. altogether or to space out the treatment with A.C.T.H.—were achieved by resorting to chlorambucil or to cyclophosphamide; when using A.C.T.H. to treat arthritics, we consider it indispensable, in fact, to add one of these immunosuppressive drugs to the regimen at the very earliest opportunity. I must point out, however, that these immunosuppressive agents are found to exert a beneficial effect in only about 50% of cases; in other words, one also has to reckon with failures, and for this reason we are currently treating one series of patients with D-penicillamine.

R. SCHUPPLI: Have you observed any differences between the various immunosuppressive drugs—e.g. between methotrexate, azathioprine, and cyclophosphamide?

P. MASSIAS: I'm afraid I have only had experience with cyclophosphamide, which, as I have just mentioned, has yielded favourable results in roughly 50% of cases.

D. GROSS: With immunosuppressants one is trying to combat the disease as such, whereas the aim of corticosteroid therapy is to control the secondary inflammatory reaction. The drugs employed for these two purposes may act either synergistically or antagonistically. There doesn't seem to be much point, for example, in giving corticosteroids in combination with gold salts, because—as demonstrated by WEISSMANN*, and also by PERSELLIN and ZIFF**—the two antagonise each other. But a combination of corticosteroids or A.C.T.H. with antimetabolites appears to result in a synergistic action. In rheumatoid arthritis and collagen diseases, I regard a combination of corticosteroids or A.C.T.H. with an immunosuppressive drug as the treatment of choice.

P. MASSIAS: There is certainly a great deal to be said for these combinations of A.C.T.H. plus an immunosuppressant. But it must be borne in mind that immunosuppressive agents do not produce any clinical effects until the patient has been receiving them for several weeks; sometimes, indeed, one even has to wait several months. Consequently, during the initial period of treatment, the patient still requires relief from his pain and inflammation. This is the reason why I consider it quite essential to administer a corticosteroid or A.C.T.H. in addition. The argument in favour of additional treatment with A.C.T.H. applies particularly to patients who are corticoid-dependent and in whom corticosteroids no longer produce an adequate response. Sometimes, indeed, we find that a patient in receipt of corticoid therapy is already suffering from adrenocortical insufficiency. In such cases, one is faced—perhaps for several months— with a real therapeutic dilemma, and this is an instance in which A.C.T.H. can render very valuable service.

G. GEYER: During this symposium we have heard a great deal about the favourable effect of Synacthen in asthma, and I should therefore like to ask whether anyone here

---

*WEISSMANN, G.: Lysosomes and joint disease. Arthr. and Rheum. 9, 834 (1966)
**PERSELLIN, R.H., ZIFF, M.: The effect of gold salt on lysosomal enzymes of the peritoneal macrophage. Arthr. and Rheum. 9, 57 (1966)

has the impression that in asthmatics treatment with A.C.T.H. does in fact constitute something more than a mere indirect form of corticoid therapy. Can anyone offer any suggestions concerning the mechanism of action of A.C.T.H. in this indication? One possibility I should like to submit for consideration is that A.C.T.H. may perhaps intervene in the cyclic adenosine-monophosphate system—in which case its mechanism of action would have something in common with that of glucagon or the prostaglandins, whose use in the treatment of asthma is currently under discussion.

J. AUBERT: I shall say something about the mode of action of A.C.T.H. in asthma in the paper I shall be presenting later on, in which I also refer to the cyclic adenosine-monophosphate system.

Synthetic corticotrophin or prednisolone in the treatment of chronic aggressive hepatitis: preliminary data on a controlled trial

by G. Giusti, P. E. Lucchelli, B. Galanti, F. Piccinino, G. Ruggiero, G. G. Balestrieri, E. Sagnelli, and R. Utili*

Introduction

Among the various drugs employed in the treatment of chronic aggressive hepatitis (sometimes referred to as "chronic active hepatitis"), the anti-inflammatory steroids (prednisolone and prednisone), 6-mercaptopurine, and azathioprine are those most extensively studied in clinical trials[3,10,15,17,23,26]. Trials on the combined use of steroids and immunosuppressive drugs have also been carried out[17,23,26]. The usefulness of treatment with 6-mercaptopurine or azathioprine, administered either alone or together with anti-inflammatory steroids, is still controversial[1,5,9,11,14,17,26]. Steroids have been reported to be beneficial inasmuch as they may improve the results of liver function tests and may prolong survival[3,17,26]. Only a few authors indicate that such treatment may also improve the hepatic histological picture[2,17,26]. No treatment, however, has yet been reported which induces a constant and marked improvement in both the liver histological picture and the prognosis of the disease.

The purpose of the present study was to compare the efficacy of prednisolone with that of corticotrophin in the management of chronic aggressive hepatitis. It is well known that some chronic diseases which may be treated with immunosuppressive drugs are controlled by corticotrophin more successfully than by steroids. Moreover, the undesirable side effects provoked by long-term treatment with corticotrophin may well prove less serious than those encountered during prolonged steroid therapy. Since controlled clinical trials had already shown that prednisolone or prednisone are more effective than placebo treatment[3,26], we decided not to include a placebo group in the present trial.

This report deals with the preliminary results of a controlled trial on the treatment of chronic aggressive hepatitis with either prednisolone or a synthetic corticotrophin depot preparation.

Materials and methods

Patients with chronic aggressive hepatitis hospitalised in the Clinic for Infectious Diseases, University of Naples 1st Medical School, have been included in this study. In each case the diagnosis was established on the basis of the case history, biochemical and clinical evidence of liver disease, and histological findings according to the criteria reported in the literature[4,7,21]. None of the patients included in this study had ascites, portal hypertension, or encephalopathy, nor

* Clinica delle Malattie Infettive della 1ª Facoltà di Medicina, Università degli Studi di Napoli, Naples, Italy.

did any of them show histological evidence of liver cirrhosis. Excluded from the trial were patients with peptic ulcer, tuberculosis, diabetes, or psychosis, those with a history of high alcohol intake, pregnant women, and children under seven years of age. Before selection for the trial, none of the patients had ever undergone prolonged treatment with steroids, immunosuppressive drugs, or corticotrophin.

Our study began in January 1971; since then, a total of 40 patients have been admitted to the trial and have been assigned at random, but not on a double-blind basis, to either prednisolone or corticotrophin treatment.

Three of the patients were subsequently withdrawn from the trial for incidental reasons (in the first case, because the patient became pregnant; in the second, because of a traumatic fracture of the tibia; and in the third, because the patient moved to a different town); a fourth patient was withdrawn owing to the development of a duodenal ulcer; and two interrupted treatment of their own accord. Finally, nine cases were treated for less than six months, i.e. not long enough to enable us to make a preliminary assessment of the therapeutic effects.

The present report will therefore be limited to 11 patients treated with prednisolone and 14 treated with corticotrophin.

Treatment schedules

The two drugs tested in this trial were administered as follows:

Prednisolone*: 40 mg. daily for two weeks; 30 mg. daily for two weeks; 25 mg. daily for two weeks; 20 mg. daily for six weeks; and 15 mg. daily as a maintenance dose. Patients ranging in age from seven to 14 years received approximately two-thirds of these doses.

Long-acting synthetic corticotrophin**: 1 mg. daily for three days by the intramuscular route; 1 mg. i.m. every three days for two weeks; and 1 mg. i.m. once a week as a maintenance dose.

Patient follow-up

At monthly intervals, a physical examination was carried out in the out-patient department and the following laboratory tests performed: serum bilirubin, serum flocculation tests, and S.G.O.T. measured according to KARMEN's method [8]. At six-month intervals, the patients were hospitalised again and the following additional tests were performed: electrophoretic determination of the serum proteins, measurement of the immunoglobulins by the method of MANCINI et al.[12], detection of "hepatitis B associated antigen" (Australia antigen) by electro-osmophoresis [20, 22], chest and digestive-tract radiography, and liver biopsy obtained using a Menghini needle [13].

The histological findings were always evaluated by two pathologists working independently of each other. For each liver biopsy the histological changes in

---

*®Meticortelone (Schering Corporation, U.S.A.).
**®Synacthen Depot (CIBA-GEIGY S.p.A., Italy), a synthetic β1–24 corticotrophin (zinc-phosphate complex).

the portal tract were assessed independently of the changes affecting the parenchymal areas.

The severity of the histological changes observed in each initial biopsy prior to the start of treatment was graded on a scale ranging from 0 to 8.

To evaluate the histological modifications that occurred during treatment, histological findings from subsequent biopsies of each patient were compared with the findings obtained prior to treatment. These comparative assessments were also graded by means of an arbitrary scale in which 0 indicated no change, +1 to +3* an improvement, and −1 to −3** a deterioration. The scores from the two histologists were almost always identical; where they disagreed, however, the arithmetic mean of the two scores was used.

The influence of the two treatments on pituitary-adrenocortical function was investigated by determining the circadian rhythm of cortisol secretion and by measuring the plasma cortisol levels after administration of A.C.T.H. as well as after insulin-induced hypoglycaemia. These tests were carried out in the majority of patients treated for longer than six months. The circadian rhythm of cortisol secretion was determined by recording the plasma cortisol concentrations at 8 a.m. and at 4 p.m.; the normal rhythm was considered inverted if the plasma cortisol level in the afternoon was approximately 60% higher than the morning level. The A.C.T.H. test was performed by administering 0.25 mg. of short-acting synthetic corticotrophin intravenously in the morning and then determining the rise in the plasma cortisol levels. An increase in these levels of 50% or more was considered normal.

For the insulin test, 0.15 units of insulin per kg. body-weight was administered intravenously. After 15, 30, 45, and 60 minutes the blood sugar concentrations and the plasma cortisol levels were measured. The test results were regarded as normal if, during the hypoglycaemia, the plasma cortisol level rose by at least 50%. The plasma cortisol levels were all determined by the method based on competitive protein binding[16]. In the prednisolone group, the drug was not given on those days on which tests of pituitary-adrenocortical function were performed. In the corticotrophin group, the tests in question were carried out four days after the day on which the patient had received his weekly dose of the drug.

Statistical analysis

When comparing the parametric data from the two groups, the following statistical analyses were employed: Student's t test, Student's t test for paired data, split-plot factorial analysis of variance, and analysis of covariance[27]. The non-parametric data were evaluated using the fourfold-table test, the chi-square test, and the Mann and Whitney U test[24, 27].

For a preliminary comparison of the two treatments we have considered only the results obtained at the sixth and 12th month of treatment. The data

---

*+1 = slight improvement; +2 = moderate improvement; +3 = marked improvement.
**−1 = slight deterioration; −2 = moderate deterioration; −3 = marked deterioration.

recorded at the 18th and 24th month have not been included because the number of patients followed up for more than one year is not yet large enough to allow a statistical comparison.

Comparability of the two groups before treatment
The present paper deals with the data obtained from 25 patients, 14 of whom were treated with corticotrophin and 11 with prednisolone. All 25 cases were followed up for six months; six patients from each of the two groups have been followed up for as long as 12 months.
The initial pre-treatment data from the 25 cases and the statistical comparison of the two groups are given in Table 1. These data show that the two groups were comparable with each other and that in both groups young patients and males predominated.

Table 1. Initial data prior to the start of treatment.

		All cases	Prednisolone group	Corticotrophin group	Statistical comparison
Number of cases		25	11	14	
Sex	Male	19	9	10	$\chi^2 = 0.017$
	Female	6	2	4	n.s.**
Age	Mean	16.64	16.00	17.14	
(years)	(± S.D.)	(±8.34)	(±6.83)	(±9.62)	$t = 0.333$
	Median	14.0	14.0	14.5	
	Range	7–39	8–30	7–39	n.s.
S.G.O.T. (I.U./litre)					
	Mean	110.04	86.00	128.93	$t = 1.252$
	(± S.D.)	(±83.32)	(±45.34)	(±105.99)	n.s.
Serum albumin (g.%)					
	Mean	3.24	3.07	3.37	$t = 1.163$
	(± S.D.)	(±0.62)	(±0.67)	(±0.60)	n.s.
Serum globulins (g.%)					
	Mean	4.00	3.96	4.04	$t = 0.437$
	(± S.D.)	(±0.44)	(±0.47)	(±0.43)	n.s.
IgG (mg.%)					
	Mean	1,930.64	2,090.36	1,805.14	$t = 1.173$
	(± S.D.)	(±590.84)	(±520.25)	(±660.51)	n.s.
Number of cases with total bilirubinaemia >1.5 mg.%		6	3	3	$\chi^2 = 0.115$ n.s.
Number of H.B. Ag.-positive* cases		14	7	7	$\chi^2 = 0.465$ n.s.
Severity of histological changes in the portal tract		5.17	5.00	5.30	U = 65.5 n.s.
Severity of histological changes in the parenchyma		4.11	4.20	4.04	U = 64.5 n.s.

* H.B. Ag. = "hepatitis B associated antigen"
**n.s. = not significant

Results

Table 2 shows the laboratory test results obtained from the two groups before drugs were started, as well as at the sixth and 12th month of treatment.

Figures 1 and 2 indicate the S.G.O.T. changes that were observed during the first six or 12 months of treatment, given as percentages of the respective initial values.

Shown in Figure 3 are the serum albumin, total serum globulins, and serum IgG (immunoglobulin G) values measured during treatment.

The data indicate that in both groups, jaundice, when present at the beginning, eventually disappeared during treatment; the S.G.O.T. values also showed a significant decrease (analysis of variance: $P < 0.01$). During the first year of therapy, no significant changes in the serum proteins were observed in either of the two groups, nor did the percentage of patients in whom hepatitis B associated antigen was detected in the serum show any evident variation.

Figures 4 and 5 show the histological changes observed in each individual case during treatment. The degree of improvement or worsening was graded as detailed in the method section. The data indicate that the parenchymal lesions showed an improvement in the majority of cases from each of the two groups, both at the sixth and at the 12th month of treatment. The changes in the portal-tract histology, however, were far less pronounced in both groups; most of the patients, in fact, showed no important changes, whereas in the remainder the number of improvements and deteriorations was roughly the same.

Table 2. Laboratory data from the 25 patients with chronic aggressive hepatitis, before and during treatment with prednisolone or corticotrophin.

	Prednisolone group			Corticotrophin group		
Duration of treatment (months)	0	6	12	0	6	12
Number of cases	11	11	6	14	14	6
S.G.O.T. (I.U./litre)						
Mean	86.00	32.82	23.33	128.93	49.14	63.29
(± S.D.)	(±45.34)	(±12.71)	(±10.54)	(±105.99)	(±36.34)	(±55.57)
Serum albumin (g.%)						
Mean	3.07	3.39	3.58	3.37	3.14	3.39
(± S.D.)	(±0.67)	(±0.44)	(±0.63)	(±0.60)	(±0.58)	(±0.37)
Serum globulins (g.%)						
Mean	3.96	3.78	3.78	4.04	3.87	3.82
(± S.D.)	(±0.47)	(±0.62)	(±0.41)	(±0.43)	(±0.37)	(±0.56)
IgG (mg.%)						
Mean	2,090.36	1,858.20	1,811.50	1,805.14	1,773.69	1,716.00
(± S.D.)	(±520.25)	(±522.88)	(±271.62)	(±660.51)	(±280.34)	(±306.22)
Number of cases with total bilirubinaemia >1.5 mg.%	3	0	0	3	0	0
Number of H.B. Ag.- positive cases	7 (63%)	6 (54%)	3 (50%)	7 (50%)	8 (57%)	3 (50%)

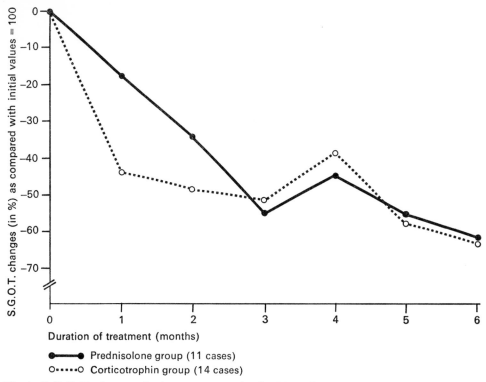

Fig. 1. S.G.O.T. changes during treatment in the 25 patients.

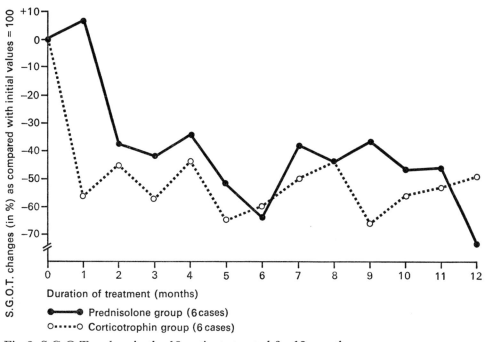

Fig. 2. S.G.O.T. values in the 12 patients treated for 12 months.

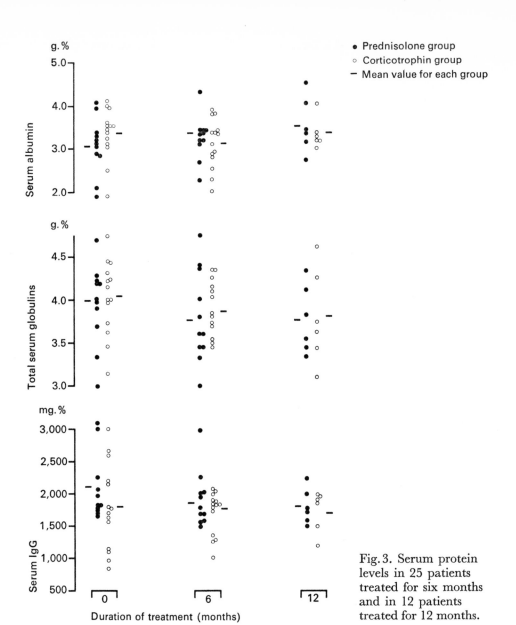

Fig. 3. Serum protein levels in 25 patients treated for six months and in 12 patients treated for 12 months.

The relative effectiveness of the two different treatments was evaluated by comparing the two groups with respect to the laboratory test results as well as to the histological findings. The laboratory test results obtained at the sixth month of treatment were compared by covariance analysis; no significant difference was found. For patients from the two groups followed for at least 12 months, the split-plot analysis of variance was used: here, too, no significant treatment-by-time interaction was observed. Finally, the Mann and Whitney test showed no significant difference between the histological changes in the prednisolone group and those in the corticotrophin group.

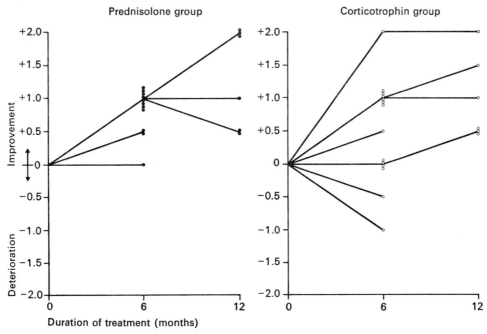

Fig. 4. Changes in parenchymal lesions during treatment. The degree of the histological alterations was graded as stated in the method section.

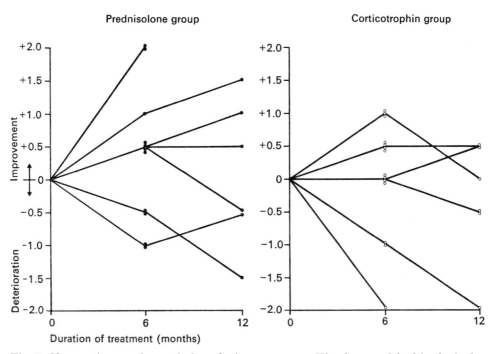

Fig. 5. Changes in portal-tract lesions during treatment. The degree of the histological alterations was graded as stated in the method section.

Table 3. Hypothalamo-pituitary-adrenocortical function in nine patients treated with prednisolone and eight treated with corticotrophin. The fourfold-table test was used for statistical comparisons.

Circadian rhythm		Inverted	Normal	Total	
	Prednisolone group	9	0	9	
	Corticotrophin group	0	8	8	
					P <0.01
		9	8	17	

A.C.T.H. test		Pathological	Normal	Total	
	Prednisolone group	5	4	9	
	Corticotrophin group	0	8	8	
					P = 0.05
		5	12	17	

Insulin test		Pathological	Normal	Total	
	Prednisolone group	7	2	9	
	Corticotrophin group	2	6	8	
					P = 0.10
		9	8	17	

Effect of the two treatments on hypothalamo-pituitary-adrenocortical function
Function of the pituitary-adrenocortical axis was studied in patients treated for longer than six months, i.e. in nine with prednisolone and eight with corticotrophin. From the results presented in Table 3 it is clearly evident that prednisolone caused an inversion of the circadian rhythm of cortisol secretion in all nine cases. In the majority of the patients receiving prednisolone, the adrenal response to A.C.T.H. was absent and the pituitary-mediated adrenal response to hypoglycaemia was likewise impaired. On the other hand, in the patients treated with synthetic corticotrophin, no alterations were observed either in the circadian rhythm of cortisol secretion or in the adrenal response to A.C.T.H. The insulin test showed normal results in six out of the eight patients from this group. The difference between the results of the hormone tests in the two groups was statistically significant.

Side effects of the treatment
Two patients included in this trial developed intolerance to the synthetic corticotrophin zinc-phosphate complex (one at the ninth month, the other at the 12th month of therapy). The first, a 30-year-old male, reported that immediately after the drug had been injected a feeling of malaise and prostration set in and then subsided spontaneously within about 30 minutes. The second, an 18-year-old male, stated that the injection had been followed at once by the appearance of a papular rash which was associated with itching and which completely cleared again within roughly two hours. In both cases, skin-sensitivity tests were negative; however, the next administration of 1 mg. of the drug caused the same reactions as before. Corticotrophin was therefore discontinued, and the two patients were placed on prednisolone instead. In the

present report, only the data relating to the period when these two patients were still receiving corticotrophin are included. Intolerance to the cortico-trophin zinc-phosphate complex has also been reported by others[6, 18, 19, 28].

In the corticotrophin-treated group, one patient with a previous non-ulcerative duodenitis developed clinical and radiographic evidence of an uncomplicated duodenal ulcer at the third month of treatment. This patient was therefore excluded from the trial. Mild acne of the face was seen in another case.

In the prednisolone group, the following side effects were observed: marked obesity and mooning of the face in three cases; hypertension in one case (a boy aged 13 years); and severe acne of the face and trunk in three cases.

Conclusions

The findings presented in this paper indicate that an improvement in the results of some laboratory tests occurred in the course of treatment both with pred-nisolone and with corticotrophin. In particular, the initial jaundice, when present, disappeared (Table 2), and the S.G.O.T. values also decreased (Table 2, Figures 1 and 2).

The liver histology data showed that, in the majority of the patients from both groups, the liver parenchyma improved (Figure 4) mainly because of a decrease in the degenerative and necrotic lesions. But the histological picture of the portal tract exhibited a great variability in response to both drugs tested; only a small percentage of the patients in either group showed a slight but definite improve-ment ranging from $+1$ to $+2$ in the scale which we adopted (Figure 5).

Given the limited number of cases studied, no significant difference between the efficacy of prednisolone and that of corticotrophin could be found, although our data do suggest that prednisolone was a little more effective than corticotrophin in improving some biochemical and histological parameters. In the light of the data presented here, we have meanwhile changed the corticotrophin main-tenance dosage and are now administering one injection of 0.5 mg. twice a week. This modification is aimed at checking whether more frequent administra-tion of the drug, albeit in smaller doses, may perhaps result in an enhanced therapeutic effect.

It is by no means easy to compare the preliminary data from this study with the results of similar controlled trials[3, 26], especially since we did not admit to our trial any patients showing histological evidence of liver cirrhosis or clinical signs of portal hypertension and ascites.

We should like to stress that, although some clinical, laboratory, and histo-logical data have shown an improvement in patients from both groups, no patient has yet recovered nor has control of the disease yet been achieved in any of these cases. This is indicated particularly by the fact that in the majority of our patients the histopathological picture of the portal areas has either remained unchanged in the course of treatment or has actually tended to deteriorate. On the other hand, it should also be emphasised that in none of our cases have we so far observed any clinical signs of worsening or any histological evidence of cirrhosis.

References

1 ARTER, W.J., PERKINS, K.W., BLACKBURN, C.R.B.: Experience with the use of 6-mercaptopurine and "Imuran" in the treatment of progressive hepatitis (active chronic hepatitis). Aust. Ann. Med. *15*, 222 (1966)

2 BAGGENSTOSS, A.H., SOLOWAY, R.D., SUMMERSKILL, W.H.J., ELVEBACK, L.R., SCHOENFIELD, L.J.: Chronic active liver disease: the range of histologic lesions, their response to treatment, and evolution. Hum. Path. *3*, 183 (1972)

3 COOK, G.C., MULLIGAN, R., SHERLOCK, S.: Controlled prospective trial of corticosteroid therapy in active chronic hepatitis. Quart. J. Med., N.S. *40*, 159 (1971)

4 GEALL, M.G., SCHOENFIELD, L.J., SUMMERSKILL, W.H.J.: Classification and treatment of chronic active liver disease. Gastroenterology *55*, 724 (1968)

5 GEENEN, J.E., HENSLEY, G.T., WINSHIP, D.H.: Chronic active hepatitis treated with 6-mercaptopurine – sustained remission. Ann. intern. Med. *65*, 1277 (1966)

6 GOT, A.: Severe reaction from tetracosactrin. Med. J. Aust. *59/i*, 493 (1972)

7 GROOTE, J. DE, DESMET, V.J., GEDIGK, P., KORB, G., POPPER, H., POULSEN, H., SCHEUER, P.J., SCHMID, M., THALER, H., UEHLINGER, E., WEPLER, W.: A classification of chronic hepatitis. Lancet *ii*, 626 (1968)

8 KARMEN, A.: A note on the spectrophotometric assay of glutamic-oxalacetic transaminase in human blood serum. J. clin. Invest. *34*, 131 (1955)

9 KRAWITT, E.L., STEIN, J.H., KIRKENDALL, W.M., CLIFTON, J.A.: Mercapto-purine hepatotoxicity in a patient with chronic active hepatitis. Arch. intern. Med. *120*, 729 (1967)

10 MACKAY, I.R.: Chronic hepatitis: effect of prolonged suppressive treatment and comparison of azathioprine with prednisolone. Quart. J. Med., N.S. *37*, 379 (1968)

11 MACKAY, I.R., WEIDEN, S., UNGAR, B.: Treatment of active chronic hepatitis and lupoid hepatitis with 6-mercaptopurine and azathioprine. Lancet *i*, 899 (1964)

12 MANCINI, G., CARBONARA, A.O., HEREMANS, J.F.: Immunochemical quantita-tion of antigens by single radial immunodiffusion. J. Immunochem. *2*, 235 (1965)

13 MENGHINI, G.: One-second needle biopsy of the liver. Gastroenterology *35*, 190 (1958)

14 MISTILIS, S.P., BLACKBURN, C.R.B.: The treatment of active chronic hepatitis with 6-mercaptopurine and azathioprine. Aust. Ann. Med. *16*, 305 (1967)

15 MISTILIS, S.P., BLACKBURN, C.R.B.: Active chronic hepatitis. Amer. J. Med. *48*, 484 (1970)

16 MURPHY, B.E.P.: Some studies of the protein-binding of steroids and their application to the routine micro and ultramicro measurement of various steroids in body fluids by competitive protein-binding radioassay. J. clin. Endocr. *27*, 973 (1967)

17 PAGE, A.R., GOOD, R.A., POLLARA, B.: Long-term results of therapy in patients with chronic liver disease associated with hypergammaglobulinemia. Amer. J. Med. *47*, 765 (1969)

18 PATRIARCA, G.: Desensitisation to tetracosactrin-depot. Lancet *ii*, 822 (1971)

19 PAVLATOS, F., KELAIDIS, E., BENOS, S.: Adrenal function tested with tetracosac-trin-depot. Lancet *i*, 807 (1971)

20 PESENDORFER, F., KRASSNITZKY, O., WEWALKA, F.: Immunoelektrophoretischer Nachweis von «Hepatitis-associated-antigen» (Au/SH-antigen). Klin. Wschr. *48*, 58 (1970)

21 POPPER, H., SCHAFFNER, F.: The vocabulary of chronic hepatitis. New Engl. J. Med. *284*, 1154 (1971)

22 PRINCE, A.M., BURKE, K.: Serum hepatitis antigen (SH): rapid detection by high voltage immunoelectroosmophoresis. Science *169*, 593 (1971)

23 SCHIMMELPFENNIG, W., WAGNER, K., THEUER, D., SCHNEIDER G., HECHT A., SCHIMMELPFENNIG, R.: Die Langzeittherapie der chronisch progredienten (aggressiven) Hepatitis mit einer Kombination von Imuran und Prednison. Dtsch. Gesundh.-Wes. *26*, 1965 (1971)

24 SIEGEL, S.: Nonparametric statistics for the behavioral sciences (McGraw-Hill, New York/Toronto/London 1956)

25 SJÖBERG, K.-H., WELIN, G.: Treatment of active chronic hepatitis with 6-mercaptopurine. Acta hepato-splenol. (Stuttg.) *14*, 157 (1967)

26 SOLOWAY, R.D., SUMMERSKILL, W.H.J., BAGGENSTOSS, A.H., GEALL, M.G., GITNICK, G.L., ELVEBACK, L.R., SCHOENFIELD, L.J.: Clinical, biochemical, and histological remission of severe chronic active liver disease: a controlled study of treatment and early prognosis. Gastroenterology *63*, 820 (1972)

27 STEEL, R.G.D., TORRIE, J.H.: Principles and procedures of statistics (McGraw-Hill, New York/Toronto/London 1960)

28 TAN, D.B.P.: Severe reaction from tetracosactrin. Med. J. Aust. *59/i*, 387 (1972)

Discussion

C. VAN DER MEER: May I ask Dr. GIUSTI if the daily dosage of prednisolone was given as a single dose in the morning or in the form of fractional doses divided over the day.

G. GIUSTI: It was administered in fractional doses after meals.

C. VAN DER MEER: And when was the drug given on the days upon which you carried out analyses in order to investigate the hypothalamo-pituitary-adrenocortical function?

G. GIUSTI: In the prednisolone-treated group, no prednisolone was given on the day on which we performed these tests. In the corticotrophin-treated group, the last dose of corticotrophin had been administered five days previously.

C. VAN DER MEER: Just one small point concerning the circadian rhythm: I believe that in Italy you have a siesta in the afternoon; do the patients sleep during this siesta?

G. GIUSTI: Yes, they usually do. Down in the south of Italy where I live, everyone takes a nap for an hour or two in the afternoon.

C. VAN DER MEER: What, then, is the normal circadian rhythm in the south of Italy?

G. GIUSTI: To answer that question, allow me to show you a slide in which the circadian rhythms are plotted both for the corticotrophin group and for the prednisolone group (Figure 1). You can see that in the corticotrophin group the rhythm is similar to that reported as normal by JAMES and LANDON*, despite the afternoon siesta, whereas all the patients we studied in the prednisolone group showed a loss of circadian rhythm.

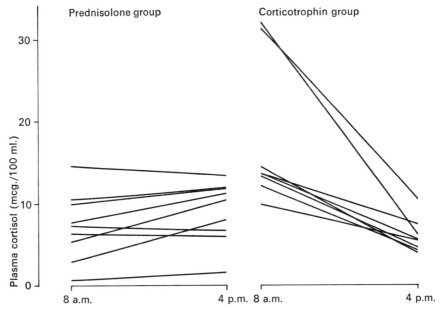

Fig. 1. Circadian rhythm of cortisol secretion in patients treated for longer than six months with either prednisolone (nine cases) or corticotrophin (eight cases).

---

*JAMES, V.H.T., LANDON, J.: Hypothalamic-pituitary-adrenal function tests (CIBA LABORATORIES LIMITED, Horsham, Sussex 1971)

C. van der Meer: I note that, when determining the circadian rhythm, you recorded the plasma cortisol levels at 8 a.m. and at 4 p.m., but sometimes I have the impression that it is preferable to take the samples at 8 o'clock in the morning and at 9 o'clock in the evening.

G. Giusti: As some of the tests were performed in out-patients, this would have been rather difficult in our case.

C. van der Meer: Oh! I see. Yes. I understand that. Thank you.

G. Geyer: I should like to ask whether all these patients of yours, Dr. Giusti, were cases that had developed from acute infective hepatitis.

G. Giusti: Our patients were hospitalised in the Clinic for Infectious Diseases and frequently the reason for their admission to hospital was the appearance of jaundice. But it was seldom, if ever, possible to determine whether these were episodes of jaundice occurring incidentally in the course of chronic aggressive hepatitis or jaundice due to the onset of viral hepatitis. As you may know, throughout the whole of Italy hepatitis B associated antigen (Australia antigen) is found in a very high percentage of cases of chronic aggressive hepatitis. This percentage (70 to 80%) is much higher than in other countries.

G. Geyer: And the biopsies you performed, Dr. Giusti, were blind liver biopsies obtained with a Menghini needle?

G. Giusti: Yes. I should perhaps add that the patients were admitted to the trial only if their liver disease dated back over a period of at least six months. In all our patients a histological examination of the liver was carried out *before* their admission to the trial; after the diagnosis had been confirmed by the histological findings, they were assigned at random to one of the two treatment groups.

G. Geyer: And was it only on the basis of the histological findings that you differentiated between cirrhosis and hepatitis?

G. Giusti: It is not easy to distinguish between initial cirrhosis and chronic hepatitis by means of Menghini's needle liver biopsy. Soloway et al.*, for instance, have demonstrated how difficult it is to make such a distinction. I should like to emphasise, however, that none of the patients in our trial ever showed any clinical signs of cirrhosis—such as portal hypertension, etc.—or any histological evidence of cirrhosis. Moreover, since in these patients we have performed liver biopsies every six months, with the result that some of them have had as many as three, four, or even five biopsies, I think it very unlikely that our series includes cases of cirrhosis misdiagnosed as chronic active hepatitis.

K. F. Weinges: I gather, Dr. Giusti, that your cases consisted mainly of children and adolescents. Do children with chronic aggressive hepatitis respond better to steroids than adults? In adults, treatment with steroids alone does not prove successful; this is the reason why we prefer to administer them in combination with immunosuppressive agents.

G. Giusti: As is apparent from the median age of our patients, as opposed to their mean age, the majority of them ranged in age from 13 to 25 years. Children thus accounted for only a small percentage of our case material. Most of the patients were young males, whereas in the relevant literature it is young females who predominate. However, as can be seen from Table 1 in my paper, the age distribution was similar in

---

* Soloway, R. D., Baggenstoss, A. H., Schoenfield, L. J., Summerskill, W. H. J.: Observer error and sampling variability tested in evaluation of hepatitis and cirrhosis by liver biopsy. Amer. J. digest. Dis. *16*, 1082 (1971)

both treatment groups. Finally, we did not observe any age-related differences in the response to treatment in either group.

E. Polli: Dr. Weinges, what is your opinion about the use of 6-mercaptopurine and azathioprine in chronic active hepatitis? Do you think that they yield satisfactory results? It seems to have been demonstrated that treatment with 6-mercaptopurine sometimes proves dangerous for the liver. I myself have also seen a number of patients in whom this antimetabolite appeared to have exerted a harmful influence on the liver.

R. Schuppli: About three years ago a conference was held in Turin on the use of immunosuppressive drugs in chronic hepatitis and nephritis and in other chronic diseases. According to the majority of the reports presented on that occasion, the medium and long-term results of treatment with these drugs in chronic hepatitis were disappointing.

G. Giusti: So far as I know, the most recent paper on the treatment of chronic active liver disease with immunosuppressive drugs was that published by Soloway et al.* in 1972. In the studies reported by these authors—which differed to some extent from our own trial in that a large number of the patients were suffering from active liver cirrhosis, whereas our cases did not include cirrhosis—prednisone proved much more effective than azathioprine alone or placebo. Combined treatment with azathioprine and prednisone was found to have roughly the same therapeutic effect as treatment with prednisone alone. But, since the group of patients treated with a combination of prednisone and azathioprine received 10 mg. prednisone daily, it is conceivable that the therapeutic effect of the combined regimen might have been attributable solely to the prednisone.

R. Schuppli: What sort of medium and long-term results have you obtained, Dr. Weinges?

K. F. Weinges: We have abandoned treatment with steroids alone in favour of combined therapy. But the problem which arises here is that of deciding when to commence treatment. We do not make a start until we have satisfied ourselves that the patient really is suffering from chronic aggressive hepatitis—and by then it is perhaps a little late. A diagnosis of chronic aggressive hepatitis implies transaminase values of over 40 and a corresponding histological picture. Our therapeutic results have, I regret to say, been meagre—and such favourable responses as we have obtained were achieved with combined therapy.

R. Schuppli: The results of your long-term studies are of interest to me as a dermatologist because we also employ methotrexate in the treatment of psoriasis; in such cases there is a danger that even a patient with a healthy liver may develop cirrhosis after ten to 15 years.

G. Geyer: Dr. Giusti, is the rise that occurs in the plasma cortisol levels in response to A.C.T.H. prolonged in patients with chronic liver disease? One would expect this to be the case, because in these patients cortisol is eliminated at a considerably slower rate.

G. Giusti: In none of our patients was impairment of liver function so severe as to interfere with the metabolism of cortisol. This is apparent from the results obtained with the insulin test in the group treated with corticotrophin; here the height and duration of the plasma cortisol levels recorded in response to the hypoglycaemia-induced stress were the same as those reported in the literature for healthy controls.

---

*Soloway, R.D., Summerskill, W.H.J., Baggenstoss, A.H., Geall, M.G., Gitnick, G.L., Elveback, L.R., Schoenfield, L.J.: Clinical, biochemical, and histological remission of severe chronic active liver disease: a controlled study of treatment and early prognosis. Gastroenterology 63, 820 (1972)

D. GROSS: Is there any objective evidence to show that immunosuppressive agents do indeed exert an effect on the immunological "apparatus", i.e. that they are in fact capable of suppressing immunological processes? I don't think any such evidence is forthcoming in the rheumatological field, because here, although we may see an improvement in the clinical picture under treatment with immunosuppressants, this treatment has no positive influence on the rheumatoid factors. What about immunological changes in the liver in response to immunosuppressive drugs?

K. F. WEINGES: Immunological studies have certainly been carried out before and after treatment with steroids and immunosuppressants in cases of chronic aggressive hepatitis; but I cannot recall here and now any details of the findings, nor do I remember whether they proved of any clinical value. Similar investigations are at present also being undertaken on a fairly large scale in patients with chronic nephritis. A distinction has to be drawn, however, between humoral immunological processes, such as those in which rheumatoid factors are involved, and tissue-mediated immunological processes; the changes occurring in the tissues undoubtedly have a more important bearing on the course of the disease.

G. GIUSTI: We studied several auto-antibodies in our patients, and we observed no significant changes in them during the course of treatment. FINLAYSON et al.* report that in their cases there was a significant separation into those with auto-antibodies but without hepatitis B associated antigen, those with hepatitis B associated antigen but without auto-antibodies, and those with neither. In our cases a similar differentiation could not be found.

H. JESSERER: I think it should be pointed out that cytotoxic agents exert an immunosuppressive effect only indirectly via their cytotoxic activity. But they do, of course, also produce an effect in many other pathological processes in which immunological factors play no aetiological role at all. In this connection it seems to me that the term "immunosuppressive" has become something of a catchword.

---

* FINLAYSON, N. D. C., KROHN, K., ANDERSON, K. E., JOKELAINEN, P. T., PRINCE, A. M.: Interrelations of hepatitis B antigen and autoantibodies in chronic idiopathic liver disease. Gastroenterology *63*, 646 (1972)

Corticotrophin and corticosteroid treatment in cerebrovascular accidents: a multicentre comparative study

by E. POLLI*

1. Introduction

The use of adrenocortical steroids in the treatment of cerebral oedema has now gained wide acceptance. Several papers—some published only recently[21]—have clarified many aspects of the mechanism by which these steroid hormones act in experimental and clinical brain oedema. In particular, the effects of steroids on cerebral oedema occurring secondarily to acute cerebrovascular accidents have been discussed by PATTEN et al.[13], who demonstrated in a double-blind trial that high doses of dexamethasone exert a beneficial influence on the functional status of patients with cerebral lesions of vascular origin.

Other authors, most of them French[1-5, 7-12, 14], believe that in cerebral oedema even better results can be achieved with A.C.T.H. Although these authors obtained more consistently favourable responses in cases of cerebral oedema secondary to tumours or to neurosurgery, they nevertheless also agree in ascribing to A.C.T.H. a primary role in the treatment of acute stroke.

The increase in the average life span of people today, and in the prevalence of arteriosclerosis as well, has resulted in a higher incidence of cerebral lesions of vascular origin, which in turn poses major public health and rehabilitation problems. Any therapeutic advance in this area is thus of great interest.

Since, so far as I know, no comparative studies had ever been carried out in this field with corticosteroids and A.C.T.H., it was decided to run a preliminary controlled trial with corticosteroids versus synthetic corticotrophin in acute cerebrovascular accidents, in order to discover whether any possible differences could be discerned between the effects of the two forms of treatment.

2. Material and methods

2.1. Investigators

The investigators participating in the trial are all members of the "*Gruppo di Farmacologia Clinica Regionale Lombardo*" (Clinical Pharmacology Group of the

* Prof. E. POLLI is in charge of Clinica Medica I at the University of Milan, Italy. The investigators participating in this study were: E. POLLI (chief investigator), M. CASTELFRANCO (Palazzolo sull'Oglio), P. F. CROSTI (Milan), E. DE MICHELI (Passirana di Rho), V. FIERRO (Bollate), P. FRANZOSI (Angera), E. GIULIANI (Casorate Primo), A. LIMENTANI (Limbiate), P. D. LUCCHELLI (Milan), F. LUCIONI (Tradate), M. MANDELLI (Varese), L. MASCARETTI (Sarnico), G. F. MELLONI (Romano Lombardo), A. M. MONTI (Mariano Comense), G. RATTI (Busto Arsizio), D. RIVA (Vimercate), and P. E. LUCCHELLI (Milan), who was responsible for planning and statistical analysis.

Lombard Region), which is made up of physicians working in the Internal Medicine Divisions of several hospitals located in the region of Lombardy. They hold regular medical meetings and cooperate as a team in conducting therapeutic studies. A number of reports on work which they have undertaken in this context have already been published[15-20].

2.2. Trial plan

The multicentre trial to be described in the present paper was planned as a single-blind between-patient study. In order to obtain balanced groups of cases, the patients were assigned to corticosteroid or corticotrophin therapy within each centre on the basis of a randomisation list. The decision to admit a patient to the trial was taken before his allocation to one of the two treatments.

2.3. Treatments

The scheduled duration of the study was ten days. The patients assigned to corticosteroid treatment were given 4 mg. betamethasone (®Bentelan) twice daily by intramuscular injection, i.e. at 8 a.m. and 8 p.m.; the other group of patients received 1 mg. ®Synacthen Depot daily i.m. at 8 a.m. Depending on the individual clinical condition, fluids, cardiac glycosides, antibiotics, and insulin were added, but no diuretics, theophylline, or papaverine were administered. After the ten-day course of medication some of the patients were followed up until their discharge from hospital or their death; in no case was corticosteroid or corticotrophin therapy continued beyond the tenth day.

2.4. Criteria of admission

It was decided to adopt fairly "loose" criteria of admission and evaluation which would cover not only patients treated in hospital—irrespective of staff, equipment, and facilities—but also patients treated at home by general practitioners. Patients of either sex, aged over 35 years, in whom a cerebrovascular accident had occurred within the last 48 hours, were eligible for inclusion in the trial. Those with a history of peptic ulcer, a diastolic pressure exceeding 120 mm. Hg, or severe diabetes were excluded. No specific instrumental or radiological diagnostic procedures were employed for the purpose of deciding whether or not a patient was eligible for admission; such procedures as lumbar puncture and cerebral angiography were resorted to only in cases where the patient's condition indicated that they were necessary. Whenever a patient in whom lumbar puncture had been deemed advisable was found to have blood in his C.S.F., he was excluded from the trial.

2.5. Criteria of evaluation

The criteria of evaluation adopted for assessing the effectiveness of treatment consisted of a physical and neurological examination, together with certain other simple clinical parameters.
The neurological examination included:
– level of consciousness, which was categorised as follows: a) full consciousness; b) vigilant coma (patient able to regain consciousness and to react coordinately

221

to painful stimuli); c) coma (patient unconscious and reacting uncoordinately to painful stimuli); d) deep coma (patient unresponsive to stimuli);
– behaviour: orderly (patient cooperative, quiet, able to carry out simple orders) or disorderly;
– convulsions: present or absent;
– focal brain lesions: a score was assigned to each of the following: speech, ocular mobility, impairment of the remaining cranial nerves (i.e. in addition to the optic and abducent nerves), limb mobility, sensitivity to touch and pain, and the triceps, patellar, and plantar reflexes;
– sphincter control;
– neck rigidity: present or absent;
– overall assessments made on the tenth day and upon the patient's discharge from hospital.
The other clinical parameters included: pulse rate, blood pressure, respiration, maximum daily temperature, daily urine excretion, blood urea nitrogen, blood sugar, and state of the eyegrounds.
A check-up of the physical and neurological signs, together with recordings of the blood pressure, pulse rate, respiration, daily urine volume, and temperature, were made each day throughout the treatment. The other examinations were performed before and after the trial.

2.6. Statistical methods
The statistical analysis of the results was carried out with the aid of non-parametric tests (chi-square test, Mann and Whitney U test, and fourfold-table test) [6, 22].

3. Results

The total number of patients treated was 122. Since in this multicentre study the same trial plan was adopted throughout, and the criteria of evaluation had been discussed and defined by the investigators themselves at a joint meeting, the results obtained in the various centres were pooled and no attempt was made to analyse them separately centre by centre.

Table 1. Main features of the sample, totalling 122 patients.

	Patients on betamethasone	Patients on Synacthen Depot	Total
Number of cases	60	62	122
Median age (years)	61.9	62.6	62.2
Sex: male	31	31	62
female	29	31	60
Previous cerebrovascular episodes	16	15	31
History of other cardiovascular diseases	23	24	47

3.1. Description of the sample

The main features of the sample are listed in Table 1. As illustrated by the data contained in this table, the two treatment groups displayed a satisfactory degree of homogeneity.

Table 2. Investigators' overall assessment of the results of treatment.

	Patients on betamethasone	Patients on Synacthen Depot	Total
Improved	38	38	76
Unchanged or worsened	12	14	26
Deceased	9	4	13
Deceased within 12 hours of the start of treatment*	1	2	3
Treatment withdrawn*	0	4	4
Total	60	62	122

* These cases were disregarded in the statistical analysis.

Table 3. Results relating to some indirect signs of cerebral oedema.

	Patients on betamethasone	Patients on Synacthen Depot	Total
a) *Level of consciousness*			
Deranged at beginning of treatment	24	26	50
Improved	14	18	32
Unchanged	2	5	7
Worsened	3	0	3
Deceased	5	3	8
Mann and Whitney test: U = 265.5; z = 0.903, not significant			
b) *Behaviour*			
Disorderly at beginning of treatment	22	22	44
Improved	11	15	26
Unchanged	5	5	10
Worsened	1	0	1
Deceased	5	2	7
Mann and Whitney test: U = 295; z = 1.244, P $\simeq$ 0.25			
c) *Convulsions*			
Present before treatment	3	2	5
Improved	1	1	2
Deceased	2	1	3
d) *Neck rigidity*			
Present before treatment	7	6	13
Improved	3	5	8
Unchanged	0	1	1
Worsened	1	0	1
Deceased	3	0	3

3.2. Clinical results

The overall assessment made by the investigators at the end of the ten-day trial is summarised in Table 2.

Three of the patients died within 12 hours of the start of treatment. In the remaining nine deceased patients belonging to the betamethasone group, death occurred on the second, third (two cases), fourth, fifth (two cases), seventh, ninth, and tenth days; the four deceased patients receiving Synacthen Depot died on the second, fifth, sixth, and ninth days, respectively.

Although fewer patients died in the Synacthen Depot group than in the group treated with betamethasone, the difference between the two treatments in this respect was not statistically significant (chi-square 2 d.f. = 2.0).

In order to make a closer investigation of the effect of treatment on indirect signs of cerebral oedema, the following parameters were selected: level of consciousness, behaviour, convulsions, and neck rigidity. The results recorded are outlined in Table 3.

In 75 cases, additional follow-up data obtained after the ten-day trial period were provided. These data reveal that, of 38 patients who had received betamethasone, 31 showed a continuing improvement, three either remained unchanged or deteriorated, and four died (on the 13th, 15th, 30th, and 40th days, respectively). Of the 37 patients treated with Synacthen Depot, 30 continued to improve, three showed either no change or a worsening, and four died (on the 16th, 17th, 20th, and 24th days, respectively).

4. Tolerability

In the group receiving Synacthen Depot, the medication was withdrawn in three patients for reasons unrelated to the drug, while in a fourth patient the treatment was discontinued owing to the onset of severe psychomotor excitation on the fourth day.

Particular attention was paid to the detection of possible differences between the effects of the two trial preparations on blood pressure (Table 4) and on the daily volume of urine excreted (Table 5).

Patients with a diastolic pressure exceeding 95 mm. Hg were classified as hypertensive, and those whose excretion of urine amounted to less than 700 ml./24 hours were considered to be suffering from oliguria. In connection with the problem of oliguria, it should be added that administration of fluids was resorted to wherever necessary.

Although the number of patients showing an increase in blood pressure during treatment was higher in the group receiving Synacthen Depot, the difference between the two groups in this respect was not significant. As for the 24-hour urine volumes, oliguria disappeared in more patients under Synacthen Depot than under betamethasone (fourfold-table test, $P \simeq 0.05$).

Among the side effects reported, in which a connection with the trial preparation cannot be ruled out, were the following: firstly, in the betamethasone group, severe and prolonged ankle oedema in one case, severe hyperglycaemia (up to 373 mg./100 ml.) in one case, and moderate transient hyperglycaemia in eight

Table 4. Blood pressure before and on the tenth day of treatment.

Before treatment On tenth day	Normal ↓ High	Normal ↓ Normal	Total	High ↓ Normal	High ↓ High	Total	Total number of recordings
Betamethasone	1	27	28	15	13	28	56
Synacthen Depot	6	24	30	10	14	24	54
Total	7	51	58	25	27	52	110

Table 5. Daily excretion of urine before and on the tenth day of treatment.

Before treatment On tenth day	Normal ↓ Reduced	Normal ↓ Normal	Total	Reduced ↓ Normal	Reduced ↓ Reduced	Total	Total number of recordings
Betamethasone	2	31	33	9	7	16	49
Synacthen Depot	3	26	29	14	1	15	44
Total	5	57	62	23	8	31	93

cases; secondly, in the Synacthen Depot group, fluid retention and acute cardiac insufficiency in one case, acute pulmonary oedema in one case, and moderate transient hyperglycaemia in eight cases.

5. Concluding observations

The overall mortality rate during the ten-day trial period, irrespective of which of the two forms of treatment was employed, amounted to 11%, and an improvement in the patients' general condition occurred in 66% of cases—which on the whole can be regarded as a satisfactory outcome. The majority of the focal brain lesions either disappeared or showed an improvement.

Administered in a daily dose of 1 mg., Synacthen Depot displayed the same degree of therapeutic efficacy as betamethasone injected in a dosage of 8 mg. daily.

Despite the fact that the statistical analysis failed to disclose any significant differences between the responses in the two groups, it must be pointed out that the results, judged by reference to the overall assessment and to the signs of cerebral oedema, were somewhat better in the group treated with Synacthen Depot.

The mortality rate was 7% in the corticotrophin group and 15% in the betamethasone group; in the patients receiving Synacthen Depot, the level of consciousness improved in 69% of cases and never underwent a deterioration, whereas in those treated with the corticosteroid it improved in 58% of cases and worsened in three cases. Although high blood-pressure levels were recorded more frequently in the corticotrophin group, no particular problems arose with regard to side effects. Fewer cases of fluid retention were reported under Synacthen Depot than under betamethasone.

In conclusion, our clinical study has confirmed the observations of other authors who have found corticotrophin therapy to be effective in acute cerebrovascular accidents. The direct comparison made between Synacthen Depot and betamethasone yielded evidence in favour of the former—evidence which trials conducted on a broader and deeper basis might well serve to confirm.

Summary

A single-blind multicentre trial was carried out in order to compare the effectiveness of a corticosteroid (betamethasone) and a synthetic corticotrophin (Synacthen Depot) in the treatment of acute cerebrovascular accidents. The patients, totalling 122, were treated for ten days. Although no statistically significant differences between the two treatments were found, the overall outcome of the study and the responses assessed by reference to certain indirect signs of cerebral oedema did indicate that the corticotrophin therapy had yielded better results. Both preparations were well tolerated.

References

1 BERNARD-WEIL, E., DAVID, M.: Traitement hormonal de l'œdème cérébral. Inform. thér. *7*, 52 (1969)
2 BOUCHARD, C., SINDOU, M., TIMBAL, Y.: L'hypertension intra-cranienne. France méd. *32*, 195 (1969)
3 CLAISSE, R., DALAYEUN, J., FONTAINE, C., LESSIEUX, G.: L'ACTH de synthèse dans les affections neurologiques médicales graves. Gaz. méd. Fr. *77*, 6739 (1970)
4 COSSA, P., DARCOURT, G., BOUCEBCI, M., CAPDEVILLE, C., BECLE, J., ALBARANES, S.: Le traitement des accidents vasculaires cérébraux par la méthode de Bernard-Weil (d'après une série de 117 cas). Gaz. méd. Fr. *75*, 3451 (1968)
5 DARCOURT, G., ALBARANES, S., BECLE, J., CAPDEVILLE, C., COSSA, P.: La corticothérapie dans le traitement des accidents vasculaires cérébraux. Bilan actuel. Nice méd. *6*, 177 (1968)
6 DOCUMENTA GEIGY: Scientific tables, 7th Edition (Basle 1970)
7 FAÇON, E., SCHWARTZ, B.: Le traitement hormonal de l'œdème cérébral des accidents cérébrovasculaires. Presse méd. *72*, 2377 (1964)
8 FERRARI, E., RAGONESE, G.: L'associazione A.C.T.H.-ossitocina nel trattamento delle affezioni cerebrali edemigene. Acta neurol. (Naples) *25*, 435 (1970)
9 GOUTELLE, A., BRUNON, J., RAVON, R.: Place du Synacthène dans le traitement de l'œdème cérébral. Gaz. méd. Fr. *76*, 6462 (1969)
10 GUIOT, G., LANGIE, S.: Le traitement médical de l'œdème cérébral. Rev. Prat. (Paris) *19*, 3389 (1969)
11 JAVALET, A.: Indications thérapeutiques dans les tumeurs cérébrales. Feuill. Prat. *35*, 597 (1970)
12 PAILLAS, J.E., PELLET, W., MANELLI, J.-C., RAKOTOBÉ, A.: A.C.T.H.-thérapie en neuro-chirurgie. In: A.C.T.H.-thérapie moderne, Coll. thér. CIBA, Marseilles 1969, p. 139 (Kapp & Lahure, Vanves 1970)
13 PATTEN, B.M., MENDELL, J., BRUUN, B., CURTIN, W., CARTER, S.: Double blind study of the effects of dexamethasone on acute stroke, loc. cit.[21], p. 259
14 PERTUISET, B.: L'hypertension intra-cranienne et son traitement. Méd. int. *4*, 61 (1969)

15 POLLI, E.: Sperimentazione multicentrica con differenti metodi di terapia nella leucemia acuta dell'adulto. Minerva med. *57*, 1116 (1966)

16 POLLI, E.: Le fasi della sperimentazione clinica di un nuovo farmaco. Recenti Progr. Med. *42*, 1 (1967)

17 POLLI, E., BARBIERI, D., BONOMO, E., BUSSI, L., CASTELFRANCO, M., CHIRICO, M., CROSTI, P.F., DE MICHELI, E., FERRARI, A., FRANZINI, P., GIRELLI, M., MARUBINI, E., MAZZOLENI, L., MELLONI, G., NOCCA, G., RATTI, G., SALA, G., SELVINI, A., TERRUZZI, L.: Sperimentazione clinica controllata di tre trattamenti diuretici nella cirrosi epatica con ascite. Sperimentazione policentrica. Minerva med. *58*, 2189 (1967)

18 POLLI, E., BARBIERI, D., BONOMO, E., BUSSI, L., CASTELFRANCO, M., CHIRICO, M., CROSTI, P.F., DE MICHELI, E., FRANZINI, P., LUCCHELLI, P.E., MAZZOLENI, L., MELLONI, G., RATTI, G., SALA, G., SANTARATO, E., SELVINI, A., STABILINI, G., TERRUZZI, L.: Sperimentazione policentrica pianificata con diuretici nella cirrosi epatica ascitogena. Atti Accad. med. lombarda *18*, 1065 (1963)

19 POLLI, E., BONOMO, E., CASTELFRANCO, M., CHIRICO, M., DE MICHELI, E., FRANZINI, P., MARUBINI, E., MAZZOLENI, L., NOCCA, G., PILOTTI, A., TERRUZZI, L.: La terapia cortisonica dell'epatite virale – sperimentazione policentrica controllata. In: Symp. Epatite virale, p. 232 (Minerva med., Turin 1969)

20 PRAGA, C.: Cooperative clinical study on Adriamycin in advanced lung tumors. In Carter, S.K., et al. (Editors): Int. Symp. on Adriamycin, p. 173 (Springer, Berlin/Heidelberg/New York 1972)

21 REULEN, H.J., SCHÜRMANN, K. (Editors): Steroids and brain edema (Springer, Berlin/Heidelberg/New York 1972)

22 SIEGEL, S.: Nonparametric statistics for the behavioral sciences (McGraw-Hill, New York/Toronto/London 1956)

Discussion

H.J.BAUER: I think your study, Dr. POLLI, raises the fundamentally important question as to whether it is permissible to evaluate such a heterogeneous group of cases as cerebrovascular accidents on the basis of the symptomatology. This is not a criticism, especially as I am only too well aware of the circumstances one is often confronted with when dealing with patients of this kind. Our own experience is that it is extremely difficult to evaluate a drug such as a corticosteroid or A.C.T.H. in the hectic clinical situation of a cerebrovascular accident—a situation in which cardio-vascular therapy, correction of the fluid and electrolyte balance, and all the other measures that have to be taken play such an important role and compel one to do a lot of things that simply cannot be as carefully controlled as in a chronic disease. I have three brief questions I should like to ask you. Firstly, in your group of 122 patients did you try to differentiate between cerebral haemorrhage and encephalo-malacia? Secondly, did you manage to establish any relationship between the presence of hypertension and the prognosis? Thirdly, you quote median ages for the two groups of patients which are almost identical, but this does not necessarily mean that the age range in the two groups is strictly comparable. Could you give us some more data on this point?

E.POLLI: The question of differentiating between encephalomalacia and cerebral haemorrhage is certainly an important one. As I mentioned in my paper, we did not resort in every case to such diagnostic procedures as lumbar puncture or cerebral angiography. The investigators participating in the trial were no doubt dealing with both types of cerebrovascular accident, i.e. stroke due to encephalomalacia as well as stroke due to cerebral haemorrhage. Common to all cases, however, was injury to brain tissue and especially cerebral oedema. It is our impression that the oedema can be improved by administering steroids or corticotrophin. But, to revert to your three questions, we did not distinguish between encephalomalacia and cerebral haemor-rhage, nor did we establish any correlation between hypertension and the prognosis; as for the ages of the patients in the two groups, I can only add that their ages ranged from 37 to 80 years in the betamethasone group and from 40 to 77 years in the Synacthen Depot group.

Incidentally, I must confess that one problem which has quite often worried me con-cerns the equivalence of dosages—particularly in acute conditions, such as cerebral oedema, status asthmaticus, and other immunological diseases, where you can some-times obtain good therapeutic results with doses of prednisolone, dexamethasone, or betamethasone that are simply not comparable with the doses of A.C.T.H. that would be employed. Perhaps this is not simply a question of equivalence of dosage, and perhaps the mechanisms of action by which corticosteroids and A.C.T.H. produce their therapeutic effects differ somewhat.

R.DEGUILLAUME: It has been reported in the literature that patients who have suffered an acute stroke already show elevated plasma cortisol levels from the very outset. Other authors have also tried to establish a correlation between the initial plasma cortisol levels and the prognosis. You didn't make any reference to this in your paper, so may I ask if you have any further findings that might be relevant in this connection?

E.POLLI: No, I'm afraid I haven't.

Synthetic A.C.T.H. preparations in respiratory diseases

by J. Charpin, J. Aubert, J. Boyer, and P. Vague*

In this paper the following three questions will be dealt with:
1. What is at present known about the mode of action of A.C.T.H. in asthma?
2. What are the indications for A.C.T.H. in the treatment of asthma and chronic respiratory failure?
3. What immunological complications are liable to occur in response to β1–24 corticotrophin, i.e. complications in the form of either allergic reactions or the appearance of antibodies directed against A.C.T.H.?

1. Mode of action of A.C.T.H. in cases of asthma

Viewing the problem of treatment for status asthmaticus from the clinical aspect, we have always had the impression[42] that there were genuine advantages to be gained from administering A.C.T.H. in addition to corticosteroid infusions. After the year 1962, when the high incidence of allergic reactions provoked by non-purified A.C.T.H. extract-preparations[16, 20] induced us to omit A.C.T.H. from the infusions we were using in cases of asthma—or, at least, only to employ A.C.T.H. with extreme caution—the treatment forfeited some of its efficacy. As clinicians we suspect in fact, if only intuitively, that in the management of asthma A.C.T.H. may well constitute more than a mere link in the chain of command governing adrenocortical secretion. We do not propose to re-examine here the mechanism or mechanisms by which A.C.T.H. and the glucocorticoids act upon the various types of allergic phenomena, since these have been expertly analysed only recently by Jasani[38]. Instead, we shall simply consider briefly the direct action which A.C.T.H. appears to exert on the smooth muscle of the bronchi.

In 1970, Svedmyr et al.[53] published evidence showing that, when employed in a dose of 0.1–1.2 units/ml., A.C.T.H. has a relaxing effect on human bronchial muscle *in vitro* and that this effect, which attains a maximum with the synthetic 1–39 derivative, disappears when only the 1–14 fragment of the molecule is used; the same authors also found that this bronchodilator action was potentiated by theophylline and inhibited by beta-blockers. In another study, Andersson et al.[4] reported that the relaxing effect exerted by A.C.T.H. on the rabbit colon was accompanied by an increase in the production of cyclic adenosine monophosphate. A similar increase in cyclic adenosine monophosphate was also observed by the same group of authors[3] in human bronchial muscle under the

* Clinique de Pneumo-Phtisiologie, Faculté mixte de Médecine et de Pharmacie, Université Aix-Marseille, Marseilles, France.

influence of a synthetic A.C.T.H. of human type containing the full complement of 39 amino acids.

2. Indications for A.C.T.H. in the treatment of asthma and chronic respiratory failure

2.1. In patients suffering from *status asthmaticus,* we administer two infusions per day, each containing:
- 0.5 mg. tetracosactide (®Synacthen);
- 20 mg. methylprednisolone or triamcinolone (in the first few days we also add one ampoule of a rapid-acting corticosteroid, i.e. either 4 mg. betamethasone or 4 mg. dexamethasone); in certain cases of very severe status asthmaticus, in which treatment has been delayed or the patient is already in a state of collapse, we replace the methylprednisolone or triamcinolone during the first few critical days by 100–500 mg. hydrocortisone hemisuccinate;
- 1 g. chloramphenicol hemisuccinate, because some degree of secondary infection is also present in all these cases;
- often an agent serving to correct acidosis, e.g. T.H.A.M. (trihydroxymethyl-aminomethane).

To this cocktail some physicians, of course, also add aminophylline (500 mg.) and a sympathomimetic drug such as terbutaline.

If cardiac stimulants, e.g. ®Cedilanid, prove necessary, these should not be added to the infusion solution in the flask—since mixing them with the latter may result in their inactivation—but should be injected into the tube.

Though such infusions constitute the basic treatment for status asthmaticus, it is often advisable to supplement them by other measures, i.e.:
- continuous administration, via a nasal catheter, of oxygen at a low rate of two litres per minute;
- β_2-bronchodilators, provided the patient has not already developed tolerance to them;
- endoscopic removal of plugs of mucus, plus assisted respiration in grave cases of coma.

2.2. In acute attacks of asthma, in severe asthmatic crises, or in acute bouts of decompensation occurring in patients with respiratory failure, twice-daily infusions as described above can likewise be given, provided the patient has been admitted to hospital; if he is being treated at home, recourse may be had to ®Synacthen Depot—administered in a dosage of 1 mg. daily i.m. for two or three days and then every other day for four to ten days—together with broad-spectrum antibiotics.

In order to avoid the onset of status asthmaticus, it is absolutely essential in such cases to discontinue all the customary forms of medication—including in particular β_2-bronchodilators and theophylline, of which the patient will probably have been using excessive quantities—and to resort at once to treatment either with antibiotics and corticosteroids or with antibiotics and A.C.T.H.

The same applies to all asthmatic crises of any violence occurring in the course of an asthmatic illness that has responded reasonably well to causal therapy.

Any sudden exacerbation that is at all serious should preferably be treated with a brief course of antibiotic + corticosteroid or antibiotic + A.C.T.H. therapy.

2.3. In asthmatics suffering from persistent dyspnoea despite long-term treatment with corticosteroids, we have endeavoured to determine what benefit might be derived from use of the less allergenic forms of A.C.T.H. that are now available. Our research along these lines has served to answer two different questions:
– Can A.C.T.H. help in weaning a patient from corticoids (A)?
– Can A.C.T.H. prevent suppression of pituitary-adrenocortical function in the course of continuous (B) or intermittent treatment with corticoids (C)?

A. In the initial study which we carried out with Synacthen Depot, we made an attempt at the *withdrawal* of corticosteroids in 15 hospitalised patients who had been receiving prolonged steroid therapy; in these cases we replaced the corticosteroid medication by first injecting 1 mg. Synacthen Depot daily i.m. and then successively prolonging the interval between injections to 48 hours and to three, four, or five days. In 14 out of the 15 patients it did indeed prove possible to substitute Synacthen Depot for the corticosteroid, but during this trial—which lasted from three weeks to four months, depending on the case—it was found that the side effects (cushingoid syndrome, pigmentation of the face and hands) were more pronounced than those observed during long-term corticosteroid therapy.

This problem of withdrawing corticosteroids has been very carefully studied by other authors. WOLFROMM and HERMAN[62] in particular have undertaken prolonged trials in which, during withdrawal of the corticosteroids, adrenocortical function was monitored by repeated Thorn tests. These authors conclude that injection treatment with Synacthen Depot can prove a valuable aid in solving the invariably difficult problem of corticosteroid withdrawal, provided the following dosage schedule is adopted: one injection of 1 mg. Synacthen Depot daily for three days, followed by one injection every two days for a further week, the interval between injections then being successively prolonged by 24 hours every week. In other words, one has to proceed fairly quickly with the progressive prolongation of the interval between injections; where this is not done, i.e. where the injections are repeated for some length of time at the rate of one every two or three days, very disagreeable side effects are liable to occur, associated in particular with high plasma cortisol levels of a cushingoid type which show no nyctohemeral fluctuations. A similar observation has also been reported by BRICAIRE and LUTON[9].

It therefore appears that, although in asthmatics suffering from persistent dyspnoea the use of Synacthen Depot may well help in completely weaning the patient from corticosteroids in those very rare cases where a definitive withdrawal of the steroid therapy proves possible at all, such substitution treatment with Synacthen Depot can only serve as a temporary aid in this connection. It would seem neither possible nor advisable on a long-term basis to replace steroid therapy by injections of Synacthen Depot that have to be administered indefinitely every two or three days.

In this respect, the approach adopted by chest specialists appears to differ somewhat from that of French and British rheumatologists[40, 47], who evidently find it easier in their rheumatic patients than we do in our asthmatics to achieve genuine withdrawals or to inject depot A.C.T.H. every three to seven days without encountering troublesome side effects.

B. In patients receiving prolonged treatment with *daily doses of corticosteroids*, does the periodic administration of A.C.T.H. serve in the long run to maintain adrenocortical function? BOYER and CODACCIONI[8], as well as DEGUILLAUME[22], emphasise that, even in patients already undergoing steroid therapy for a very long time, doses of A.C.T.H. are still capable of reactivating the adrenal cortex to a certain extent and that, consequently, such periodic reactivation would *a priori* appear worth while as a means of maintaining adrenocortical function. But what does this mean in practice? Hardly any convincing quantitative data are to be found in the literature. We ourselves are at present engaged upon a long-term study in which we are monitoring adrenocortical secretion over 48-hour periods (using the method of Cope and Black) in a group of asthmatics receiving prolonged steroid therapy, some of whom are also being given Synacthen Depot "boosts" of 1 mg. every fortnight. Our impression—for the moment at least—is that, except where adrenocortical secretion is measured within the three days following the administration of Synacthen Depot, there does not seem to be much difference in "basic" secretion between the patients receiving supplementary Synacthen Depot therapy and those treated with corticosteroids alone. Thus, although we cannot yet draw any final conclusions, we are already beginning to wonder, like LANDON et al.[39] and TURIAF et al.[56], whether A.C.T.H. boosts really do serve any purpose in patients subjected to continuous treatment with corticosteroids.

C. There are in fact other dosage schedules which would seem to offer better prospects. It has now been well established, for example, that *intermittent* steroid medication, in which the fractional doses previously administered over a 48-hour period are given in one large dose every two days, causes less interference with pituitary-adrenocortical function than continuous treatment (REICHLING and KLINGMAN[46]; HARTER et al.[33]; AKOUN[1]; PORTNER et al.[43]); this is also true even in cases where the dose employed is greater than the sum of the two daily doses prescribed hitherto (FALLIERS et al.[24]).
It would appear that additional treatment with A.C.T.H. makes it easier for a patient to switch to this type of intermittent steroid medication. For instance, when an attempt was made to institute intermittent treatment in a group of 71 adult patients who had been undergoing long-term corticosteroid therapy for at least a year[14], it was found possible to do so without increasing the dosage and without administering any A.C.T.H. supplement in 19 cases; in 23 cases, however, an injection of 1 mg. Synacthen Depot had to be given periodically, i.e. either once or twice a month.
A similar method is adopted by HERMAN (personal communication) in asthmatics whom it has proved impossible to wean from corticosteroids; in these

cases he administers combined treatment in the form, for example, of one injection of A.C.T.H. on the first day of the week, followed by corticosteroids on the last three days.

In the field with which we are concerned, it is therefore, we feel, probably along the following lines that a solution may be found to the problem of eliminating continuous steroid therapy as far as possible: recourse to a combination of intermittent steroid therapy plus injections of depot A.C.T.H. given with an interval of at least one week between injections.

3. Immunological reactions: allergy to tetracosactide and formation of antibodies directed against A.C.T.H.

3.1. Experimental data

FELBER et al.[26] have demonstrated that synthetic 1–39 corticotrophin has the same antigenic potential as purified A.C.T.H. of animal origin and that β1–24 corticotrophin, though displaying very little antigenicity, may nonetheless enter into competition with the whole molecule and thus bind antibodies directed against A.C.T.H., whereas the amino acid sequences 1–10 and 11–24 are both incapable of doing this.

IMURA et al.[36] have studied the biological and immunological activity of three corticotrophins obtained by extraction (ovine, human, and porcine) and of six amino acid chains prepared by synthesis (i.e.: three sequences containing the first 17, 19, and 24 amino acids of A.C.T.H., respectively; human 1–26 A.C.T.H.; porcine 1–39 A.C.T.H.; and the 22–39 fragment of ovine A.C.T.H.). They found that, whereas the A.C.T.H. extract-preparations and the synthetic chains of 24, 26, and 39 amino acids displayed identical *biological activity*, the biological activity of the chain containing 19 amino acids was reduced by one-half; neither the chain consisting of 17 amino acids nor the 22–39 ovine amino acid sequence exhibited any biological activity. The *immunological activity*, on the other hand, proved to be strong in the case of the 1–39 sequence and less marked in the case of the 1–26 and 1–24 sequences, whereas the chains of 17 and 19 amino acids were immunologically inactive; the 22–39 sequence exhibited strong immunological activity.

SALVIN and LIAUW[48] have shown that both the 39 amino acid molecule and the 24 amino acid molecule are capable of inducing a delayed form of hypersensitivity. Studies undertaken with fragments of the 24 amino acid chain disclosed that only the 11–24 portion is antigenic, its antigenicity being concentrated chiefly in the amino acid fragment 17–24.

The investigations conducted by SALVIN and LIAUW indicate that the immunogenic potential of the 39 amino acid A.C.T.H. molecule is mainly accounted for by the C-terminal sequence 25–39; compared with the intact molecule, the immunogenic potential of the 1–24 sequence is far weaker, and *such immunogenic activity as it does display seems to be essentially due to the 17–24 fraction.*

Although these experimental studies reveal that the antibodies evoked by A.C.T.H. cannot be assigned to the category of reagins, they do shed interesting light on the clinical problem of immunological reactions to A.C.T.H.

3.2. It will be remembered that non-purified A.C.T.H. preparations obtained by extraction have frequently been the cause of allergic accidents. Such complications were already described by TRAEGER[54] in 1950, and were subsequently also encountered by, for example, BROWN and HOLLANDER[11], STEVENSON[52], ARBESMAN et al.[5], BRODWALL[10], and ARNOLDSSON[6]. In a report of ours published in 1961[20], we too referred to 43 allergic reactions which had occurred in a series of 113 asthmatics treated with A.C.T.H. It was these complications, the characteristics of which we have already outlined elsewhere[16], that induced us progressively to restrict the use of non-purified A.C.T.H. extract-preparations in asthmatic patients. The impurities present in these preparations were evidently the main factor responsible for the allergic reactions in question[16,17,19], and the advent of purified A.C.T.H. extracts accordingly marked a step in the right direction[41]. Nevertheless, we personally have observed one fatality in a patient receiving a purified A.C.T.H. extract-preparation by infusion, as well as six confirmed allergic reactions among 168 asthmatics who had been given a total of 1,267 injections of purified A.C.T.H.

3.3. In connection with the use of *synthetic A.C.T.H. polypeptides*, including β1–24 corticotrophin in particular, two points have to be considered: firstly, their allergenicity (A) and, secondly, the possibility that they may provoke the appearance of antibodies directed against A.C.T.H. without actually giving rise to signs and symptoms of allergy (B).

A. In man the problem of allergenicity can be studied along various lines. In the first place, one can select patients known to be allergic to A.C.T.H. extract-preparations, test them to ensure that they still show a positive reaction to A.C.T.H. of animal origin, and then perform cutaneous tests with a synthetic polypeptide; here, as revealed by a study undertaken on controls who were not allergic to A.C.T.H., it is important to note that, to avoid obtaining false positive results, only concentrations of 1:100 should be employed.
When we adopted this method in 58 patients known to be allergic to A.C.T.H., 48 of whom still showed a positive reaction to A.C.T.H. when re-tested, we found only one case in which the patient reacted positively to tetracosactide diluted 1:100.
A second criterion of allergenicity can be obtained by giving treatment with a synthetic A.C.T.H. polypeptide to these same patients exhibiting a known allergy to A.C.T.H. For this purpose, 43 of the 58 patients mentioned above were treated with the short-acting form of β1–24 corticotrophin, the total dosage ranging from *0.125 mg. to 45 mg.* The results were as follows:
– In 39 cases the medication was excellently tolerated.
– Four allergic reactions, which prompted us to withdraw the treatment, were encountered:
  a) pruritus and oedema of the face accompanied by an asthmatic crisis
  b) asthmatic crisis unaccompanied by any other signs of allergy
  c) generalised erythema
  d) pruritus of the face and hands.

On the other hand, 21 patients of this same type (including 14 from the aforementioned series) were treated with depot tetracosactide (total dosage per patient: 6–13 mg.) without developing any allergic complications.

Finally, a third criterion of allergenicity may be provided by a study of the way in which subjects prone to allergy, but not allergic to A.C.T.H., react to a synthetic polypeptide. In an investigation of this kind, 107 patients were treated with β1–24 corticotrophin, which was administered in the short-acting form in 21 cases and in the depot form in the remaining 86 cases.

In ten of these patients, the following signs of intolerance were observed:

On three occasions, infusions of β1–24 corticotrophin repeated over a prolonged period led to the appearance of *acne punctata* on the face and chest; when the acne had cleared, *minute pigmented spots* remained visible at the sites of the lesions. This minor side effect did not necessitate withdrawal of the drug.

In four cases, the patients felt a sensation of *generalised warmth* immediately after the start of the infusion accompanied by reddening of the face, but not by oedema or pruritus; in two of these four patients, the reaction was associated with an—admittedly mild—aggravation of dyspnoea. This type of phenomenon might conceivably be attributable to a liberation of histamine, as observed by JAQUES and BRUGGER [37] in experimental studies with β1–24 corticotrophin.

In the three other cases, details of which are given below, typical allergic reactions occurred:

Case 1: A 56-year-old woman suffering from asthma marked by persistent dyspnoea and undergoing long-term corticosteroid therapy. She was also receiving an injection of 1 mg. Synacthen Depot once a month. Whereas the ninth injection, administered on 8th November 1968, was well tolerated, the tenth injection (on 8th December 1968) was followed 15 minutes later by the onset of itching, a generalised skin rash, and dyspnoea. As the patient omitted to report this incident, she was given her 11th injection on 8th January 1969; this immediately provoked another generalised rash together with very severe dyspnoea lasting 48 hours. These allergic manifestations did not completely subside until the 12th day.

When sensitivity tests were carried out on 13th March 1969, the patient showed a positive cutaneous reaction to two different forms of corticotrophin (i.e. a purified A.C.T.H. preparation obtained by extraction and the synthetic polypeptide containing 24 amino acids).

It is interesting to note that skin tests performed in 1965 on the same patient and with the same preparations had proved negative. When she had to be admitted to hospital on 10th December 1969 to receive treatment for an acute attack of asthma, she was given a different synthetic A.C.T.H. product composed of 25 amino acids, and the latter provoked no allergic reactions.

Case 2: A 53-year-old woman in receipt of long-term corticosteroid therapy for asthma with persistent dyspnoea. From 15th September 1967 to January 1969 she received a total of 16 injections of 1 mg. Synacthen Depot, administered once a month. The dosage was then raised to one injection every fortnight. The

21st injection, given on 10th March 1969, was followed by pains in the lumbar region and vomiting, but no cutaneous symptoms. On 24th March, an injection of 0.25 mg. Synacthen Depot caused the same manifestations, followed on the next day by angioneurotic oedema and generalised urticaria. Skin tests subsequently performed with tetracosactide (1:100) and purified A.C.T.H. (1:100 and 1:1,000) proved positive.

Case 3: A 58-year-old woman undergoing prolonged corticosteroid therapy as treatment for asthma of late onset with persistent dyspnoea. Prior to 24th June 1970, when she was admitted to hospital suffering from an attack of asthma, she had apparently never been treated with A.C.T.H. On 3rd July 1970, at the start of an infusion of short-acting Synacthen, she complained of a sensation of warmth, which was followed by generalised pruritus, a skin eruption confined to the legs, and increased dyspnoea. The infusion was broken off and intravenous corticosteroid medication given instead. Skin tests carried out on 4th July showed a positive reaction to tetracosactide 1:10 and a negative reaction to a dilution of 1:100. Afterwards, however, the patient suffered no ill effects when first 25 units and then 100 units of another synthetic A.C.T.H. preparation (consisting of 25 amino acids) were administered intravenously.

Similar observations have also been made by PEPYS (personal communication), as well as by UZZAN et al.[58], who describe a case in which fatal anaphylactic shock occurred in a 77-year-old man in whom two previous allergic reactions had passed unheeded.

The three reactions referred to in detail above, including the first two in particular, were of quite a different kind from the other side effects observed by us; that they were in all probability of a genuinely allergic nature is suggested by the fact that the injections were perfectly well tolerated to begin with, but that the adverse reactions then became progessively more severe (Cases 1 and 2), one injection merely provoking a minor disturbance whereas the next injection gave rise to very severe manifestations.

Likewise clearly indicative of an allergic aetiology are the results obtained in the cutaneous tests carried out with weak dilutions of 1:100 and 1:1,000.

Thirdly and lastly, the fact that in two of the cases no untoward incidents occurred when the patient was given another synthetic 25 amino acid polypeptide (in which the sequence of three amino acids differed as compared with tetracosactide) also points in the same direction.

B. In connection with the possibility that synthetic A.C.T.H. polypeptides may provoke the formation of antibodies directed against A.C.T.H., reference has already been made to the findings obtained by FELBER et al.[26] in animals.

In a study undertaken in collaboration with J. VAGUE at the Endocrinological Clinic in Marseilles, we have been employing a radioimmunological technique in order to investigate the occurrence of antibodies directed against β1–24 corticotrophin. Of 35 adult asthmatics treated with Synacthen or Synacthen Depot for periods ranging from a minimum of six months to a maximum of

51 months (2–106 injections), nine have shown allergic reactions to the injections. Also in nine of the 35 patients, antibodies directed against tetracosactide have been detected (positive tests having been obtained in all nine cases with dilutions of 1:10 and 1:50, and in six of them with dilutions of 1:100). Antibodies against Synacthen, however, were traced in only two of the nine patients who showed allergic reactions to the preparation. In three of the patients in whom antibodies had been detected we studied the patients' reactions to fragments of the corticotrophin chain (1–10 and 11–24): all three of them showed negative reactions to the 1–10 fragment and positive reactions to the 11–24 fragment. This investigation—which is still in progress and which would appear for the moment to indicate that the presence of antibodies directed against tetracosactide is not necessarily associated with the presence of specific reagins— is also to be supplemented by a study on the functional significance of the anti-tetracosactide antibodies, in which an attempt will be made to discover whether any disturbances in the Thorn test occur in patients with these antibodies.

Conclusions

1. In the management of asthma and chronic respiratory failure, Synacthen and Synacthen Depot are capable of playing an important role as treatment for status asthmaticus, severe attacks of asthma, and acute asthmatic crises, as well as for acute bouts of decompensation occurring in patients with respiratory failure. In the great majority of asthmatics suffering from persistent dyspnoea, however, Synacthen Depot cannot be employed on a long-term basis as a substitute for corticosteroid therapy; nor has it yet been clearly established that intermittent doses of Synacthen Depot serve to attenuate the depressant effect exerted by continuous corticosteroid therapy on pituitary-adrenocortical function. On the other hand, it would appear profitable to study the possibility of employing dosage schedules in which A.C.T.H., given with an interval of at least one week between injections, is administered in combination with discontinuous corticosteroid therapy.

2. Immunological reactions to A.C.T.H. of synthetic origin:

– Though allergy to tetracosactide does occur, it is very rare and must be distinguished from complications due to different mechanisms (histamine liberation, spasmophilia); in practice it proves little obstacle to the use of Synacthen or Synacthen Depot, even in patients already prone to allergic reactions.

– Antibodies directed against tetracosactide, which probably differ from reagins, are quite frequently encountered. Their functional significance, which has not yet been precisely determined, would appear at present to be relatively minor.

References

1   Akoun, G.: La prescription à jour alterné de la corticothérapie au long cours en pneumo-phtisiologie. Lille méd. *14*, 644 (1969)
2   Akoun, G., Vachon, J., Muon, Brocard, H.: La prescription à jour alterné de la corticothérapie au long cours. Sem. Hôp. Paris *44*, 3141 (1968)

3 ANDERSSON, R., BERGH, N.P., SVEDMYR, N.: Metabolic actions in human bronchial muscle associated with ACTH induced relaxation. Scand. J. resp. Dis. 53, 125 (1972)

4 ANDERSSON, R., MOHME-LUNDHOLM, E., SVEDMYR, N., VAMOS, N.: Relaxing and metabolic actions of ACTH in rabbit colon. Acta physiol. scand. 81, 11 (1971)

5 ARBESMAN, C.E., SCHNEIDER, M.A., GREENE, D.G., OSGOOD, H.: Intravenous ACTH and oral cortisone in the treatment of bronchial asthma. J. Allergy 23, 293 (1952)

6 ARNOLDSSON, H.: Allergische Reaktionen auf ACTH. Acta allerg. (Kbh.) 8, 369 (1955)

7 AUBERT, L., FELBER, J.-P.: Studies on ACTH-binding antibodies: characterization of immunological specificities. Acta endocr. (Kbh.) 62, 521 (1969)

8 BOYER, J., CODACCIONI, J.-L.: A.C.T.H.-thérapie, compagnon, rival, ou successeur de la corticothérapie. In: A.C.T.H.-thérapie moderne, Coll. thér. CIBA, Marseilles, 1969, p. 215 (Kapp & Lahure, Vanves 1970)

9 BRICAIRE, H., LUTON, J.-P.: Les tests de stimulation de la cortico-surrénale, fonction aldostérone exceptée, loc. cit.[8], p. 21

10 BRODWALL, E.K.: Sensibilisering fremkalt av corticotropin (Allergic reactions due to corticotropin). Nord. med. 51, 301 (1954)

11 BROWN, E.M., Jr., HOLLANDER, J.L.: Allergy to ACTH and the use of beef ACTH. In Mote, J.R. (Editor): Proc. IInd Clin. ACTH Conf., Vol. II – Therapeutics, p. 391 (Blakiston, New York/Philadelphia/Toronto 1951)

12 CHARPIN, J.: Les corticostéroides dans le traitement de l'allergie. In Rose, B., et al. (Editors): Allergology, Proc. VIth Congr. Int. Ass. Allerg., Montreal 1967. Int. Congr. Ser. No. 16, p. 447 (Excerpta med. Found., Amsterdam etc. 1968)

13 CHARPIN, J.: L'asthme bronchique et son traitement (Maloine, Paris 1968)

14 CHARPIN, J., AUBERT, J.: Corticothérapie alternative dans l'asthme bronchique. Gaz. Hôp. (Paris) 29, 787 (1969)

15 CHARPIN, J., AUBERT, J.: Allergie au tétracosapeptide. Marseille-méd. 106, 881 (1969)

16 CHARPIN, J., AUBERT, J.: Allergy to ACTH and its prevention. In Serafini, U., et al. (Editors): New concepts in allergy and clinical immunology, Proc. VIIth Int. Congr. Allerg., Florence 1970. Int. Congr. Ser. No. 232, p. 224 (Excerpta med., Amsterdam 1971)

17 CHARPIN, J., AUBERT, J.: Accidents provoqués par l'ACTH et les polypeptides synthétiques. Méd. et Hyg. (Geneva) 29, 38 (1971)

18 CHARPIN, J., AUBERT, J., BOUTIN, C.: The allergenic properties of the newer adrenocorticotrophic hormones. Acta allerg. (Kbh.) 22, 289 (1967)

19 CHARPIN, J., ZAFIROPOULO, A., AUBERT, J., OHRESSER, P., BOUTIN, C.: Données actuelles concernant l'allergie à l'ACTH. Presse méd. 72, 3025 (1964)

20 CHARPIN, J., ZAFIROPOULO, A., BLANC, M.: Accidents allergiques dûs à l'A.C.T.H. In Charpy, J. (Editor): Thérapeutique dermatologique et allergologique, VIIᵉ Colloque Filiale marseillaise Soc. franç. Derm., p. 153 (Masson, Paris 1961)

21 DEGUILLAUME, R.: Etat actuel du traitement par un peptide corticotrope de synthèse, le tétracosactide-retard. Presse méd. 79, 233 (1971)

22 DEGUILLAUME, R.: Quelle est la valeur de l'ACTH dans la prévention et le traitement de l'insuffisance surrénale post-cortisonique? Presse méd. 79, 965 (1971)

23 DUCHAINE, J., SPAPEN, R., JACQUES, M.: L'allergie à l'A.C.T.H. – étude expérimentale. Rev. franç. Allerg. 2, 15 (1962)

24 FALLIERS, C.J., CHAI, H., MOLK, L., BANE, H., CARDOSO, R.R. DE A.: Pulmonary and adrenal effects of alternate-day corticosteroid therapy. J. Allergy 49, 156 (1972)

25 FELBER, J.-P., ASHCROFT, S.H.J.: The relationship between structure and antigenicity and properties of ACTH. In: Abstr. Europ. Biochem. Soc., Vienna 1965, p. 225

26 Felber, J.-P., Ashcroft, S.H.J., Villanueva, A., Vannotti, A.: Antibodies to synthetic corticotrophin. Nature (Lond.) 211, 654 (1966)

27 Fleischer, N., Givens, J.R., Abe, K., Nicholson, W.E., Liddle, G.W.: Studies of ACTH antibodies and their reactions with inactive analogues of ACTH. J. clin. Invest. 44, 1047 (1965); abstract of paper

28 Fournier, A.: Etat fonctionnel de l'axe hypothalamo-hypophyso-corticosurré-nalien après corticothérapie prolongée. Rev. Prat. (Paris) 16, 1698 (1966)

29 Frouchtman, R.: Premiers résultats cliniques obtenus avec une nouvelle corti-costimuline de synthèse d'action retard: Synacthen Retard. Praxis 57, 845 (1968)

30 Gelzer, J.: Immunochemical study of β-corticotropin-(1–24)-tetracosa-pep-tide. Immunochemistry 5, 23 (1968)

31 Graber, A.L., Ney, R.L., Nicholson, W.E., Island, D.P., Liddle, G.W.: Natural history of pituitary-adrenal recovery following long-term suppression with corticosteroids. J. clin. Endocr. 25, 11 (1965)

32 Halpern, B.N., Jacob, M., Binaghi, B., Macquet, V.: Etude clinique et expérimentale de l'allergie provoquée par la corticostimuline hypophysaire A.C.T.H. Rev. franç. Allerg. 1, 188 (1961); abstract of paper

33 Harter, J.G., Reddy, W.J., Thorn, G.W.: Studies on an intermittent corti-costeroid dosage regimen. New Engl. J. Med. 269, 591 (1963)

34 Hill, B.H.R., Swinburn, P.D.: Death from corticotrophin. Lancet i, 1218 (1954)

35 Imura, H., Sparks, L.L., Grodsky, G.M., Forsham, P.H.: Immunologic studies of adrenocorticotropic hormone (ACTH): dissociation of biologic and immunologic activities. J. clin. Endocr. 25, 1361 (1965)

36 Imura, H., Sparks, L.L., Tosaka, M., Hane, S., Grodsky, G.M., Forsham, P.H.: Immunologic studies of adrenocorticotropic hormone (ACTH): effect of carboxypeptidase digestion on biologic and immunologic activities. J. clin. Endocr. 27, 15 (1967)

37 Jaques, R., Brugger, M.: Synthetic polypeptides related to corticotrophin acting as histamine liberators. Pharmacology (Basle) 2, 361 (1969)

38 Jasani, M.K.: Possible modes of action of ACTH and glucocorticoids in allergic diseases. Clin. Allergy 2, 141 (1972)

39 Landon, J., Wynn, V., Wood, J.B.: Adrenal response to infused corticotropin in subjects receiving glucocorticoids. J. clin. Endocr. 25, 602 (1965)

40 Massias, P.: A.C.T.H.-thérapie en rhumatologie, loc. cit.[8], p. 41

41 Panzani, R.: Une nouvelle ACTH purifiée dans le traitement de la maladie asthmatique. Etude clinique. Rev. franç. Allerg. 6, 93 (1966)

42 Pasteur Vallery-Radot, Wolfromm, R., Charpin, J., Halpern, B.N.: Maladies allergiques (Flammarion, Paris 1963)

43 Portner, M.M., Thayer, K.H., Harter, J.G., Rayyis, S., Liang, T.C., Kent, J.R.: Successful initiation of alternate-day prednisone in chronic steroid-dependent asthmatic patients. J. Allergy 49, 16 (1972)

44 Quarles van Ufford, W.J.: Sudden death during prolonged treatment with ACTH. Int. Arch. Allergy 3, 229 (1952)

45 Rajka, G.: On the prophylactic possibilities in ACTH allergy. Acta allerg. (Kbh.) 16, 159 (1961)

46 Reichling, G.H., Klingman, A.M.: Alternate-day corticosteroid therapy. Arch. Derm. 83, 980 (1961)

47 Savage, O., Copeman, W.S.C., Chapman, L., Wells, M.V., Treadwell, B.L.J.: Pituitary and adrenal hormones in rheumatoid arthritis. Lancet i, 232 (1962)

48 Salvin, S.B., Liauw, H.L.: Hypersensitivity to peptide fragments. Allergy appl. Immunol. 31, 366 (1967)

49 Schwyzer, R., Sieber, P.: Total synthesis of adrenocorticotrophic hormone. Nature (Lond.) 199, 172 (1963)

50 SCHWYZER, R., SIEBER, P.: Synthetic peptides with ACTH activity. Amer. Rev. Biochem. *33*, 374 (1964)

51 SERAFINI, U.: In tema di diagnosi e terapia dell'asma bronchiale. Rif. med. *83*, 67 (1969)

52 STEVENSON, C.R.: Discussion on Brown, E.M., Jr., Hollander, J.L., loc. cit.[11], p.394

53 SVEDMYR, N., ANDERSSON, R., BERGH, N.P., MALMBERG, R.: Relaxing effect of ACTH on human bronchial muscle in vitro. Scand. J. resp. Dis. *51*, 171 (1970)

54 TRAEGER, C.H.: Discussion on Clark, W.S.: Changes produced by the administration of ACTH and cortisone in rheumatoid arthritis. In Mote, J.R. (Editor): Proc. Ist Clin. ACTH Conf., p. 356 (Blakiston, Philadelphia/Toronto 1950)

55 TREADWELL, B.L.J., SAVAGE, O., SEVER, E.D., COPEMAN, W.S.C.: Pituitary-adrenal function during corticosteroid therapy. Lancet *i*, 355 (1963)

56 TURIAF, J., BASSET, G., GEORGES, R., JEANJEAN, Y., BATTESTI, J.-P.: Complications et répercussions hormono-sécrétoires de la cortisonothérapie au long cours appliquée au traitement de l'asthme à dyspnée continue. Bull. Soc. med. Hôp. Paris *114*, 10 (1963)

57 UZZAN, D.: Discussion on Charpin, J., Aubert, J., loc. cit.[8], p. 127

58 UZZAN, D., CHEBAT, J., OLLIERO, H., ISRAEL-ASSELAIN, R.: Traitement des bronchopathies obstructives par le tétracosapeptide retard (corticostimuline synthétique). Presse méd. *77*, 1485 (1969)

59 WILSON, L.A.: Protein shock from intravenous A.C.T.H. Lancet *261*, 478 (1951)

60 WILTNER, W.: L'effet de l'ACTH synthétique à 28 éléments amino-acides, sur les fonctions de la glande surrénale et sur l'asthme bronchique. In: VIIth Int. Congr. Allerg., Florence 1970, Abstr., Int. Congr. Ser. No. 211, p. 122 (Excerpta med., Amsterdam 1970)

61 WOLFROMM, R., HERMAN, D.: L'allergie médicamenteuse à l'ACTH: ses manifestations cliniques, ses moyens de prévention. Sem. Hôp. Paris *43*, 1252 (1967)

62 WOLFROMM, R., HERMAN, D.: La β^{1-24}corticotropine ou tétracosactide dans l'asthme et les maladies allergiques. Thérapeutique (Sem. Hôp. Paris) *45*, 131 (1969)

Discussion

M. GIORDANO: One question concerning the skin sensitivity test: is the corticotrophin or Synacthen injected intracutaneously or subcutaneously? And is the test likely to give rise to any dangerous reactions?

J. AUBERT: When performing skin tests with a view to detecting allergy to A.C.T.H., it is our practice to give the injection intracutaneously. In a preliminary study, in which we carried out several series of skin tests in healthy controls, we came to the conclusion that the only tests to which any significance can be ascribed are those in which the subject shows a positive reaction to a dilution of 1:100; I don't think that such tests are liable to give rise to dangerous allergic reactions of the type sometimes observed with penicillin, for example.

J. GELZER: I should also be interested to hear from Dr. AUBERT at what time he recorded the results of these skin tests, since this might shed some light on the type of antibodies involved.

J. AUBERT: When testing for immediate allergic reactions, we record the response to the intracutaneous injection within the first 20 minutes, and we take no account of delayed reactions observed at the 24th or the 48th hour.

T. B. BINNS: Despite the advent of disodium cromoglycate and of betamethasone-dipropionate aerosols, asthma is still a major indication for Synacthen Depot in the United Kingdom, where it is usually treated with intramuscular doses of about 0.5 mg. once or twice a week—or half this dose in children, who accept and tolerate it very well. Sometimes the interval between injections is even longer, because asthma is one of the conditions in which the clinical benefit outlasts the plasma cortisol response by quite a considerable margin. Now this is a phenomenon which interests me, because this does not seem to happen with prednisolone, the effect of which lasts

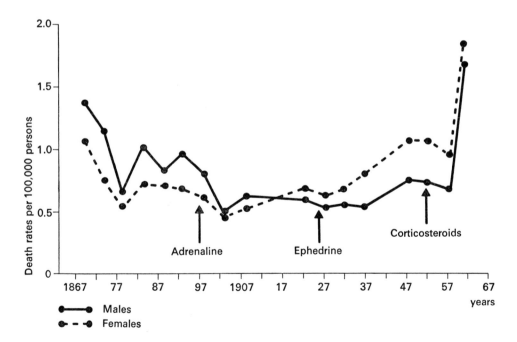

Fig. 1. Death rates from asthma in England and Wales (1867–1966) among males and females aged 5–34 years.

241

Table 1. Plasma cortisol levels before (zero column) and 1, 4, 8, and 24 hours after administration of 1.0 mg. Synacthen Depot in five patients with severe asthma.

Patient No.	Sex	Age	Plasma cortisol—mcg./100 ml. at (hr)				
			Zero	1	4	8	24
16	F	16	20	43	57	75	69
17	F	58	18	52	60	90	110
18	M	49	16	30	68	68	48
19	M	56	16	25	49	82	54
20	F	21	18	43	57	76	42
	Mean		17.6	39	58	78	65
	(± S.E.M.)		(0.74)	(4.88)	(3.05)	(3.68)	(12.20)

only for 8–12 hours. I should therefore like to ask whether anyone here can offer an explanation for this prolongation of the clinical response to Synacthen Depot as compared with the plasma cortisol response.

I have two slides which may be of interest in this connection. Both of them were kindly loaned to me by Dr. T. CLARK of Guy's Hospital in London. The first one (Figure 1) shows the death rates from asthma in England and Wales over the past 100 years. It is surprising to observe that the advent of adrenaline, ephedrine, and the corticosteroids evidently had remarkably little influence on the mortality. The enormous peak at the end has been ascribed to the misuse of aerosols containing isoprenaline; it has been estimated, in fact, that during the years 1961 to 1967 the deaths of some 3,500 patients may well have been due to the excessive use of these aerosols. As soon as this was realised, warnings were addressed both to members of the medical profession and to the public, with the result that the death rate from asthma has since rapidly declined again.

Shown in the next slide (Table 1) are data from a study, carried out at the Brompton Hospital and at Guy's Hospital, in which Dr. CLARK and Dr. COLLINS employed various forms of treatment in patients suffering from severe asthma, most of whom could more or less be described as cases of status asthmaticus. In this slide we have data on five patients who, upon their admission to hospital, were given treatment with Synacthen Depot. In the zero time column the mean figure for their plasma cortisol was 17.6 mcg./100 ml. Their plasma cortisol was thus hardly elevated at all, whereas one might have expected to find quite a marked increase under the stress of severe asthma. This, I think, is rather surprising. On the other hand, the patients reacted very well to Synacthen Depot, in terms both of their plasma cortisol levels and of the clinical response. In fact, their response to this regime was every bit as good as the response to intravenous steroids. Incidentally, I should like to add that infusion treatment with A.C.T.H., which used to be given at one time, can now be regarded as quite outmoded. As Dr. GRANT* in Glasgow pointed out in a brief note published in the Lancet, the response to intramuscular Synacthen Depot is just as rapid as the response to ordinary Synacthen given intravenously.

R. SCHUPPLI: Have you any idea, Dr. BINNS, what the precise causes of death were in all these asthma patients who died in the 1960s?

T. B. BINNS: I cannot say for certain, but it seems probable that the abuse of these isoprenaline-containing aerosols gave rise to cardiac arrhythmias. Though various other possibilities have been suggested, I think that this is the most likely explanation.

242   *GRANT, J. K.: Response to tetracosactrin. Lancet i, 371 (1969)

The use of A.C.T.H. in the treatment of neurological diseases

by R.-J.Wüthrich*

It is not surprising that neurology should be one of the branches of medicine in which treatment with adrenocortical hormones and with A.C.T.H. continues to command keen interest. For many diseases of the peripheral and central nervous systems no form of causal therapy has so far been discovered—usually for the simple reason that not enough research has yet been done on the aetiology and pathogenesis of the conditions in question. Hence the eagerness with which clinicians have seized upon the possibility of attenuating or improving the clinical course of these diseases by recourse to non-specific forms of treatment; from the very beginning, empirical studies in this connection have embraced quite a wide field of pathology, the main emphasis, however, being placed on those diseases that are associated with inflammatory processes and immunological reactions.

Although A.C.T.H. has already been employed in the treatment of neurological diseases for more than 20 years, we still do not seem to have come to the end of the stage of empirical investigation. This is bound up with the difficulties encountered in demonstrating significant and reproducible therapeutic effects in chronic diseases of the nervous system, some of which are also relatively uncommon. A review of the current status of A.C.T.H. therapy in this domain must therefore inevitably be somewhat tentative and incomplete. On the other hand, the excessive optimism with which the advent of A.C.T.H. was first greeted has meanwhile given way to a more critical evaluation, thanks to which—in some areas at least—a broad consensus of opinion and certain acceptable guidelines have emerged. It is with these aspects of practical importance that I chiefly propose to deal here.

In the course of the years, attempts have also repeatedly been made in the realm of neurological diseases to draw distinctions between the indications for A.C.T.H. and those for the glucocorticoids. This, too, is a task that has not yet been completed, and a great deal of further fundamental research will no doubt be required before this problem can be adequately clarified. In none of the diseases to which I shall be referring here has it been really convincingly demonstrated that with A.C.T.H. it is possible to achieve therapeutic results which are clearly superior to those yielded by corticosteroids. The choice in favour of A.C.T.H. therapy has tended, to some extent at least, to be dictated by extraneous reasons, such as the fact that previous authors may have recommended it for a given disease. Although a greater body of critical experience has been acquired with A.C.T.H. than with other drugs of relevance in this

---

* Neurologische Universitätsklinik, Basle, Switzerland.

context, this should not tempt us to overlook the imperfect nature of our basic knowledge concerning A.C.T.H. therapy.

Treatment with A.C.T.H. is now widely resorted to in the following neurological diseases:

Multiple sclerosis, including retrobulbar neuritis
Myasthenia gravis
Hypsarrhythmia
Bell's palsy
Guillain-Barré syndrome
Cerebral oedema.

To this list must be added a few other conditions which, strictly speaking, do not fall within the compass of neurology, i.e. the neurological manifestations of collagen diseases (lupus erythematosus, dermatomyositis, and periarteritis nodosa), neurological features of the various rheumatic and rheumatoid illnesses, and infections involving the central nervous system (encephalomyelitis). In the present paper, the principal emphasis will be placed on multiple sclerosis and myasthenia gravis, the remaining indications being touched upon only briefly.

Multiple sclerosis

There is probably no other neurological syndrome in which it is more difficult to evaluate the effect of treatment than in demyelinating processes. The chronicity of the disease, the extreme variability of the clinical course, and the high spontaneous remission rate during the early stages of the illness pose almost insuperable problems for an investigator responsible for the conduct of a clinical trial. The fact that these problems have nevertheless been tackled time and again is no doubt a reflection of the feeling of impotence and desperation stemming from previous attempts at treatment, coupled with the expectation or hope—prompted by theoretical considerations and the results of animal experiments—that A.C.T.H. might indeed exert a positive effect. Since inflammatory processes, immunopathological mechanisms, and reparative reactions are predominant features of the pathology of multiple sclerosis, it was a logical step to resort to a symptomatic form of treatment which combats inflammation and exudation, suppresses immune responses, and inhibits mesenchymal reactions. Moreover, in the experimental model of multiple sclerosis, i.e. allergic encephalomyelitis induced in animals by the injection of cerebral antigens, it was soon discovered[9] that A.C.T.H. did in fact produce a beneficial effect.

Early clinical studies, including those of ALEXANDER et al.[1, 2] in particular, appeared at first to confirm the expectations that had been placed in A.C.T.H., and only a few sceptics raised their voices to dampen the optimism which such publications initially aroused. These earlier reports, some of which were based on trials involving large numbers of cases, will not be discussed in detail here. Suffice it to say that they had two main shortcomings: firstly, insufficient attention was paid to the fact that in patients suffering from multiple sclerosis

A.C.T.H. therapy also produces effects which have no direct bearing on the disease process as such; and, secondly, the results were assessed without having made provision for adequate controls.

The non-specific effects of treatment with A.C.T.H. may assume a wide variety of forms in multiple sclerosis. In certain patients, for example, the pronounced euphoria induced by A.C.T.H., one of the salient features of which is enhancement of drive, may sometimes create the erroneous impression that an improvement has actually occurred in the neurological symptoms. A beneficial influence on muscle spasm and on secondary changes affecting the locomotor system in immobilised patients can also repeatedly be observed in cases of multiple sclerosis treated with A.C.T.H. The possibility of a placebo effect must likewise be borne in mind, since in chronic cases the adoption of an active approach to therapy may be sufficient in itself to produce strong psychological repercussions. Another point to be considered in this connection is the fact that, when a course of A.C.T.H. therapy is decided upon, the patient is often admitted to hospital to receive the treatment, and that here various other therapeutically effective measures are taken which would perhaps otherwise have been omitted.

Only in rare cases of multiple sclerosis would these various "positive side effects" of A.C.T.H. in themselves justify recourse to the drug's use, because the same effects can also be achieved with other forms of treatment.

But it is not only for the reasons I have just outlined that controlled trials with A.C.T.H. are necessary in order to obtain valid data on the therapeutic efficacy of such medication; another reason is that so little is known about the spontaneous clinical course of multiple sclerosis in a given group of patients that only a comparison between treated and untreated cases bearing as close as possible a resemblance to one another can be expected to yield findings that are at all reliable. To date, eight controlled studies of this kind have been published [1, 2, 5, 7, 17, 18, 23, 25-27].

Seven of them deal with short-term therapy administered chiefly during acute exacerbations of multiple sclerosis, and only one describes the results of long-term treatment.

The "cooperative study in the evaluation of therapy in multiple sclerosis" which was carried out by ten large American hospitals and published in 1970 [26, 27] can at present be regarded as providing the most authoritative verdict on short-term treatment. The results obtained in this large-scale investigation tally fairly closely with the findings reported in the other controlled trials.

In this study, 103 cases of multiple sclerosis treated with A.C.T.H. during acute exacerbations were compared and contrasted with 94 controls. The treatment, which lasted two weeks, took the form of A.C.T.H. gel given in daily intramuscular doses of 80 units for one week, followed by 40 units for a further four days and 20 units on the last three days.

Before, during, and after this course of treatment, the condition of the patients was recorded and statistically evaluated on the basis of a sophisticated system of tests and examinations.

In the tests performed at weekly intervals after the start of therapy, a significantly higher improvement rate was observed in the A.C.T.H.-treated patients during the first three weeks. As was to be expected, however, the control group also showed quite a high improvement rate: for example, an improvement—in terms of the global clinical impression—was registered in approximately one-half of the controls after one week of placebo treatment, as compared with an improvement in 70% of the patients who had been receiving A.C.T.H. for one week. From week to week the improvement rates increased in both the A.C.T.H. group and the control group, though among the controls the increase occurred more abruptly. By the end of the fourth week after the start of the fortnight's course of treatment, the difference between the two groups was no longer statistically significant with respect to all the criteria of assessment employed. Looking back over the study in retrospect, the authors very much regret that they did not make provision for more prolonged follow-up periods. Consequently, although the acute exacerbations evidently subsided more rapidly in the patients treated with A.C.T.H., the investigation failed to shed any light on the possible value of the treatment with regard to the overall course of the illness.

In this connection, reference should also be made to the very carefully controlled trial conducted by RAWSON et al.[23], in which treatment was given for retrobulbar neuritis. Here, in 25 patients treated for 30 days with daily intramuscular injections of 40 units of A.C.T.H. gel, a significantly better and more rapid improvement in vision was observed than in 25 untreated cases. In this study too, however, the findings obtained in the two groups showed a progressive tendency to coincide as the trial continued. Consequently, the results reported merely indicate once again that treatment with A.C.T.H. is capable of cutting short the duration of acute exacerbations. That A.C.T.H. also exerts a beneficial influence on the long-term repercussions of these acute bouts of inflammation must therefore remain pure supposition.

It is from the study undertaken in Ireland by MILLAR et al.[17] that the best impression of the effects of long-term A.C.T.H. therapy in multiple sclerosis can be gained. In this trial, 181 patients treated with daily intramuscular doses of 15–25 units of A.C.T.H. gel for 18 months were compared with 169 untreated controls. The A.C.T.H. therapy proved unable to reduce either the frequency or the severity of fresh acute attacks, and the condition of the treated patients at the end of their long-term medication was no better than that of the controls. Moreover, such were the side effects of the treatment that MILLAR et al. consider long-term A.C.T.H. therapy to be unjustified in this indication. After the 18-month period of treatment had been completed, however, the withdrawal of A.C.T.H. at least had no adverse effects on the subsequent course of the disease[16].

Although the problem of tolerability plays, of course, a bigger role in patients receiving prolonged treatment, A.C.T.H. is also liable to provoke side effects even when given on a short-term basis and even when the customary measures have been taken to avoid them. On the other hand, psychotic episodes, peptic ulcers, gastric haemorrhages, and complications due to infection are such rare occurrences that, in my opinion, the benefit to be derived from short-term A.C.T.H. therapy outweighs the risk of these side effects.

The current status of A.C.T.H. therapy for multiple sclerosis can be summed up as follows:

Experience indicates that short-term treatment with A.C.T.H. is justified during acute exacerbations, since there is reason to hope that such therapy may shorten the duration of the exacerbation and attenuate its residual effects. In mild exacerbations showing a tendency towards rapid spontaneous regression, however, A.C.T.H. is not necessary. The more severe an acute attack, and the longer it persists, the greater the justification for A.C.T.H. therapy becomes. Although yet to be confirmed by evidence from controlled trials, the impression nevertheless exists that in cases of multiple sclerosis where the disease is rapidly worsening, or where severe exacerbations are failing to regress satisfactorily, treatment with A.C.T.H. may bring about a turn for the better.

Long-term A.C.T.H. therapy involves a greater element of risk and is seldom, if ever, justified. A.C.T.H. is probably unsuitable for use in cases in which the disease is either stationary or progressing only slowly. The mode of action of A.C.T.H. in acute exacerbations of multiple sclerosis has not yet been adequately investigated[3]. Whether the drug merely acts by combating oedema[17], or whether the other effects exerted by A.C.T.H. also enter into play in this connection, is still a moot point. Treatment with A.C.T.H. is unlikely to entail a much lower incidence of side effects than treatment with brief courses of corticosteroid medication. The claim made by certain authors[18] that A.C.T.H. proves more effective in multiple sclerosis than corticosteroid therapy has, in my view, yet to be satisfactorily substantiated.

As regards the approach to be adopted in practice when administering treatment with A.C.T.H., there are various possible alternatives. But the choice of preparation, the dosage schedule selected, and attempts to adapt the medication to the patient's circadian rhythm appear to have relatively little influence on the overall effect of the therapy.

The dosage scheme which we ourselves employ is as follows: 1 mg. ®Synacthen Depot daily by the intramuscular route for ten days, followed by reduction of the dosage over a period of two to three weeks, care being taken at the same time to adhere to the precautions which should always be observed when administering A.C.T.H.

Myasthenia gravis

Following earlier, somewhat discouraging attempts to treat myasthenia gravis with A.C.T.H., it is only during recent years that the drug's use in certain types of case and under certain carefully defined conditions has gained acceptance. Only in large centres is it possible to acquire sufficient experience to enable a verdict to be reached on the value of A.C.T.H. in this disease [6, 12, 13, 19-22, 28].

Curiously enough, in those cases which respond to the treatment, therapeutically adequate doses of A.C.T.H. initially produce a deterioration in the clinical picture. On or around the third day of medication with daily doses of 100–200 units of A.C.T.H., the patient develops increased muscular weakness and shows a diminished response to cholinesterase inhibitors. Not until the A.C.T.H. is withdrawn does the patient's condition undergo an improvement—an improvement which in many cases contrasts very favourably with the clinical picture prior to the treatment. The amelioration, however, is usually of limited duration, i.e. it persists only for a few weeks or months. A renewed therapeutic effect can be achieved by repeating the course of treatment; and it may sometimes also prove possible to prolong partial remissions by resorting to intermittent doses of A.C.T.H.[6, 12].

The initial deterioration under treatment with A.C.T.H. is an almost invariable prelude to a good response in cases of myasthenia gravis. This deterioration, as well as the subsequent improvement, appears to some extent to be related to the severity of the clinical picture prior to the start of medication: the more severe the illness, the greater the likelihood of its responding favourably to the treatment[20, 21].

In the light of experience acquired in the studies already mentioned, it has come to be accepted that A.C.T.H. therapy is indicated in those severe and very severe cases of myasthenia in which other forms of treatment are unable to elicit any improvement. In such cases the initial worsening of the patient's condition quite often leads to respiratory failure, with the result that artificial respiration proves necessary, not only while the A.C.T.H. treatment is actually in progress but usually also for a certain time after it has been terminated. For this reason, A.C.T.H. therapy should be attempted only in very well-equipped hospitals in which all possible intensive-care facilities are available.

Why patients with myasthenia gravis show an initial deterioration in response to A.C.T.H. is a question about which no more is known than about the reasons for the partial remission that occurs when the treatment is withdrawn. Electrophysiological studies[11, 19] have merely revealed that A.C.T.H. exerts an effect on the actual mechanism of neuromuscular transmission, an effect which may possibly be due to its influence on the resynthesis of acetylcholine. It has long been known from experience that in severe cases of myasthenia the complete withdrawal of cholinesterase inhibitors—under cover of artificial respiration—may result in some degree of remission, or at least may make it possible subsequently to manage with smaller doses of cholinesterase inhibitors. At this point, however, it should be added that patients reacting favourably to A.C.T.H. therapy have also included cases which had previously shown no improvement in response to an interruption of treatment with cholinesterase inhibitors under cover of artificial respiration[21].

In myasthenia gravis, a therapeutic effect at least partially comparable with that of A.C.T.H. can likewise be achieved with glucocorticoids; but I am not aware that any major studies have been conducted with high dosages of glucocorticoids.

A summary review of results obtained with A.C.T.H. therapy in myasthenia gravis has been published by NAMBA et al.[21], according to whom some temporary improvement can be expected to occur in 87% of cases. Neither the previous duration of the illness nor the pathological findings obtained at a thymectomy appear to have much bearing on the response to treatment with A.C.T.H. Patients who have already undergone thymectomy have still been found to derive benefit from A.C.T.H. In addition, A.C.T.H. is also suitable for use as preparatory medication prior to thymectomy in particularly severe cases.

Hypsarrhythmia

The syndrome referred to as "lightning seizures", "infantile spasms", or "propulsive petit mal" is characterised among other things by electro-encephalographic findings indicative of hypsarrhythmia—a distinctive form of reaction on the part of the infantile brain to various types of noxa. Experience has shown that these seizures respond favourably to A.C.T.H. therapy and probably also just as well to treatment with glucocorticoids. The therapeutic effect of such hormone therapy appears to be attributable, not so much to the influence it may exert on the underlying disorder itself, but rather to the fact that it reduces the child's susceptibility to the attacks. The prognosis in cases of hypsarrhythmia depends primarily upon the severity of the brain disease as such and only secondarily upon the nature of the epileptic manifestations. Hormone therapy is indicated in cases where the prognosis does not seem to be all that bad, but where other forms of treatment have failed to eliminate the seizures [8]. A.C.T.H. medication should be commenced with a high dosage and, following cessation of the attacks, continued for a period of weeks to months with gradually diminishing doses[10, 15]. It must be given in combination with anti-epileptic drugs. Since the introduction of the diazepam derivatives, the indications for A.C.T.H. in the treatment of hypsarrhythmia have become more restricted.

Bell's palsy

Opinions still differ as to the value of corticosteroid or A.C.T.H. therapy in Bell's palsy (idiopathic facial paralysis). Data from a recent statistical study[29], however, would appear to bear out the claim that, provided A.C.T.H. therapy is instituted early on after the onset of the paralysis, such treatment is indeed justified. But in this indication it is very doubtful whether A.C.T.H. is superior to oral corticoid medication.

Guillain-Barré syndrome

Patients with Guillain-Barré syndrome (acute polyradiculoneuritis) often recover spontaneously, provided there are no grave complications, such as respiratory paralysis, to blight the victim's prospects of survival. Consequently, in mild cases there is no need to resort to treatment with corticosteroids or A.C.T.H., especially since such treatment is hardly likely to speed recovery and involves a relatively high risk of provoking complications. In severe cases, on the other hand, there is more to be said for instituting hormone therapy; particularly in cases where the disease runs a slowly progressive course, such therapy may—as in multiple sclerosis—occasionally bring about a decisive turn for the better[14].

Cerebral oedema

Corticosteroids have now assumed a role of major practical importance in the treatment of cerebral oedema. In many cases it is possible with their aid to keep even critically dangerous cerebral-compression syndromes under control and to produce responses similar to those achieved with injections of hypertonic solutions and with other specific measures designed to eliminate excess fluid. The use of A.C.T.H. in combination with oxytocin, as advocated by BERNARD-WEIL and BUISSON-FEREY[4] in particular, seems to offer no appreciable advantages over treatment with glucocorticoids in this indication, since in most instances it is in any case only short-term medication that is required; there is still a need, however, for controlled comparative trials in order to differentiate between the relative merits of these two forms of treatment[4, 24].

References

1 ALEXANDER, L., BERKELEY, A.W., ALEXANDER, A.M.: Multiple sclerosis. Prognosis and treatment (Thomas, Springfield, Ill. 1961)
2 ALEXANDER, L., CASS, L.J.: The present status of ACTH therapy in multiple sclerosis. Ann. intern. Med. *58*, 454 (1963)
3 ALEXANDER, L., CASS, L.J.: ACTH-induced adrenocortical response patterns in multiple sclerosis and their relation to the clinical effectiveness of ACTH therapy. Confin. neurol. (Basle) *33*, 1 (1971)
4 BERNARD-WEIL, E., BUISSON-FEREY, J.: Effects of an association between oxytocin and ACTH on the EEG and clinical evolution of some cerebral diseases. Electroenceph. clin. Neurophysiol. *21*, 601 (1969)
5 BLOMBERG, L.H.: Comments on treatment of multiple sclerosis with ACTH. Acta neurol. scand. *41*, Suppl. 13/Part II: 485 (1965)
6 CAPE, C.A., UTTERBACK, R.A.: Treatment of myasthenia gravis with adrenocorticotropic hormone (ACTH): massive short-term and maintenance treatment. J. Neurol. Neurosurg. Psychiat. *32*, 290 (1969)
7 CENDROWSKI, W.S.: Follow-up study on corticotrophin treatment of multiple sclerosis. Psychiat. et Neurol. (Basle) *154*, 65 (1967)
8 CHEVRIE, J.J., AICARDI, J.: Le pronostic psychique des spasmes infantiles traités par l'ACTH ou les corticoïdes. J. neurol. Sci. *12*, 351 (1971)
9 FIELD, E.J., MILLER, H.: Experimental allergic encephalomyelitis: comparison of protective effects of prednisolone and corticotrophin. Brit. med. J. *i*, 843 (1962)
10 GAMSTORP, I.: Pediatric neurology, p. 102 (Butterworths, London 1970)
11 GANDIGLIO, G., PINELLI, P.: EMG analysis of myasthenic ACTH deterioration. Europ. neurol. *1*, 2 (1968)
12 GIBBERT, F.B., NAVAB, F., SMITH, C.L.: Treatment of ocular myasthenia with corticotrophin. J. Neurol. Neurosurg. Psychiat. *34*, 11 (1971)
13 GROB, D., NAMBA, T.: Corticotropin in generalized myasthenia gravis. Effect of short, intensive courses. J. Amer. med. Ass. *198*, 703 (1966)
14 HELLER, G.I., DE JONG, R.N.: Treatment of the Guillain-Barré syndrome. Use of corticotrophin and glucocorticoids. Arch. Neurol. (Chic.) *8*, 179 (1963)
15 KRUSE, R.: Epilepsie-Therapie im Kindesalter. Pädiat. Fortbild. Prax. *26*, 85 (1969)
16 MILLAR, J.D.H., RAHMAN, R., VAS, C.J., NORONHA, M.J., LIVERSEDGE, L.A., SWINBURN, W.R.: Effect of withdrawal of corticotrophin in patients on long-term treatment for multiple sclerosis. Lancet *i*, 700 (1970)

17 MILLAR, J. D. H., VAS, C. J., NORONHA, M. J., LIVERSEDGE, L. A., RAWSON, M. D.:
Long-term treatment of multiple sclerosis with corticotrophin. Lancet *ii*, 429
(1967)

18 MILLER, H., NEWELL, D. J., RIDLEY, A.: Multiple sclerosis. Treatment of acute
exacerbations with corticotrophin (A.C.T.H.). Lancet *ii*, 1120 (1961)

19 NAMBA, T.: Corticotropin therapy in patients with myasthenia gravis. Arch.
Neurol. (Chic.) *26*, 144 (1972)

20 NAMBA, T., SHAPIRO, M. S.: Corticotrophin therapy in patients with myasthenia
gravis: steroid metabolism and histology of skeletal muscle and thymus. J. Neurol.
Sci. *16*, 165 (1972)

21 NAMBA, T., SHAPIRO, M.S , BRUNNER, N. G., GROB, D.: Corticotropin therapy
in myasthenia gravis: indications and limitations. Neurology (Minneap.) *20*,
385 (1970); abstract of paper

22 OSSERMAN, K. E., GENKINS, G.: Studies in myasthenia gravis. Short-term massive
corticotropin therapy. J. Amer. med. Ass. *198*, 699 (1966)

23 RAWSON, M. D., LIVERSEDGE, L. A., GOLDFARB, G.: Treatment of acute retrobulbar neuritis with corticotrophin. Lancet *ii*, 1044 (1966)

24 REULEN, H. J., SCHÜRMANN, K. (Editors): Steroids and brain edema (Springer,
Berlin/Heidelberg/New York 1972)

25 RINNE, U. K., SONNINEN, V., TUOVINEN, T.: Corticotrophin treatment in multiple sclerosis. Acta neurol. scand. *44*, 207 (1968)

26 ROSE, A. S., KUZMA, J. W., KURTZKE, J. F., NAMEROW, N. S., SIBLEY, W. A.,
TOURTELLOTTE, W. W.: Cooperative study in the evaluation of therapy in mul-
tiple sclerosis: ACTH vs placebo. Final report. Neurology (Minneap.) *20*,
No. 5/Part 2 (1970)

27 ROSE, A. S., KUZMA, J. W., KURTZKE, J. F., SIBLEY, W. A., TOURTELLOTTE, W. W.:
Cooperative study in the evaluation of therapy in multiple sclerosis; ACTH vs
placebo in acute exacerbations. Preliminary report. Neurology (Minneap.) *18*,
No. 6/Part 2 (1968)

28 SHAPIRO, M. S., NAMBA, T., GROB, D.: Corticotropin therapy and thymectomy
in management of myasthenia gravis. Arch. Neurol. (Chic.) *24*, 65 (1971)

29 TAVERNER, D., COHEN, S. B., HUTCHINSON, B. C.: Comparison of corticotrophin
and prednisolone in treatment of idiopathic facial paralysis (Bell's palsy). Brit.
med. J. *iv*, 20 (1971)

Discussion

H. J. BAUER: First of all, I would like to compliment Dr. WÜTHRICH on his critical selection of what he considers to be valid evidence for A.C.T.H. therapy in neurological disease. He has already said the essential things; permit me to make only some marginal comments:

Dr. WÜTHRICH summarised the cooperative A.C.T.H. study carried out in the U.S.A. by ten of the finest neurological centres in the world and supported by the N.I.H. It was perhaps the most perfectionistic, expensive, and time-consuming study of this type ever conducted, but, with respect to its ultimate results, it remained somewhat delphic. I quote from the final report published in Confinia neurologica*: "Short-term, high-dosage use of ACTH hastened the evidences of improvement of symptoms and signs, but it cannot be stated from the data of this study that the ultimate extent of improvement was greater than that attained by placebo."

The N.I.H. study may possibly have been a futile investment, because the course of A.C.T.H. therapy was too brief. It may well be, moreover, that many other neurological endeavours to influence multiple sclerosis by corticotrophin therapy have likewise been unsuccessful because certain basic prerequisites were not fulfilled. After having listened to the contributions at this meeting, I am beginning to feel that our own attempts might fall into this category.

In his endocrinological laboratory, Prof. REISERT carried out measurements on some of our neurological patients and demonstrated that the daily injection of 1 mg. of synthetic A.C.T.H. led to a therapeutically effective elevation of endogenous cortisol production over a period of about six hours, and that under this treatment the diurnal rhythm of the adrenotrophic system and the endogenous stress reactions were maintained. In view of the problematic nature *per se* of A.C.T.H. therapy in M.S., this reassured us, and we felt that treatment of this type should be tried. Accordingly, for the past three years we have been treating most of our hospitalised M.S. patients suffering from acute bouts or exacerbations with a four-week course of Synacthen given in a dosage of 1 mg. every morning. This was not a controlled study, but it may serve to indicate what sort of results can be attained with Synacthen in the treatment of M.S. in a reasonably well-equipped neurological department.

The 123 cases treated with Synacthen comprised approximately one-third of the total number of consecutive cases of M.S. admitted to the neurological department of the University of Göttingen during the past four years. They were classified according to certainty of diagnosis as clinically definite, probable, confirmed by autopsy, and questionable (Table 1). The 17 clinically questionable cases were omitted from the following evaluation. A patient was considered as improved if there was a gain of at least one point on the disability scale graded 0–10. Patients with only subjective improvement were not classified as improved.

By these criteria almost two-thirds of the patients (37 out of 57) with bouts and remissions improved in response to a four-week course of Synacthen and 20 did not improve; by contrast, only 17 out of the 49 chronic cases showed improvement (Table 2). There was a similar correlation with regard to duration of the disease (Table 3): 14 out of 17 patients with M.S. of less than one year's standing improved, whereas subsequently the figures were almost evenly distributed; four cases of very long standing—over 20 years—showed no improvement. With respect to the degree of disability, the mild forms responded well, while the majority of the severe forms did not improve (Table 4). This series thus reflects the well-established experience that early cases with a course of bouts and remissions respond more favourably to Synacthen therapy than the chronic, long-standing, severe cases.

---

* ALEXANDER, L., CASS, L. J.: ACTH-induced adrenocortical response patterns in multiple sclerosis and their relation to the clinical effectiveness of ACTH therapy. Confin. neurol. (Basle) *33*, 1 (1971)

Table 1. Cases of multiple sclerosis treated with Synacthen. Patients classified according to certainty of diagnosis.

Total number of cases		123
comprising:	Clinically definite	55
	Clinically probable	49
	Confirmed by autopsy	2
	Clinically questionable	17

Table 2. Course of the disease and result of treatment with Synacthen in 106 cases* of multiple sclerosis.

	Improved		Not improved	
Bouts and remissions	37		20	
Chronic-progressive:				
Initially bouts and remissions, then chronic progressive	8	} 17	14	} 32
Chronic progressive from the outset	9		18	

* Clinically definite, probable, or confirmed by autopsy

Table 3. Duration of disease and result of treatment with Synacthen in 106 cases* of multiple sclerosis.

Duration of disease (years)	Improved	Not improved
0– 1	14	3
2– 4	18	16
5– 9	18	20
10–19	8	5
>20	0	4

* Clinically definite, probable, or confirmed by autopsy

Table 4. Degree of disability and result of treatment with Synacthen in 106 cases* of multiple sclerosis.

Degree of disability	Improved	Not improved
0– 2	19	8
3– 5	29	25
6–10	9	16

* Clinically definite, probable, or confirmed by autopsy

Our most serious complication during treatment with Synacthen was a case of death due to fulminating pulmonary embolism. In two cases the medication had to be discontinued because an allergic reaction developed. In another patient, treatment was interrupted because of severe vertigo. Fresh bouts and exacerbations were seen in three cases during the four-week course of Synacthen therapy. Mild diabetes became manifest in two patients, but this disturbance was transient. ®Lioresal appeared to be the more likely cause of improvement in five cases. In two patients with previous

253

severe tuberculosis—one of whom had had a lung resection—Synacthen was given together with tuberculostatic drugs. In five patients who did not respond to Synacthen, subsequent administration of corticosteroids produced an improvement.

The C.S.F. was examined in all but three patients in our series. Typical alterations, found in 92 patients prior to treatment with Synacthen, were mononuclear pleocytosis and/or a left shift in the colloidal curve and an increase in the IgG quotient with normal or only slightly elevated total protein. Eleven patients had normal or non-specific C.S.F. findings.

In 53 of the 106 patients with multiple sclerosis classified as clinically definite, probable, or confirmed by autopsy, the C.S.F. was examined before and after the four-week course of Synacthen therapy (Table 5). The most conspicuous and most frequent alteration was a decrease in pleocytosis, which was observed in 22 out of 40 cases (reduction of cells by at least $20/3 = 7$ per cu. mm.); 13 patients had no pleocytosis.

A decrease in the IgG concentration ($\downarrow Q > 0.5$) was seen in 10 cases. Prior to treatment, 38 of the 53 patients had an IgG quotient of more than 1.5, so that there was a significant reduction in this quotient in roughly one-quarter of them following A.C.T.H. therapy.

It is a well-known fact that clinical improvement in M.S. is not synonymous with an abatement of the inflammatory reaction. Let me cite an example:

The majority of cases of retrobulbar neuritis are early, monosymptomatic forms of M.S., in which the C.S.F. changes are initially restricted to mononuclear pleocytosis; the typical increase in the IgG concentration in the C.S.F. has not yet developed.

The IgG response was studied in 1,178 patients, of whom 303 had M.S. and 22 retrobulbar neuritis. The majority of the M.S. cases, but not a single case of retrobulbar neuritis, exhibited an increased IgG quotient. In this group we were very careful to include only early acute monosymptomatic forms of retrobulbar neuritis. Most of them were successfully treated with A.C.T.H. Since the series started, however, several patients have progressed to a disseminated symptomatology typical of M.S., including characteristic alterations in the C.S.F., with pronounced IgG elevation.

There is a clear-cut indication for steroids or A.C.T.H. in the treatment of chemical meningitis provoked by isotope cisternography and in the management of toxic encephalopathies accompanied by inflammatory reactions and oedema.

Dr. WÜTHRICH did not discuss the question of A.C.T.H. therapy in encephalitis; perhaps he was wise not to meddle with such a controversial topic. Fragmentary evidence seems to indicate that:

a) In varicella encephalitis, the use of steroids and A.C.T.H. is not warranted. The same can be said of poliomyelitis, which fortunately has nowadays become a rare disease.

b) In mumps encephalitis, steroids and A.C.T.H. have proved beneficial, especially in cases with accompanying orchitis.

c) In herpes encephalitis, steroids and corticotrophin used to be considered as contra-indicated by many paediatricians and neurologists, particularly after the advent of

Table 5. Comparison of C.S.F. findings* in 53 cases of multiple sclerosis** before and after four weeks of treatment with Synacthen.

Clinical status only improved	15
C.S.F. findings only improved	10
Both improved	12
Neither improved	16

* Cell count, total protein, colloidal reaction, and IgG quotient
** Clinically definite, probable, or confirmed by autopsy

idoxuridine. Since the hopes placed in this drug have not been fulfilled, there is again a tendency to use steroids and A.C.T.H. in herpes infections of the nervous system. In S.S.P.E. (subacute sclerosing panencephalitis) it is possible to prolong life with steroids or A.C.T.H.

Abacterial meningo-encephalitis, whatever that may be, deserves to be considered as a possible indication for A.C.T.H. therapy. We neurologists have repeatedly seen cases of persisting meningitis of undetermined aetiology in which steroids or A.C.T.H., employed as a last resort, proved successful.

RADL* has recently claimed that para-infectious encephalitis is becoming more frequent. He mentions that para-infectious encephalitis as a complication of measles has increased from 0.5 to 3.3%, with sequelae in 80% of the cases.

As regards the use of A.C.T.H. therapy in such conditions, there are in my opinion two factors to be borne in mind:

Firstly, the administration of A.C.T.H. in preference to corticosteroids—i.e. the stimulation of endogenous cortisol production—obviates the problem of blood-brain barrier penetration. We have quite a bit of information on various corticosteroids, indicating that we have to administer fairly high doses if we wish to achieve therapeutic effects within the parenchyma of the central nervous system; dexamethasone therapy in neurosurgery is a good example of this. However, it would also be very important to know more concerning the blood-brain barrier permeability of endogenous cortisol. I would be extremely grateful for any information on this from experts in the audience.

Secondly, the central lesions may interfere with the production of corticotrophin-releasing factor; the use of A.C.T.H. in this situation could represent a more physiological and better overall method of replacing impaired function than the use of steroids.

In a very noteworthy article that appeared some three years ago in the Annals of Internal Medicine**, the pathophysiology of an epidemic of St. Louis encephalitis was analysed. The brain lesions in many of the cases led to: an inappropriate secretion of antidiuretic hormone; an impairment of pituitary-adrenocortical function; and disturbances in blood flow and metabolism.

I will refer only to the first two of these problems. Hyponatraemia, deficient urinary dilution (attributed to partial impairment of antidiuretic hormone function), and the loss of physiological circadian fluctuations in the 17-hydroxycorticosteroid levels were often observed.

Administration of A.C.T.H. proved that adrenocortical function was intact; there was a normal response to dexamethasone suppression, and insulin challenge produced a rise in the plasma concentrations of 17-hydroxycorticosteroids and growth hormone. The ®Metopirone test caused the plasma 11-desoxycorticosteroids to increase. All the anomalies found indicated a reaction to severe stress.

Hence, there is in my opinion a double indication for A.C.T.H. in such cases, because it not only combats inflammation and oedema, but also compensates for the functional impairment resulting from lesions in the hypothalamus.

Finally, it seems to me that we neurologists have not been insistent enough in demanding technical facilities and laboratory capacity for the analysis of endocrine functions in certain diseases of the nervous system. Our own studies with A.C.T.H., and especially what I have heard at this symposium, have convinced me that this is an urgent problem.

---

* RADL, H.: Zur Häufigkeit und Prognose parainfektiöser Enzephalitiden. Wien. klin. Wschr. *84*, 21 (1972)

**WHITE, M.G., CARTER, N.W., RECTOR, F.C., SELDIN, D.W., DREWRY, S.J., SANFORD, J.P., LUBY, J.P., UNGER, R.H., KAPLAN, N.M., SHAPIRO, W., EISENBERG, S.: Pathophysiology of epidemic St. Louis encephalitis. Ann. intern. Med. *71*, 691 (1969)

K. F. Weinges: May I ask if anyone here can offer an explanation for the mechanism of action of steroids in cerebral oedema, or can indicate to what extent steroid therapy differs from injection treatment with hypertonic solutions or from other forms of treatment designed to remove excess fluid?

R.-J. Wüthrich: I can't give a definite answer to this question, nor do I know whether any detailed studies on the mechanism of action of steroids have been undertaken in this connection. But I can state that—in comparison with diuretic medication, treatment with hypertonic solutions, or even glycerin—corticosteroids do at all events offer distinct advantages, both as regards the problem of rebound phenomena and from the standpoint of practicability. It is for this reason that corticosteroid therapy has gained widespread acceptance in the field of neurosurgery, where cerebral oedema is most frequently encountered.

H. J. Bauer: As a general rule, hypertonic solutions are also administered in addition to dexamethasone in all these neurosurgical cases. It is thought that the corticoid may possibly have the effect of reducing membrane permeability; but I don't know whether pharmacologists can confirm this assumption. I do at any rate believe that treatment with high doses of dexamethasone has ushered in a new era in the management of cerebral oedema. In my opinion, treatment for oedema occurring in post-operative states, or in patients undergoing radiotherapy for inoperable or only partially excised cerebral tumours, might well constitute a further field in which the possibility of using A.C.T.H. instead of steroids ought to be investigated. Radiotherapy has to be continued over a fairly prolonged period, and in these patients—who are already in a very poor condition—treatment with steroids in a dosage high enough to prove effective must presumably impose a severe strain; I could therefore imagine that in such cases A.C.T.H. might perhaps have advantages to offer.

P. A. Desaulles: It can be assumed that corticosteroids reduce membrane permeability in the brain in just the same way as they do in other tissues. From the nature of the processes occurring in the cerebral blood vessels it can likewise be assumed that the behaviour of corticosteroids administered from without, as well as of corticosteroids secreted from within in response to corticotrophin injections, is essentially similar in the brain to what it is in the periphery. But hardly any experimental studies have yet been carried out with a view to comparing and quantifying the changes in permeability produced in the brain by corticosteroids or corticotrophin preparations.

J. Girard: In this connection, I should like to ask a question concerning pseudotumour cerebri. Have we any idea as to what is responsible for the occurrence of pseudotumour cerebri in patients treated with steroids? Is there any risk of a pseudotumour developing under treatment with A.C.T.H.?

R.-J. Wüthrich: It is something of a paradox that we employ corticoids to treat cerebral oedema, despite the fact that pseudotumour cerebri has been known to develop following steroid medication. All one can say here is that the conditions leading to pseudotumour cerebri vary greatly and are difficult to analyse in a given case; to what extent steroid therapy constitutes the decisive factor is often a moot point.

H. Jesserer: So far as I know, pseudotumour cerebri occurs in such cases, not as a consequence of treatment with corticosteroids, but as a form of withdrawal syndrome after cessation of the medication.

H. J. Bauer: Nothing is really known about the precise causes of this disorder. It may develop as a withdrawal syndrome following corticosteroid therapy, and it also occurs, though very rarely, as a consequence of the treatment itself. In most cases, however, the pseudotumour has nothing to do with either corticosteroid or corticotrophin medication. In these patients, in whom the clinical picture of pseudotumour cerebri is characterised by papilloedema, headache sometimes so severe as to cause vomiting, and life-threatening signs of cerebral compression, it is impossible to detect any changes by means of angiography or scintigraphy. In a very small number of cases, examination of the C.S.F. reveals pleocytosis. As treatment for such conditions we prefer spironolactone to steroid therapy.

And now I should like to revert to the topic of myasthenia. Dr. WÜTHRICH made it clear in his paper that monotherapy with A.C.T.H. is not a very satisfactory form of treatment in this indication. A.C.T.H. is indicated chiefly after thymectomy—and it is thymectomy which, when resorted to in appropriate cases, yields the most lasting results. It is capable of effecting an improvement both in hyperplastic and in non-hyperplastic forms of the disease. Following the operation, treatment with a combination of cytotoxic agents and steroids has been given in a large number of cases. Allow me briefly to quote an example from among my own patients. This woman was subjected to thymectomy at an age when, according to the statistics, the operation is no longer permissible, i.e. at the age of 46 years. She has now been receiving cytotoxic drugs for the past six years, and her condition can be described as tolerable. Tracheotomy has had to be performed on three occasions, on one of which respiratory standstill had occurred during a period of A.C.T.H. therapy. Treatment with A.C.T.H. is currently enjoying popularity again, but its long-term results in myasthenia gravis are still unsatisfactory.

R. SCHUPPLI: Myasthenia has occasionally also been observed as an accompaniment to certain immunological disorders, such as Hashimoto's goitre, as well as in pemphigus. This might possibly be a reason for giving treatment with A.C.T.H. and immunosuppressants.

R.-J. WÜTHRICH: I think I should perhaps emphasise that in myasthenia treatment with A.C.T.H., which entails considerable risks, particularly in the shape of respiratory failure, should be attempted only where all other measures have proved of no avail. In other words, it is an *ultima ratio*, but one which quite often deserves consideration in severe cases of myasthenia. Despite thymectomy, treatment with immunosuppressive agents, radiotherapy, and the use of very high doses of cholinesterase inhibitors, some patients continue to deteriorate, and in these instances one is obliged to exhaust all the possibilities that are available—and A.C.T.H. is one of these possibilities.

H. J. BAUER: There is quite a body of evidence indicating that immunopathological factors are involved in myasthenia. Antibodies directed against muscle substance have been detected, for example, although no causal relationship can be established between these antibodies and the severity of the disease. Possibly of greater relevance are the results of clinical experiments on the lymph. In response to drainage of the thoracic duct, patients show a striking, although only temporary, improvement. After termination of the drainage, the patient reverts to his previous condition. The re-infusion of cell-free lymph has been found to produce a sudden worsening of myasthenia—a finding which resurrects the old question as to the existence of a circulating "myasthenia factor". We know that lymphocytic infiltrates are present in the muscle tissues of patients with myasthenia, even after thymectomy has been performed, and it seems reasonable to postulate that these infiltrates might be the source of the factors responsible for weakening the muscles. It is to be hoped that studies now being undertaken in this direction will help to shed further light on the whole problem.

Closing addresses

R. SCHUPPLI: In the course of our symposium it has, I think, become clear that synthetic A.C.T.H. has enabled progress to be made in certain branches of medicine. This applies, for example, to my own field, which is that of dermatology. Here, I would remind you that at one time pemphigus had a 90% mortality, whereas now – thanks to treatment with A.C.T.H.—the mortality has dropped to 5% and, moreover, in at least 50% of cases we are able to achieve permanent cures, i.e. the patients effect a complete clinical recovery and no longer require any treatment. In addition, in the patients we treat with Synacthen Depot we no longer encounter vertebral fractures, which used to be one of the side effects most feared in the course of corticoid therapy.

Another area in which the progress achieved strikes me as self-evident is that of juvenile asthma. In asthmatic children treated with synthetic A.C.T.H. in lieu of corticosteroids, the absence of growth inhibition should prove of major practical importance.

Whether treatment with Synacthen also marks a genuine advance in the domain of rheumatology is a question which, in the light of the papers presented at this symposium, I cannot answer. Possibly a combination of this drug with immunosuppressive agents may be the key to future therapy for rheumatic disorders. In patients suffering from rheumatism, too, however, the choice between corticosteroids and A.C.T.H. has to be reached after due consideration has been given to the question of their respective side effects.

In the field of neurological disorders, I feel that—speaking with all the caution that it behoves one to observe here—the use of Synacthen Depot may be regarded as justified in the treatment of severe acute exacerbations of multiple sclerosis, as well as in cerebral oedema.

As regards the side effects of A.C.T.H. in comparison with those of corticosteroid therapy, it seems apparent that some of them are less common and others less severe in the case of A.C.T.H. In this context I should like to refer once again to the problem of bone fractures which has caused us so much trouble in patients receiving corticosteroids. While I do not doubt that osteoporosis is also liable to occur following treatment with A.C.T.H., I would point out that this is basically a question of degree. Much the same applies to gastric ulceration as a side effect: only a few of us have ever observed a gastric ulcer during A.C.T.H. therapy, whereas this problem of ulceration has been one of the main limiting factors encountered in the course of long-term corticosteroid medication. Elevation of the blood sugar levels may prove an unpleasant side effect of A.C.T.H., as may also oedema; still unclear is the nature of the nervous manifestations provoked by injections of A.C.T.H.—manifestations for which we have not yet managed to find a satisfactory interpretation. By and large, however, it may be concluded that the side effects of A.C.T.H. are appreciably less serious than those which prolonged corticosteroid therapy entails.

Now for a few words about the side effects of an allergic nature. The precise character of the genuine allergic side effects, which are rare, has yet to be established; it is easy to recognise them clinically in cases where they take the form of urticarial reactions. But which of the other manifestations are of an allergic or immunological type is something that we do not yet know. The problem of the formation of antibodies directed against A.C.T.H. and the clinical significance of this phenomenon have still to be clarified. One fact which strikes me as being very important is that no fatalities due to adrenal failure have been observed during treatment with A.C.T.H. Antibodies capable of blocking A.C.T.H., with the result that they might precipitate an acute adrenal crisis, are evidently extremely rare—in contrast to the insulin-blocking antibodies, which are liable to provoke an acute diabetic crisis. In this field there is an essential need for further research—research developed along the lines of the sophisticated methods about which we have already heard quite a few interesting things in the course of our symposium. Among the unresolved problems which we shall have to tackle during the next few years is the question whether long-term treatment with corticosteroids and with cytotoxic agents possibly involves a risk of inducing malignant tumours. For example, I believe there is evidence to suggest that patients with pemphigus who have been treated for years with cytotoxic drugs, with corticoids, or with A.C.T.H. show a higher incidence of carcinoma. This of course has not been statistically confirmed, but it is a possibility that should be borne in mind, particularly when treating younger patients over very long periods.

Little reference has been made during our discussions to the question of the rebound phenomenon. Which diseases become aggravated when A.C.T.H. therapy is discontinued? We have been almost exclusively concerned here with the improvements that can be achieved with such treatment, but some patients also show a worsening when A.C.T.H. is withdrawn. To quote an example from my own branch of medicine, I would point out that, after completion of a prolonged course of A.C.T.H. therapy, patients with psoriasis sometimes suffer acute exacerbations which are more severe than in previous episodes and which also respond less well than before to external treatment with chrysarobin.

Speaking as an outsider, I should at this point like to highlight one conclusion which I think the pharmaceutical company that has invited us here should draw from our deliberations. The proceedings of this symposium have clearly revealed that it would be well worth while to undertake further intensive studies in this field, particularly since research in this area also has a very important bearing on clinical problems facing us. I am sure all participants will agree with me that a new A.C.T.H. preparation displaying even better therapeutic properties and fewer side effects would be welcomed by us clinicians with open arms. Our symposium has perhaps also served to emphasise what a major contribution carefully conceived international studies, conducted along uniform lines, can make in connection with the evaluation of drugs. We have seen that in various countries of Europe the same problem has often been tackled in quite different ways. This tends to result in findings which it may well be very difficult to compare. If we were to adopt a uniform approach, I think we should be able, for example, to discover more about differences in the manner in which different populations respond. We already have some evidence which seems to indicate that in Europe various populations do in fact differ in the way they react to drugs. For instance, the side effects encountered in response to drugs in various parts of Europe often differ considerably both in their intensity and in their frequency.

This brings me to the end of the comments I wished to make concerning the purely medical aspects of our symposium. I should now like to add a brief remark on what might be called the human side of the proceedings. First of all, I want to thank you all most warmly for having come here to Dubrovnik and for having participated so actively in the discussions, throughout which the atmosphere has been such a pleasant and friendly one. The absolute fairness with which these discussions were conducted has been extremely gratifying for me as your chairman. Finally, I should like—also on behalf of you all—to express a special vote of thanks to CIBA-GEIGY, and to Dr. ADAMS and the members of his staff in particular, for the excellent organisation of this symposium, from which all of us have derived great profit.

R. OBERHOLZER: After the brilliant summing up which we have just heard, it is very difficult for me on behalf of CIBA-GEIGY to add anything that hasn't already been said. Speaking for myself, I am firmly convinced that this symposium has fulfilled its objective—which was to provide a practical review of progress to date in the field of A.C.T.H. therapy—and that, now that the meeting is over, we know quite a lot more about the indications for the two preparations Synacthen and Synacthen Depot. I think it is also important to have discussed their marginal indications, including trial indications which we shall have to follow up if possible on an international plane, as well as certain other indications which would not appear to repay further investigation. For those of us who belong to CIBA-GEIGY the searching discussions concerned with the problem of side effects were likewise of the utmost value. It is, after all, one of our responsibilities—especially *vis-à-vis* the general practitioner—not only to provide information on the possibilities inherent in treatment with our pharmaceutical products, but also to protect the doctor against the risk of committing errors in their use and, where need be, to warn him so that side effects do not come as an unpleasant surprise. In this connection, I feel we must also pay due attention to the antigenic or allergenic properties of these peptides, which, though rarely encountered, do evidently exist. You may rest assured that we shall go very thoroughly into the question as to whether the information we are now supplying to doctors fully reflects the knowledge and experience that have been acquired to date or whether this information ought to be further amplified. As previously intimated by Dr. SCHUPPLI, our research workers will certainly derive from this symposium the courage and inspiration to push ahead with their investigations, particularly since they can now be confident that A.C.T.H. preparations of this type have already established for themselves a firm place in clinical usage.

In conclusion, it only remains for me to fulfil the agreeable task of thanking all the speakers for the work they have done in preparing their contributions to the proceedings, for the papers they have presented here, and for having participated so keenly in the frank and informative discussions. In particular, I should like to thank Dr. SCHUPPLI most warmly for his excellent chairmanship, which has contributed so much to the success of this gathering.

Index

261

Tetracosactrin
  see Synacthen Depot
    Synacthen test
      Tetracosactide
Tetracosapeptide
  see Synacthen Depot
    Synacthen test
      Tetracosactide
Tetrahydro-desoxycorticosterone, urinary excretion in Metopirone test 44
− -S fraction, urinary excretion in Metopirone test 35, 39, 44
Theophylline 229, 230
Thorn test of adrenocortical function 231, 237
Thrombocytopenia 142
Thrombosis 61, 62
Thymectomy in myasthenia gravis 248, 249, 257
Thyroid hormone, effect on T.S.H. secretion 41
Thyroid-stimulating hormone
  see T.S.H.
Transcortin, binding of corticosteroids 46, 85, 89–91
− levels 89–91, 119
Triamcinolone 38, 230
−, half-life 87
Trihydroxymethylaminomethane (T.H.A.M.) 230
T.S.H., secretion in response to thyroid hormone 41
Tuberculin test 123
Tuberculosis, miliary 103
Tuberculostatics, combination with tetracosactide 254

Ulceration, gastric
  see Ulceration, peptic
−, peptic 55, 88, 95, 125, 144, 189, 213, 246, 258
Urticaria 116, 118, 119, 121–123, 125, 127, 236, 258

Vaccination reactions 144
Vasculitis, allergic or nodular, dubious effect of corticosteroids 73, 76
Vasopressin test
  see Lysine-vasopressin test
V.D.R.L. reaction 123
Ventilation disturbances 130, 132–134, 142
Ventromedial nucleus 20–23
Vertigo
  see Dizziness
Viraemia 160
Virus diseases, mode of action of A.C.T.H. 160
Vitiligo 121, 122
Vomiting 115, 236

Warmth, sensation of 124, 235, 236
Wassermann reaction 123
Waterhouse-Friderichsen syndrome 160
Weight increase 55, 102, 124, 177, 178
West's syndrome 130, 136–139
− −, factors influencing prognosis 137, 249
Whooping cough 130, 134–136, 142

Zimmermann reaction for 17-ketosteroid determination 84